OXFORD MEDICAL PUBLICATIONS

Analgesic and NSAID-induced Kidney Disease

Oxford Monographs on Clinical Nephrology

1. *Prevention of progressive chronic renal failure*
   Edited by A. Meguid El Nahas, N.P. Mallick, and Sharon Anderson
2. *Analgesic and NSAID-induced kidney disease*
   Edited by J.H. Stewart

Analgesic and NSAID-induced Kidney Disease

Edited by

J. H. STEWART

Associate Dean, Western Clinical School
University of Sydney, Australia

Oxford New York Tokyo Melbourne

OXFORD UNIVERSITY PRESS

1993

Oxford University Press, Walton Street, Oxford OX2 6DP

Oxford New York Toronto
Delhi Bombay Calcutta Madras Karachi
Petaling Jaya Singapore Hong Kong Tokyo
Nairobi Dar es Salaam Cape Town
Melbourne Auckland
and associated companies in
Berlin Ibadan

Oxford is a trade mark of Oxford University Press
Published in the United States
by Oxford University Press, New York

A catalogue record for this book is available from the British Library

Library of Congress Cataloging in Publication Data
Analgesic and NSAID-induced kidney disease / edited by J.H. Stewart.
p. cm.—(Oxford monographs on clinical nephrology) (Oxford medical publications)
Includes bibliographical references
1. Nephrotoxicology. 2. Kidneys—Effect of drugs on.
3. Analgesics—Toxicology. 4. Nonsteroidal anti-inflammatory agents—Toxicology. I. Stewart, J.H. II. Series. III. Series: Oxford medical publications.
[DNLM: 1. Analgesics—adverse effects. 2. Anti-Inflammatory Agents, Non-Steroidal—adverse effects. 3. Kidney Diseases—chemically induced. WJ 300 A5313]
RC918.N45A53 1993 616.6′1—dc20 92-22709
ISBN 0 19 261956 X

Set by Graphicraft Typesetters Ltd, Hong Kong
Printed and bound in Great Britain by
Biddles Ltd, Guildford and King's Lynn

PREFACE

Few diseases have captured the imagination of a generation of doctors in the way that analgesic nephropathy has done. For the clinician, it has demanded consummate skill, from the challenge of its protean, often calamitous, acute presentation in hospital wards at the peak of the epidemic of papillary necrosis in the 1960s, to the more subtle responsibility now of discerning surreptitious analgesic dependency, chronic interstitial nephritis, or papillary necrosis *in situ* as the cause of hypertension or mildly impaired renal function. Treatment and prevention have been equally rewarding—recovery is likely for those with acute renal failure, autonomous progression occurs less in this than in most other causes of chronic renal failure, the analgesic *habituée* generally has fared as well as her contemporaries in end-stage renal failure programmes, and when effective measures have been taken the disease has been brought under control.

While it was the introduction of the artificial kidney which enabled nephrology to separate from general medicine and cardiology, and transplantation which gave the specialty its standing in the 1960s and 1970s, analgesic nephropathy played no small part in its maturation, drawing together the new breed of scientifically trained and orientated renal physicians in the common purpose of eradicating this most superfluous of diseases. At an intellectual level, the debates were lively—chronic interstitial nephritis or papillary necrosis, ischaemia or toxicity, aspirin or phenacetin or both, education or prohibition—but the commitment to making a joint effort towards prevention of analgesic-induced kidney disease cemented the bonds forming between nephrologists as a result of the daunting task of providing dialysis and transplantation for all those with irreversible end-stage renal failure.

Having conquered analgesic nephropathy—which we may fairly claim, although not everywhere have the necessary measures been taken or the results fully accomplished—nephrology now has a new concern which is likely to entail even greater skills in clinical management and social engineering. The kidney diseases caused by non-steroidal anti-inflammatory drugs (known almost universally, and understandably, as NSAIDs) occur with pharmaceutical doses of agents providing substantial relief of pain which is difficult to mitigate by other means. It seems possible that their toxicity to the kidney arises from their mode of action, the inhibition of prostaglandin synthesis; it will, therefore, require pharmaceutical ingenuity to formulate a drug of this class acceptable alike to nephrologists, gastroenterologists, and rheumatologists. The alternative, to restrict the use of NSAIDs to only the most needy of cases, seems unduly harsh, although one's experience does suggest that there is both injudicious and excessive use of these agents.

Adding to the difficulty of controlling kidney disease arising from the NSAIDs, is that of its recognition in the individual patient. The signs are subtle and the diagnosis can be made convincingly only by biopsy, for which the accepted indications are rarely met. For these reasons, the extent of serious renal disease caused by NSAIDs is not yet known—my guess is that hypertension and mild or moderate impairment of kidney function will be common and a cause of secondary arterial disease, but that end-stage renal failure will be rare. Urothelial cancer, which loomed as a consequence of phenacetin consumption nearly as devastating as renal failure, has not been attributed to other analgesics or NSAIDs.

Questions remain for the scientist, and patients with analgesic nephropathy will continue to fascinate another generation of nephrologists. But, many of the great names in this field have reached retirement, or soon will. Sadly, I learned of Professor Zollinger's death only after writing to ask for his participation in this book. Others have contributed to the multinational list of authors, each of whom has imparted to this text a little of the distinction with which he endowed his original writings on the subject.

It has indeed been rewarding to read and collate the individual chapters. The content is the authors', but I must accept responsibility for correctness of the text and grammar. The bibliography is deliberately comprehensive, as no specialized text can answer all the needs of the inquisitive scientist, and there is currently no other one book which covers this topic fully.

Sydney J.H.S.
March 1992

CONTENTS

Contributors

Peter H. Bach
School of Science, Polytechnic of East London, Romford Road, London, E15 4LZ, England.
Staffan Björck
University of Göteborg, Department of Nephrology, Sahlgrenska Hospital, S-413 45 Göteborg, Sweden.
Giulio A. Cinotti
Istituto di Clinica Medica 2, Cattedra di Nefrologia, Università di Roma 'La Sapienza', Policlinico Umberto 1°, Viale del Policlinico, I-00161 Roma, Italy.
Marc E. De Broe
Department of Nephrology—Hypertension, University Hospital Antwerp, Wilrijkstraat 10, B-2650 Edegem/Antwerpen, Belgium.
Geoffrey G. Duggin
Department of Renal Medicine, Royal Prince Alfred Hospital, Camperdown, NSW, Australia, 2050.
Michael J. Dunn
Departments of Medicine and Physiology—Biophysics, Case Western Reserve University School of Medicine, University Hospitals of Cleveland, 2074 Abingdon Rd, Room 8124 Lakeside Building, Cleveland, Ohio, USA, 44106.
M.M. Elseviers
Department of Nephrology—Hypertension, University Hospital Antwerp, Wilrijkstraat 10, B-2650 Edegem/Antwerpen, Belgium.
Friedrich J. Gloor
Achslenstrasse 4, CH-9016 St Gallen, Switzerland.
Priscilla Kincaid-Smith
Department of Pathology, University of Melbourne, Parkville, Victoria, Australia, 3052.
D. Kleinknecht
Service de Néphrologie et de Réanimation Polyvalente, Centre Hospitalier Intercommunal de Montreuil, 56 Boulevard de la Boissière, 93105 Montreuil, France.
Hans Köhler
I. Medizinische Klinik und Poliklinik, Klinikum der Johannes Gutenberg-Universität, Postfach 3960, Langenbeckstrasse 1, D-6500 Mainz, Germany.

D. Ladewig
Psychiatrische Universitätsklinik Basel, Wilhelm-Klein-Strasse 27, CH-4025 Basel, Switzerland.
Margaret McCredie
Cancer Epidemiology Research Unit, NSW Cancer Council, PO Box 572, Kings Cross, NSW, Australia, 2011.
Michael J. Mihatsch
Institut für Pathologie der Universität Basel, Schönbienstrasse 40, CH-4056 Basel, Switzerland.
Ranjit S. Nanra
Nephrology Unit, John Hunter Hospital, Locked Bag 1, Newcastle Mail Centre, NSW, Australia, 2310.
Wolfgang Pommer
Humboldt-Krankenhaus, Innere Medizin III, Am Nordgraben 2, D-1000 Berlin 27, Germany.
Francesco Pugliese
Istituto di Clinica Medica 2, Cattedra di Nefrologia, Università di Roma 'La Sapienza', Policlinico Umberto 1°, Viale del Policlinico, I-00161 Roma, Italy.
Simin Schadmand
Institut für Klinische Strahlenkunde, Klinikum der Johannes Gutenberg-Universität, Postfach 3960, Langenbeckstrasse 1, D-6500 Mainz, Germany.
Anke Schwarz
Abteilung für Innere Medizin, Freie Universität Berlin, Klinikum Steglitz, Hindenburgdamm 30, D-1000 Berlin 45, Germany.
J.H. Stewart
University of Sydney, Western Clinical School, Clinical Sciences Building, Nepean Hospital, PO Box 63, Penrith, NSW, Australia, 2751.
J.S. Taylor
7th Floor, QBE Building, 19 Bolton Street, Newcastle, NSW, Australia, 2300.
Edward J. Zambraski
Department of Biology—Physiology Section, Bartlett Hall, Rutgers University, New Brunswick, NJ, USA, 08903.
H.U. Zollinger (posthumous)
Elisabeth Zyzik
I. Medizinische Klinik und Poliklinik, Klinikum der Johannes Gutenberg-Universität, Postfach 3960, Langenbeckstrasse 1, D-6500 Mainz, Germany.

1

Historical introduction

Friedrich J. Gloor

1.1 'Phenacetin nephritis' in Switzerland

In 1953, the clinician Otto Spühler and the pathologist Han Ulrich Zollinger observed, in 12 of 44 cases of chronic interstitial nephritis, an association with long-standing consumption of large doses of the compound analgesic Saridon (containing 0.25 g phenacetin, 0.15 g isopropylantipyrin, 0.05 g caffeine, and 0.05 g persedon) (Spühler and Zollinger 1953). Two years later, Zollinger (1955) postulated a causal relationship between phenacetin-containing analgesics and chronic interstitial nephritis, thus starting a debate in Switzerland: many clinicians and pathologists agreed with his observations (Gsell *et al.* 1957; Hensler 1957; Moeschlin 1958; Thölen 1958; Scheidegger 1958; Uehlinger 1958); others did not (Randerath 1958; Reubi 1958).

An inquiry conducted by the Swiss Health Service revealed an increasing consumption of non-narcotic analgesics in the population beginning before the Second World War (Müller and Kielholz 1957). A detailed analysis of the psychosocial and psychiatric background of analgesic abusers was performed (Kielholz 1957; Battegay 1958*a*). Most involved were middle-aged working housewives and unskilled factory workers (Horisberger *et al.* 1958).

At the same time, anaemia and cyanosis were observed by haematologists as consequences of chronic phenacetin intoxication (Schweingruber *et al.* 1955; Moeschlin 1957; Marti 1958).

Between 1955 and 1958, the first attempts to produce kidney damage experimentally with phenacetin and phenacetin-containing mixtures in animals of different species were largely unsuccessful, except that a higher susceptibility to infection was demonstrated (Studer and Zbinden 1955; Studer *et al.* 1958*a*; Miescher *et al.* 1959; Studer 1965). Therefore, the underlying disease was thought to be renal infection aggravated by consumption of phenacetin-containing drugs.

At this time, analgesic nephropathy appeared to be confined to Switzerland, and as phenacetin was the common denominator in the analgesics abused, the misleading term 'phenacetin nephritis' was applied to the disease (Moeschlin 1958).

1.2 Renal papillary necrosis in Scandinavia and Australia

A short time thereafter, the first important papers confirming and extending Swiss experience came from Scandinavia, especially from Denmark (Nissen and Pedersen 1957; Larsen and Møller 1969; Lindineg *et al.* 1959) and Sweden (Lindvall 1960; Hultengren 1961; Nordenfeldt and Ringertz 1961; Bengtsson 1962; Grimlund 1963). It was recognized at this time that renal papillary necrosis (RPN), not chronic interstitial nephritis, was the hallmark of the new kidney disease. The RPN of analgesic abusers, observed at autopsy, was of a chronic sclerotic type, quite different from the classical acute infectious type well-known in diabetes mellitus and obstructive uropathy (Schourup 1957; Gloor 1960). An increasing incidence of this new chronic type of RPN was observed in autopsy series from Switzerland (Gloor 1961), Sweden (Nordenfeldt and Ringertz 1961; Bengtsson 1962), and Australia (Burry *et al.* 1966).

In Sweden, as in Switzerland, phenacetin was thought to be the most important aetiological agent, since aspirin was not a component of the mixtures most often abused. Women were more often affected than men; the psychosocial background was the same as in Switzerland (Nissen and Pedersen 1957; Nordenfeldt and Ringertz 1961; Bengtsson 1962).

A strong epidemiological argument in favour of a causal relationship between analgesic abuse and kidney damage was the observation of a large number of renal deaths in an engineering factory with 3000 mainly male workers in the Swedish town of Huskvarna, where the reverse sex ratio, with more affected males than females (3.6 : 1) was observed. In this population of factory workers, a longstanding, heavy abuse of Hjörton powders, containing 0.5 g phenacetin, 0.5 g phenazone, and 0.15 g caffeine, was well known (Grimlund 1963).

Important for our knowledge of the disease now called analgesic nephropathy (AN), was the Australian experience (Jacobs and Morris 1962; McCutcheon 1962; Burry 1966; Kincaid-Smith 1968). In some states of Australia, per capita consumption of compound analgesics was the highest in the world (Gault *et al.* 1968*a*; Stewart 1978). The two brands mostly consumed, Bex and Vincent's contained phenacetin, caffeine, and, in contrast to mixtures in Switzerland and Sweden, aspirin. For this reason, peptic ulcers and iron-deficiency anaemia were part of the analgesic syndrome in Australia (Douglas and Johnston 1961; Dawborn *et al.* 1966).

1.2.1 The association with urothelial cancer

In 1965, Hultengren *et al.* reported for the first time on a strong association of cancers of the renal pelvis with analgesic abuse. Three years later, Bengtsson *et al.* (1968) were able to prove this relationship in a prospective study, confirming an additional serious hazard of analgesic abuse. Johansson and Wahlqvist (1977) subsequently observed a high incidence of tumours of the bladder and ureter in those taking phenacetin-containing analgesics, an association which was statistically confirmed by Mihatsch *et al.* (1980*b*). Renal pelvic cancers are frequently, but not necessarily, related to RPN or to renal impairment (McCredie *et al.* 1986).

1.3 The pathology of analgesic nephropathy

The increasing experience gained at autopsy led to the conclusion that papillary necrosis is the primary lesion, while chronic interstitial nephritis in the cortex is a secondary phenomenon resulting from obstruction of the distal nephron (Sanerkin 1966; Kincaid-Smith 1967; Burry 1967). Experimentally-induced RPN displays the same sequence of events (Murray *et al.* 1972; Davies 1968). Three stages of RPN were differentiated by Burry (1967); the earliest morphological changes appear in the inner medulla, as observed in patients with known analgesic abuse and death due to intercurrent disease (Gloor 1965, 1978*a*; Gault *et al.* 1971). Those changes, interfering with the countercurrent mechanism of urine concentration, correlate well with early clinical symptoms (Burry *et al.* 1977; Dubach *et al.* 1983).

Another pathognomonic feature of longstanding analgesic abuse is a peculiar lamellar thickening of the walls of capillaries in the mucosa of the urinary tract, so-called capillary sclerosis (Munck *et al.* 1970; Abrahams *et al.* 1976; Torhorst 1976).

The morphological picture of AN is diagnostic, and can be differentiated from other kidney diseases, especially chronic pyelonephritis (Farmer and Heptinstall 1970; Hodson 1970; Gloor 1978*b*; Heptinstall 1983).

1.4 The aetiology of analgesic nephropathy

Increasing knowledge of the disease led, in the 1970s, to world-wide acceptance of AN as an entity (Kincaid-Smith and Fairley, 1970; Haschek 1973; Gsell 1974; Kincaid-Smith 1978; Prescott 1982*a*; Mihatsch 1986). The morphological and clinical picture was now well defined; statistical data displayed a strong correlation between per capita consumption of compound analgesics in a given population and the incidence of RPN at autopsies or, more recently, the number of patients with AN entering dialysis and transplantation programmes (Stewart 1978; Brunner *et al.* 1985*a*; Drukker *et al.* 1986).

Two controlled epidemiological studies, in Switzerland (Dubach *et al.* 1973) and Australia (McCredie *et al.* 1982*a*), proved a significant association between regular intake of phenacetin-containing analgesics and subsequent development of renal disease. Elimination of phenacetin from compound analgesics in Sweden in 1961, and in Canada in 1973, was followed by a decreasing incidence of AN (Nordenfeldt 1972; Grimlund 1973; Wilson and Gault 1982).

Nevertheless, critical voices have cast doubt on the strength of the association (Gilman 1964; Sorensen 1966; Shelley 1967; Davies *et al.* 1970; Brod and Kuhn 1973; Lawson 1973). Authors from Australia, USA, and Britain, countries where compound analgesics containing phenacetin and aspirin were mainly consumed, postulated that aspirin, not phenacetin, was the agent responsible (Nanra and Kincaid-Smith 1973*b*; Lancet 1981; Prescott 1982*a*). A number of experimental studies demonstrated that it was easier to produce RPN with aspirin alone, or with aspirin and phenacetin together, than with phenacetin or paracetamol alone (Nanra *et al.* 1973; Molland 1978; Bach and Hardy 1985). Inhibition of prostaglandin synthesis in the renal medulla has been proposed as one possible mechanism of action.

While phenacetin or paracetamol are rarely abused as single ingredients, aspirin is widely prescribed to patients with rheumatoid arthritis. The question of whether therapeutic administration of aspirin over a long period of time produces renal damage is contradictory (for: Clausen and Pedersen 1961; Nanra and Kincaid-Smith 1975; Lawson and McLean 1986; against: New Zealand Rheumatism Association Study 1974; Macklon *et al.* 1974; Akyol *et al.* 1982).

1.5 Unanswered questions

The contentious history of AN is due mainly to three factors: the unusual pathogenesis of a kidney disease beginning in the papilla, great geographical variation in incidence, and the failure to produce an identical picture in animals. Many unsolved problems remain (Duggin 1980). Is a single agent, or the synergistic action of several drugs, responsible for the papillary changes? Do single ingredients consumed heavily over a long period of time produce the same renal lesions? Is RPN a direct cytotoxic effect of analgesics, due to interference with the medullary blood flow, or a combination of both? What role do genetic factors play in the development of analgesic nephropathy?

2

The biochemistry and pharmacology of antipyretic–analgesics

Geoffrey G. Duggin

The large number of drugs which share, to varying extents, analgesic, antipyretic, and anti-inflammatory properties, may also share a common mechanism of action and the potential to cause renal papillary necrosis. Derivatives of salicylic acid, the most widely used, exhibit all three pharmacological activities, as do the pyrazolons, antipyrine (phenazone) and aminopyrine (amidopyrine). The *p*-aminophenol derivatives or analids, phenacetin and paracetamol (called acetaminophen in the United States), are analgesics and antipyretics, but only weak anti-inflammatory agents; on the other hand, the newer non-steroidal anti-inflammatory drugs (NSAIDs) are used primarily for their anti-inflammatory properties, but either toxicity or relative lack of efficacy limit their use as simple analgesics or antipyretics. These NSAIDs and their effects on the kidney are described in Chapters 12, 13, and 14.

2.1 Aspirin and salicylate

Aspirin is unusual in that it is itself an effective drug, yet also a pro-drug as its hydrolysis product, salicylate, is active pharmacologically. Moreover, aspirin and salicylate inhibit the same enzyme, but by different means. Although aspirin shares many of the characteristics and properties of salicylate, it differs particularly in respect of its pharmacokinetics and mechanism of action.

2.1.1 Chemistry

Salicylic acid (*o*-hydroxybenzoic acid) may be used as one of its salts (usually sodium salicylate) or esters (Fig. 2.1). The carboxy-esters, such as methyl salicylate (oil of wintergreen) generally are too toxic for internal use (Davidson 1971), but aspirin, in which the salicyl-hydroxyl group is acetylated, is less toxic than salicylate.

Following the successful introduction of sodium salicylate in 1875 for the treatment of rheumatic fever and gout, and as an antipyretic, aspirin was

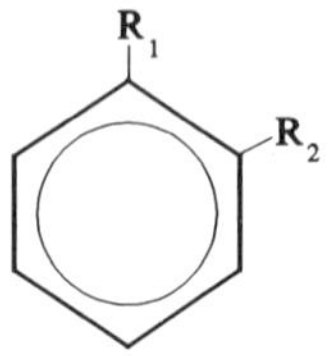

Fig. 2.1 The chemical structure of the salicylate drugs. Sodium salicylate: R_1 = –COO.Na; R_2 = –OH. Aspirin: R_1 = –COOH; R_2 = –O.$COCH_3$. Methyl salicylate: R_1 = –COO.CH_3; R_2 = –OH. Salicylamide: R_1 = –$CONH_2$; R_2 = –OH.

synthesized by Hoffman (working for Bayer) and first used clinically by Dreser in 1899 (Sneader 1985).

2.1.2 Pharmacokinetics

2.1.2.1 Absorption

Aspirin and salicylate are rapidly absorbed from the stomach and upper small intestine, the rate being dependent upon ionization and solubility (Leonards 1963). These are both affected by pH, but in opposite directions. Gastric acidity converts the drug to the absorbable, non-ionized form (pK_a of aspirin is about 3.5), but reduces its solubility in aqueous media. At neutral pH such as in intracellular fluid and blood, aspirin is largely ionized, and so moves less readily across cell membranes. Non-ionic diffusion therefore determines a particularly high concentration gradient between gastric lumen and mucosal cells. However, the vastly greater area of the small intestinal mucosa ensures that most absorption occurs from this site, despite its higher pH.

Efficient systemic absorption of aspirin is dependent on the form of administration, being best from buffered tablets; in some instances no aspirin was detected when administered in the form of plain or enteric coated tablets (Latini *et al.* 1986). The absorption of aspirin and salicylate is inhibited by the administration of activated charcoal, three doses being more effective than one (Barone *et al.* 1988).

2.1.2.2 Distribution

After absorption salicylate is distributed throughout extracellular fluid and most tissues. The distribution is in part determined by pH, and in part by active transport, for example in the kidney and choroid plexus.

In the renal cortex, the proximal tubular cells transport salicylate from the tubular lumen into the cell, principally but probably not exclusively by the organic anion transport system. Although this transport is bidirectional, the resulting renal cortex-to-plasma concentration ratio is approximately 20 (Caterson and Duggin 1980).

Within the renal papillae, the drug may concentrate further by non-ionic diffusion, for when urine within the collecting duct is acidic, salicylic acid will diffuse into the cells; when urine also is concentrated, the papillary-to-plasma ratio can be as high as 60 (Caterson and Duggin 1980).

2.1.2.3 *Metabolism*

Small doses of aspirin administered orally appear in the systemic circulation only as salicylate, being completely hydrolysed during transit through the mucosa, portal circulation and liver (Rowland *et al.* 1972). Increasing the dose results in a greater percentage of aspirin itself appearing in the systemic circulation.

In the circulation, aspirin has a short half-life of 10–15 min. Many studies on aspirin distribution and protein binding have technical flaws in that they fail to account for its rapid conversion to salicylate by transfer of the acetyl group to protein, presumably to amino-residues, and principally by a non-enzymatic process (Hawkins *et al.* 1969). Caterson *et al.* (1978) showed that there was a linear relationship between the amount of acetylated protein in tissues, and the dose of aspirin. This appears to be the only pathway for aspirin degradation, as no other metabolites have been identified.

Following hydrolysis, the metabolism of aspirin proceeds in a fashion identical to that of salicylate administered as such, chiefly in the liver, although many tissues are capable of transforming salicylate. The three principal metabolites are conjugates. The first and quantitatively greatest, salicyluric acid is formed by glycine conjugation in mitochondria, a saturable reaction at doses of about 4 mg/kg body weight. The remaining conjugation reactions, with glucuronic acid, take place in the endoplasmic reticulum and result in the formation of a phenolic (by ether linkage, also saturable) or acyl (by esterification, non-saturable) glucuronide. In addition to conjugation, small quantities of salicylate are metabolized by oxidative enzymes, such as the cytochrome p450 mixed function oxidases, to gentisic acid (2,5-dihydroxybenzoic acid), 2,3-dihydroxybenzoic acid, or 2,3,5-trihydroxybenzoic acid, which may be excreted unchanged or as their glycine conjugates. The proportions of these conjugates is dependent on two variables: the dose administered (in the case of the saturable conjugation reactions) and the rate of excretion of unmetabolized salicylate (see below).

2.1.2.4 *Excretion*

The excretion of salicylate and its conjugates is for the most part by the kidneys. However, there are negligible quantities of aspirin present in the urine unless the drug is administered parenterally in high dose.

Since salicylic acid is a weak acid with a pK_a approximately 3.5, the renal clearance of unconjugated salicylate is determined largely by the pH of the urine. The ionized form will not readily diffuse back across tubular cell membranes and so excretion rises with pH; thus clearance is increased four-fold by a change of pH from 6–8. On the other hand, when acidic urine is being excreted, non-ionized salicylate is reabsorbed in the distal nephron. However, non-ionic diffusion does not affect the distribution or excretion of the conjugates of salicylic acid.

The rate of urine flow also will influence the clearance of salicylate, but to a lesser extent than pH; high rates will decrease the concentration gradient in the collecting duct, resulting in a greater excretion of the parent molecule. Thus maximal urinary excretion of unconjugated salicylate will occur with an alkaline diuresis (Smith *et al.* 1946).

Salicylates and their conjugates also are actively secreted and reabsorbed by the proximal tubule, a transport blocked by probenecid which promotes their excretion.

2.1.3 Mode of action

As indicated above, aspirin is unique in that it and its principal metabolite, salicylate, both act on the same enzyme, prostaglandin synthase; aspirin irreversibly and non-competitively inhibits by acetylating the ε-amino-group of the lysine present at the active site of cyclooxygenase, while salicylate itself reversibly competes with arachidonic acid for its binding site. Of their various effects, it is almost impossible to determine which are exclusively those of aspirin and which are due to salicylate. Therefore their pharmacological actions will be considered together, with the exception of that on platelets.

The mechanism by which aspirin and salicylate effect pain relief in the periphery is now considered to be principally through their inhibition of prostaglandin synthase, although other biochemical effects have not been ruled out. However, there is an additional analgesic effect within the central nervous system, possibly also by inhibition of prostaglandin synthase. There is no cross-reactivity with the opioids, aspirin and salicylate being devoid of activity against endorphins.

Aspirin and salicylate exert their antipyretic activity through the temperature regulating centre in the hypothalamus, probably a direct effect of salicylate.

A third pharmacological effect is inhibition of haemostasis, which appears to be solely due to aspirin itself, not salicylate. Doses of aspirin as low as 40 mg daily will result in doubling of bleeding time, and the half-life of this inhibition is approximately seven days. The effect is mediated by irreversible inhibition of the cyclooxygenase component of platelet prostaglandin synthase (Roth and Siok 1978). The platelet, lacking a nucleus, cannot synthesize further enzyme, and thus can no longer produce thromboxane A_2, its chief product. It has been suggested that, as this small dose does not result in any systemic appearance of aspirin, the platelets are acetylated during their transit through the portal circulation (Pedersen and FitzGerald

1984). This effect has been utilized to prevent coronary artery occlusion and stroke, and may be of value in the prevention of pre-eclampsia (Uzan *et al.* 1991).

2.1.4 Toxicity

Most of the toxic effects of these compounds almost certainly are exerted by salicylate alone as, apart from bleeding, very little toxicity can be attributed directly to aspirin. However, this cannot be tested because of the lability of the aspirin molecule.

2.1.4.1 Clinical features

Salicylism is manifest as headache, dizziness, tinnitus often with decreased hearing, and blurring of vision, followed by mental confusion and drowsiness; usually sweating is profuse, the patient complaints of thirst, and there is marked hyperventilation. Nausea, vomiting and occasionally diarrhoea occur. As the severity of the poisoning increases, coma and convulsions may appear, and body temperature often is elevated. There is metabolic acidosis with an anion gap, often associated with respiratory alkalosis due to direct stimulation of the respiratory centre by salicylate over and above the drive exerted by the raised concentration of hydrogen ion. This combination of respiratory alkalosis and metabolic acidosis is almost unique to salicylate poisoning. Bleeding disorders can occur, although usually only in the most severe cases.

2.1.4.2 Biochemical basis for toxic effects

Salicylate poisoning results from its effect on oxidative phosphorylation, causing inhibition of a number of ATP-dependent reactions. The consequent accumulation of a variety of organic acids produced during intermediary metabolism is responsible for the metabolic acidosis. At high concentrations, salicylate also inhibits a variety of oxidizing enzymes such as xanthine oxidase.

Salicylate also is involved in the genesis of analgesic nephropathy. At high concentrations due to its active transport into the lumen of the proximal tubule by the organic anion transport system, and concentration in the papilla by back diffusion from an acidic urine (see 2.1.2) salicylate selectively depletes glutathione, leaving the tissue vulnerable to alkylating agents or other free radical (Duggin *et al.* 1980).

2.2 Paracetamol (acetaminophen)

Paracetamol, discovered at the Johns Hopkins University in 1877, and first used by von Mering in 1893, is now the most widely consumed antipyretic analgesic in the western world. Its popularity stems from the demonstration

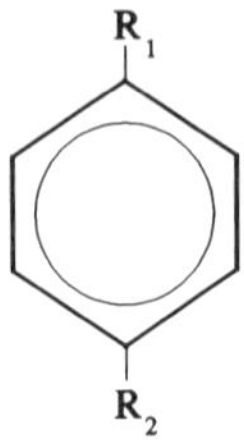

Fig. 2.2 The chemical structure of acetanilid, its derivatives, and their major metabolites. Acetanilid: R_1 = –NH.$COCH_3$; R_2 = –H. Phenacetin: R_1 = –NH.$COCH_3$; R_2 = –OC_2H_5. *p*-Phenetidin: R_1 = –NH_2; R_2 = –OC_2H_5. Paracetamol: R_1 = –NH.$COCH_3$; R_2 = –OH. *N*-acetyl-*p*-benzo-quinoneimine: R_1 = =N.$COCH_3$; R_2 = =O.

of its efficacy and metabolic relationship to phenacetin by Brodie and Axelrod in 1949 (Sneader 1985). In the USA the drug was introduced as a substitute for phenacetin in 1950; its peak use occurred in the 1970s.

The compound is a simple derivative of aniline, being *N*-acetyl-*p*-amino-phenol (Fig. 2.2).

2.2.1 Pharmacokinetics

2.2.1.1 Absorption and distribution

Paracetamol is only weakly soluble in water, but being moderately lipid soluble, migrates quickly through cell membranes. Absorption from the gastrointestinal tract therefore is rapid and complete. The drug achieves peak plasma levels ½–1 hr following oral ingestion. Plasma half-life is approximately 3 hrs in adults (Prescott 1980).

Paracetamol is distributed principally in the aqueous body fluids, the apparent volume of distribution in adults being approximately 0.7 l/kg body weight. Plasma protein binding is somewhat variable, approximately 25 per cent, the majority to albumin (Prescott 1980).

2.2.1.2 Metabolism

Several enzymes are involved, principally in the liver, but metabolism does occur in other organs, notably the kidney. However, this only becomes of significance with large ingestions, as in intentional poisoning.

The major metabolite (55–70 per cent) is the glucuronide conjugate, formed by hepatic uridine diphosphate glucuronic acid transferase, a reaction which is saturable. Approximately 25–40 per cent is conjugated by sulphate transferase using 3′-phospho-adenosine 5′-phosphosulphate as substrate. Oxidation occurs by cytochrome p450 mixed function oxidase, principally in the liver and to a lesser extent in the kidney (Duggin and Mohandas 1982), the latter being relatively unimportant except in instances of acute toxicity.

Paracetamol is thereby transformed into a radical intermediate, *N*-acetyl-*p*-benzo-quinoneimine (Fig. 2.2) which is highly reactive, but with normal therapeutic doses is deactivated by the sulphydryl group of glutathione. This reaction is probably mediated in part by glutathione-*S*-transferase, but can occur rapidly non-enzymatically. The glutathione conjugate is then broken down, with removal of the two amino acids, glycine and glutamine, and acetylation of the amine of the remaining cysteine to form the mercapturic acid derivative, which is excreted in the urine (Hart *et al.* 1980). Following a normal therapeutic dose of paracetamol, 2–5 per cent will appear in the urine in this form. Following very high doses, traces of other metabolites appear in the urine.

Two additional renal metabolic pathways have relatively little importance at therapeutic dosage, but become significant when toxic doses of paracetamol have been taken. The first is an oxidative pathway in which formation of *N*-acetyl-*p*-benzo-quinoneimine is mediated by prostaglandin synthase. The hydroperoxidase component of that enzyme oxidizes paracetamol while converting the lipid peroxide, generated by the same enzyme, to the lipid hydroperoxide (Mohandas *et al.* 1981*a*). *N*-acetyl-*p*-benzo-quinoneimine binds to sulphydryl groups, as in the liver. This pathway is predominantly in the renal medulla where there are large concentrations of prostaglandin synthase and the necessary substrates to mediate the reaction, but also occurs to a lesser extent in the renal cortex where prostaglandin synthase appears to have a similar degree of activity to cytochrome p450. The other renal pathway of metabolism, which occurs mainly in cortical cells, is deacetylation to *p*-aminophenol, which is then either reacetylated or undergoes a further oxidation to the quinoneimine, either spontaneously or mediated by prostaglandin endoperoxide synthase or cytochrome p450 mixed function oxidase (Carpenter and Mudge 1981).

2.2.1.3 Excretion

More than 90 per cent of the elimination of paracetamol and its metabolites is through the kidney; there is negligible gastrointestinal excretion.

Paracetamol itself, being poorly protein bound, readily undergoes glomerular filtration, but is in part reabsorbed by passive diffusion along the renal tubule (Duggin and Mudge 1975). The clearance of the parent compound is increased by increasing urine flow rates, but this is not quantitatively important. The glucuronide and sulphate conjugates also undergo glomerular filtration, but additionally are actively secreted by the proximal tubular organic acid transport system, which is inhibited by probenecid and other organic acids (Duggin and Mudge 1975). The renal handling of the mercapturic acid derivatives has not been studied, but it is probable that they also are transported in the same way.

2.2.2 Mechanism of action and pharmacological properties

Paracetamol has analgesic and antipyretic effects similar to those of aspirin, 500 mg of paracetamol being approximately equivalent to 300 mg of aspirin (Duggin and Mohandas 1982). The antipyretic and analgesic effects are probably mediated via the central nervous system, but the biochemical basis for this is not certain. Many have assumed that paracetamol inhibits prostaglandin synthase in a way similar to salicylate, but detailed biochemical studies have demonstrated that at therapeutic concentrations, paracetamol actually increases the activity of the enzyme, inhibition occurring only with concentrations which would be toxic. This would account for the lack of its clinical anti-inflammatory activity, and why anti-inflammatory activity is only seen in experimental animals at doses considerably in excess of those required for pain relief. Flower and Vane (1972) have suggested that the enzymes present in the central nervous system are more sensitive to the drug; on the other hand, the high concentrations of peroxides found in inflammatory tissue would make them resistant to this class of compounds (Marshall *et al.* 1987). Further evidence that paracetamol does not inhibit prostaglandin biosynthesis at therapeutic levels is that they have no effect on bleeding time or the production of thromboxane A_2 by platelets.

2.2.3 Toxicity

Paracetamol was thought to be relatively non-toxic until the late 1960s when it was realized that large overdoses produced hepatic necrosis which was associated with acute renal failure due to tubular necrosis in approximately 30 per cent of cases. The biochemical mechanisms of the hepatic toxicity have been elucidated by Mitchell *et al.* (1973*b*). Paracetamol is metabolically activated by cytochrome p450 mixed function oxidase to *N*-acetyl-*p*-benzoquinoneimine, which combines with glutathione to form a harmless metabolite. However, in overdosage, glutathione becomes depleted and the radical intermediate combines with tissue proteins, presumably sulphydryl groups. Also generated are oxygen radicals, and lipid peroxidation follows. Together, these events lead to the necrosis of the hepatocyte. The highest concentrations of cytochrome p450 occur in the centrilobular cells which are the most severely affected. As the exposure to paracetamol increases, further cells are damaged ultimately leading to total hepatic necrosis.

In the renal cortex, probably at least three enzyme systems are involved, but the toxic intermediate is the same as in the hepatocyte. The activity of cytochrome p450 mixed function oxidase in the renal cortex is only one third of that in the liver. Prostaglandin synthase is present in the renal cortex at approximately the same activity as cytochrome p450 (Mohandas *et al.* 1981*b*). The third enzyme system, deacetylase, produces *p*-aminophenol, which becomes activated by cytochrome p450 or prostaglandin synthase to the quinoneimine. These three enzyme systems result in a similar degree of covalent binding of the radical to protein, the presumed cause of damage to tissue (Mohandas *et al.* 1981*b*).

Understanding of this oxidative mechanism has led to the successful development of antidotes for paracetamol poisoning using several compounds containing sulphydryl groups (Rumack *et al.* 1981*a*). The most effective have been *N*-acetyl-cysteine and methionine, which probably work by two mechanisms: either forming an alternative substrate for the glutathione-*S*-transferase or spontaneously combining with the radical intermediate (Mohandas *et al.* 1984); or by maintaining the redox potential of the cell so as to enable the regeneration of glutathione.

2.3 Phenacetin

Phenacetin (acetophenetidin) is chemically the same as paracetamol except for ethylation of the phenolic hydroxyl group (Fig. 2.2). In the 1880s it was introduced to clinical medicine by the Bayer Company as a less toxic analogue of acetanalid, and was a popular analgesic until the 1970s when many countries restricted or banned its use (Sneader 1985). Compared to paracetamol and aspirin, there have been few studies done on phenacetin.

2.3.1 Pharmacokinetics

2.3.1.1 Absorption and distribution

Phenacetin is highly lipid soluble and relatively insoluble in aqueous media. It is rapidly and completely absorbed from the gastrointestinal tract by simple diffusion.

Being so lipid soluble, phenacetin penetrates cell membranes rapidly. It is distributed throughout the body with an apparent volume of distribution of approximately 1 l/kg body weight (Raaflaub and Dubach 1975).

2.3.1.2 Metabolism

Phenacetin is essentially a pro-drug, possibly itself being inactive as an analgesic. It undergoes extensive first-pass metabolism and, with the usual therapeutic doses, negligible quantities appear in the peripheral circulation. Metabolism in the small bowel mucosa and liver is by oxidative de-ethylation to paracetamol, catalysed by cytochrome p450 mixed function oxidase (Smith and Griffiths 1976). It is probable that paracetamol is the active metabolite (Brodie and Axelrod 1949; Prescott *et al.* 1970).

Multiple other metabolic pathways have been demonstrated, the chief being deacetylation, i.e. hydrolysis of the acetamino- bond to form *p*-phenetidine, principally in the liver and to a lesser extent in the kidney. The reaction is catalysed by a microsomal esterase (Bernhammer and Krisch

1965). *p*-Phenetidin demonstrates dose dependent metabolism. Ring hydroxylation occurs as a result of cytochrome p450 mixed function oxidase, yeilding 2-hydroxyphenacetin and 2-hydroxyphenetidine, which appear in the urine as sulphate and glucuronide conjugates (Hinson 1983). Both phenacetin and *p*-phenetidin undergo *N*-hydroxylation, catalysed by cytochrome p450, to form *N*-hydroxyphenacetin or *N*-hydroxy-*p*-phenetidine (Nelson *et al.* 1981*b*). However, only approximately 0.5 per cent of the parent drug appears in the urine in this form, some of which may bind as a reactive intermediate. *N*-hydroxyphenacetin is deacetylated to *N*-hydroxy-*p*-phenetidin (Nelson 1982), which has been shown to bind covalently to DNA, but not to cellular proteins. This latter reaction may be related to the carcinogenicity of phenacetin.

2.3.1.3 Excretion

Phenacetin itself is excreted by the kidney, being one drug whose concentration in the urine is equal to that in blood, indicating that tubular reabsorption occurs at the same rate as water (Duggin and Mudge 1976*b*). Phenacetin metabolites appear in the urine in the same proportions as following the administration of paracetamol. The half-life of phenacetin in blood is 0.7–1.25 h in man, reflecting its rapid conversion to paracetamol (Raaflaub and Dubach 1975).

2.3.2 Action

The pharmacology of phenacetin, and its therapeutic effect, appear almost identical to those of paracetamol. As paracetamol will always be present after the administration of phenacetin, it has not been possible to distinguish whether there are separate pharmacological effects. However, some human studies have indicated that phenacetin causes relaxation, drowsiness, and euphoria—it is these which have been linked with its use as a drug of habituation (Grimlund 1963).

2.3.3 Toxicity

Phenacetin toxicity appears to be similar to that of paracetamol, although there are additional effects which are thought to be mediated by its minor metabolites. Paracetamol has not been linked to carcinogenicity in the urinary tract, whereas considerable epidemiological evidence implicates phenacetin (Chapter 17). Phenacetin also produces methaemoglobin when consumed in large quantities, probably through the formation of *N*-hydroxyphenacetin, which generates redox changes within the red cell (Smith 1958).

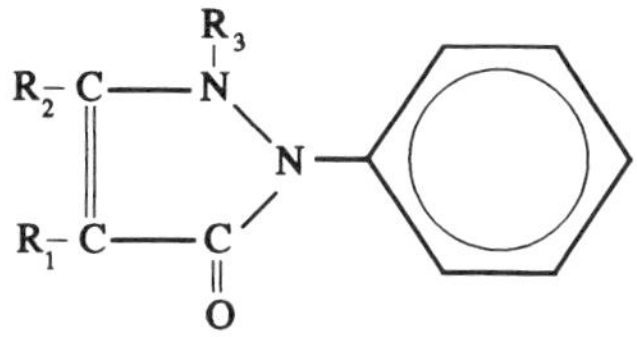

Fig. 2.3 The chemical structure of the principal pyrazolon drugs. Antipyrine: R_1 = –H; R_2 = $-CH_3$; R_3 = $-CH_3$. Isopropylantipyrine: R_1 = $-CH(CH_2)_2$; R_2 = $-CH_3$; R_3 = $-CH_3$. Aminopyrine: R_1 = $-N(CH_3)_2$; R_2 = $-CH_3$; R_3 = $-CH_3$. Phenylbutazone: R_1 = $-(CH_2)_3.CH_3$; R_2 = –H; R_3 = $-C_6H_5$. Sulphinpyrazone: R_1 = $-(CH_2)_2.SO.C_6H_5$; R_2 = –H; R_3 = $-C_6H_5$.

2.4 Pyrazolons

Antipyrine (phenazone), aminopyrine (amidopyrine; Pyramidon), and isopropylantipyrine (propyphenazone) (Fig. 2.3.) were introduced in the late nineteenth century as less toxic alternatives to salicylates, but the recognition in 1934 of often fatal agranulocytosis led to the withdrawal of aminopyrine, and possibly unfounded reservations about the continuing use of antipyrine (Sneader 1985). However, because it causes little gastric irritation, antipyrine still is a popular ingredient of proprietary analgesic preparations in continental Europe and Scandinavia.

A cogener, phenylbutazone, was in 1949 the first of the now large family of drugs introduced primarily as non-steroidal anti-inflammatory agents (NSAIDs), but it too has been abandoned because of bone marrow toxicity. Its derivative, sulphinpyrazone (Fig. 2.3), is employed mainly as a uricosuric agent because of its potent inhibition of proximal renal tubular organic anion transport.

2.4.1 Pharmacology

The pharmacokinetic properties of antipyrine have retained for it a place in investigative medicine (Vesell 1979). Firstly, its high lipid/water partition coefficient ensures rapid absorption and distribution throughout the extracellular and intracellular compartments. As it is also poorly bound to plasma proteins (less than 10 per cent), its volume of distribution is only slightly less than that of total body water, which it is used to measure. Secondly, its metabolism by cytochrome p450 mixed function oxidase is easily determined, follows first order kinetics, and is not affected by distribution or renal clearance which is negligible. Antipyrine clearance is therefore a sensitive and reliable measure of change in liver function used in monitoring the clinical status of individual patients.

Antipyrine is believed to exert its antipyretic, analgesic and anti-inflammatory effects by inhibiting prostaglandin synthesis in the central nervous system and in peripheral tissues. However, unlike the salicylates and most NSAIDs, it is not a weak acid.

No biochemical basis for its claimed nephrotoxicity (Chapter 3) or carcinogenicity (Chapter 16) has been elucidated.

2.5 Conclusions

While each of the commonly used antipyretic analgesics appears to exert its pharmacological effects through inhibition of prostaglandin synthase, this probably accounts for but a small part of the aetiology of analgesic nephropathy. The primary lesion, renal papillary necrosis, most likely is due to cytotoxic effects of metabolites of phenacetin (and probably paracetamol), to which the medullary cells are made more susceptible by depletion of glutathione (Mohandas *et al.* 1984) such as occurs when the renal papilla is exposed to high concentrations of salicylate (Duggin *et al.* 1980).

3
Experimental evidence for nephrotoxicity of analgesics

Ranjit S. Nanra and Priscilla Kincaid-Smith

3.1 Summary of experimental results

The rat is the most commonly used animal in experimental studies with analgesic nephrotoxicity. Although its kidney differs from the human in having a single papilla and a higher urine concentrating capability, the lesions induced in rats by analgesics are identical to those seen in clinical analgesic nephropathy.

3.1.1 Phenacetin

Attempts to evaluate the nephrotoxicity of phenacetin by changes in renal function have yielded conflicting results. Some studies revealed no abnormalities (Eder 1964; Ramsay and White 1965; Studer and Schärer 1965; Quintanilla and Delgado 1966; Peters *et al.* 1972; Viau *et al.* 1984). However, phenacetin given to rats and rabbits in doses of 210–3000 mg/kg body weight resulted in glomerular and tubular dysfunction. These abnormalities were: proteinuria, tubular epithelial celluria, a rise in blood urea nitrogen and serum creatinine, a fall in *p*-aminohippurate clearance (C_{PAH}), transient amino aciduria, impaired concentration and acidification, systemic acidosis, changes in urinary mucopolysaccharide composition and electrophoretic pattern, inhibition of oxygen consumption and phenol red uptake by renal cortex, and increase in urinary proximal tubular-specific antigens (Staub 1958; Clausen 1962; Angervall *et al.* 1964; Näntö *et al.* 1964; Studer and Schärer 1965; Fordham *et al.* 1965; Steele and Edwards 1970; Peters *et al.* 1972; Rosenmann *et al.* 1972) (Table 3.1).

Numerous attempts to produce renal papillary necrosis (RPN) with phenacetin in doses of 100–3000 mg/kg body weight fed to a variety of animals for 4–37 weeks were unsuccessful (Studer and Zbinden 1955; Gsell *et al.* 1957; Pletscher *et al.* *1958*; Schmidt 1958; Studer *et al.* 1958*b*; Eisalo and Talanti 1961; Keller *et al.* 1961; Eder 1964; Schnitzer *et al.* 1965; Torhorst *et al.* 1967; Brown and Hardy 1968; Kincaid-Smith *et al.* 1968*a*,*b*; Saker and Kincaid-Smith 1969; Nanra and Kincaid-Smith 1970, 1973*a*; Peters *et al.* 1972). Other studies reported only mild–intermediate grade RPN in 8–80

Table 3.1 *Renal function changes and acute tubular necrosis in analgesic-fed rats*

Function change	APC	Aspirin	Phenac -etin	Paracet -amol	Caffeine	Antipy -rine	Amino -pyrine	Phenylbut-azone	Indome -thacin
Haematuria	..	(+)	+	..	+	..	..	..	..
Epithelial celluria	..	++	+	+	(+)	+	..	..	..
Proteinuria	..	(+)	+	+	..	..	+	..	..
Glycosuria	..	..	..	..	..	..	+	..	..
β_2-microglobulinuria	..	(+)	..	+	..	..	..	..	..
Increased urinary β-*N*-acetylglucosaminidase	..	(+)	..	+	..	..	..	..	..
Enzymuria	..	++	..	..	..	..	..	..	..
Amino aciduria	..	..	+	..	..	..	..	..	..
Increased urinary acid mucopolysaccharide	..	..	+	+	..	..	..	..	..
Increased urinary renal specific antigen	..	+	+	..	..	..	..	..	..
Elevated serum urea, creatinine	..	+	+	+	..	+	+	..	..
Acute fall in *p*-aminohippurate clearance	..	+	+	..	..	..	..	..	..
Reduced phenolsulphonthalein excretion	..	(+)	..	..	..	..	..	..	+
Impaired concentration	+	+	+	+	+	+	+	..	..
Acidification defect	+	+	+	..	..	..	..	..	..
Impaired sodium conservation	+	+	+	..	..	..	..	..	..
Reduced oxygen consumption	..	..	+	+	..	..	+	..	..
Reduced cortical phenol red uptake	..	..	+	+	..	..	+	..	..
Acute tubular necrosis	..	+	..	+	+	..	..	+	+

.. Indicates no information; ( ) indicates clinical observation; Adapted from Nanra and Kincaid-Smith 1986.

per cent of rats, rabbits and mice given phenacetin in doses of 137–3000 mg/kg/day for 4–80 weeks (Clausen 1964; Abrahams *et al.* 1964; Fordham *et al.* 1965; Markovic 1971; Nanra and Kincaid-Smith 1973*a*; Molland 1978; Macklin and Szot 1980) (Table 3.2). To shorten the period of gavage feeding of phenacetin, Nanra and Kincaid-Smith (1973*a*) subjected the animals to 18 h dehydration daily as well; a constant water diuresis in the same study afforded total protection from RPN. Papillary calcification was noted in one study (Fordham *et al.* 1965) and chronic interstitial nephritis (CIN) in another (Markovic 1971); in the latter study, quartz particles were given with phenacetin.

The Gunn rat with hyperbilirubinaemia has an increased susceptibility to analgesic nephrotoxicity. Axelsen (1975) induced RPN in 7 per cent of Gunn rats with 4 weeks of feeding with phenacetin in a dose of 320–500 mg/kg/day. In a dose–response study, single doses of phenacetin of 175–720 mg/kg failed to induce renal lesions, whereas 1150 mg/kg resulted in RPN in 33 per cent of animals (Axelsen 1976) (Table 3.3).

Attempts to evaluate the effect of phenacetin on experimental pyelonephritis gave conflicting results, ranging from no effect (Dawborn *et al.* 1964; Diaz-Esquivel and Farmer 1968; Vivaldi 1968) to minor tubular degeneration, interstitial inflammation and calcification (Clausen 1962; Angervall *et al.* 1962*a*,*b*,*c*; Schourup *et al.* 1963).

3.1.2 Paracetamol

Paracetamol is the major immediate metabolite of phenacetin. In experimental studies, the renal functional defects with paracetamol in doses of 300–900 mg/kg/day given over 2–10 months were very similar to those seen with phenacetin; negative results have also been reported (Peters *et al.* 1972). The functional abnormalities reported include: proteinuria, renal tubular epithelial celluria, renal insufficiency, impaired concentration, β_2-microglobulinuria, and inhibition of renal cortical uptake of phenol red and oxygen consumption (Staub 1958; Angervall *et al.* 1964; Peters *et al.* 1972; Bernard *et al.* 1988) (Table 3.1). In studies of cadmium nephrotoxicity, paracetamol appears to render the kidney more susceptible to proteinuria and increased urinary losses of β-*N*-acetylglucosaminidase and β_2-microglobulin (Bernard *et al.* 1988).

Attempts to produce histological lesions in rats using a single dose of paracetamol, 300–7000 mg/kg, resulted in either no lesions or minor tubular changes (Boyd and Bereczky 1966; Calder *et al.* 1971; Hart *et al.* 1980); however, proximal tubular necrosis was induced with a single dose of paracetamol, 750 mg/kg, in susceptible rats (Mitchell *et al.* 1977; McMurtry *et al.* 1978). In long-term studies in various animals, paracetamol, in doses of 50–4000 mg/kg/day for periods of 4–40 weeks, failed to produce RPN, although minor tubular lesions were noted (Pletscher *et al.* 1958; Eisalo and

Table 3.2 *Renal papillary necrosis with single analgesics and NSAIDs*

Drug	Dose	Duration of feeding	Renal papillary necrosis		Chronic interstitial nephritis	Calcification
	mg/kg/day	weeks	per cent	grade	per cent	per cent
Phenacetin	137–3000	4–80	8–80	+	+	+
Paracetamol	894–3000	8–36	43–63	+	..	..
Aspirin	200–500	8–66	33–75	+ to ++	+	+
uninephrectomy	325	12–15	100	++	..	..
Caffeine	100	16	23	+	..	..
Antipyrine	1000	12–30	13	+	—	38
Aminopyrine	500–1200	7	83	+	..	..
Phenylbutazone	10	8–20	11	++	—	33
Indomethacin	12	12–30	29	++	14	43
Flufenamic acid	..	..	+	..	..	..
"	50–100	single dose	+	..	..	..
Meclofenamic acid	..	..	+	..	..	..
Mefenamic acid	100	8–20	66–67	+ to ++	—	89
Naproxen	..	..	+	..	+	..
Sudoxicam	2	..	+	..	..	..
Fenoprofen	40–305	78	+	..	+	..

.. Indicates no information.

Table 3.3 *Renal papillary necrosis in Gunn rats*

Drug	Dose	Duration of feeding	Renal papillary necrosis		Chronic interstitial nephritis
	mg/kg/day	weeks	per cent	grade	per cent
Phenacetin	320–500	4	7	+	..
	1150	single dose	33	+	..
Paracetamol	268–420	4	37	+	..
uninephrectomy	538	single dose	85	+	+
Aspirin	200–500	3–4	45–63	++	..
	175–1150	single dose	17–100	++	..
uninephrectomy	225	single dose	90	++	..
Sodium salicylate	480	single dose	50	++	..
Antipyrine uninephrectomy	471	single dose	80	++	40
APC	1190	5–18 days	100	++	..
	238	25–34	70	++	..
Aspirin plus paracetamol	1182	single dose	100	++	70
Antipyrine plus paracetamol	1260	single dose	95	++	75

.. Indicates no information.

Talanti 1961; Eder 1964; Schnitzer and Smith 1966; Boyd and Hogan 1968; Peters *et al.* 1972). Nanra *et al.* (1971) and Nanra and Kincaid-Smith (1972, 1973*a*) reported intermediate grade RPN in 43 per cent of rats given 3000 mg/kg/day paracetamol combined with 18 hours dehydration per day for 8–20 weeks. Similarly, Molland (1978) also found intermediate grade RPN in 60 per cent of animals given 894 mg/kg/day of paracetamol over 36 weeks (Table 3.2).

RPN with mild–moderate CIN has been reported in 37 per cent of Gunn rats given paracetamol orally, 268–420 mg/kg/day over 4 weeks, and in 85 per cent of uninephrectomized animals given a single intravenous dose, 3 mg/kg (Axelsen 1975; Henry and Tange 1984) (Table 3.3); the RPN was noted to be less severe than that with aspirin (Briggs *et al.* 1982).

Studies of the effect of paracetamol on experimental pyelonephritis gave conflicting results with either aggravation (Miescher and Studer 1961; Angervall *et al.* 1962*a*,*b*) or no effect (Angervall *et al.* 1962*c*; Vivaldi 1968).

3.1.3 Aspirin

In acute animal studies, aspirin readily causes renal tubular epithelial celluria (Arnold *et al.* 1973*a*), enzymuria (Raab 1969, 1970; Trnavský and Rovenský 1972), and acute tubular necrosis (Boyd 1959*a*; Fellers *et al.* 1965; Coldwell and Boyd 1966; Robinson *et al.* 1967; Szafranowa 1970; Arnold *et al.* 1973*a*,*b*,*c*). These effects are more pronounced than with phenacetin or paracetamol, and are similar to those in man; acute clinical studies with aspirin have resulted in proteinuria, haematuria, increased urinary excretion of β-*N*-acetylglucosaminidase and β_2-microglobulin, and reduced phenolsulphonphthalein excretion (Prescott 1982*a*). In long-term studies over 39–52 weeks, rats developed impaired concentration, acidification, and sodium conservation with 210–250 mg/kg/day of aspirin (Angervall *et al.* 1964; Steele and Edwards 1970) (Table 3.1). However, a lower dose of aspirin, 27 mg/kg/day over 52 weeks, had no effect on creatinine clearance, concentration, enzymuria or amino aciduria (Viau *et al.* 1984).

In 1962, Clausen reported the development of RPN in 47 per cent of rabbits fed with 1–2 g/day of aspirin for 56 weeks. Attempts to induce RPN in different animals with aspirin doses of 24–125 mg/kg/day over 4–12 weeks, or single larger doses of 250–700 mg/kg, were unsuccessful (Eder 1964; Fellers *et al.* 1965; Phillips *et al.* 1976). Similarly, pigs fed 1000 mg/kg/day of aspirin for 48 weeks also failed to develop RPN (McIver and Hobbs 1975). In separate studies, Nanra and Kincaid-Smith (1970, 1973*b*; Nanra *et al.* 1971) gavage-fed rats with 500 mg/kg/day of aspirin for 8–20 weeks and subjected the animals to 18 h dehydration daily; 33 per cent of rats developed intermediate or total RPN. Similar results were seen with a lower dose of aspirin, 200 mg/kg/day, gavage-fed over 10–66 weeks, with RPN in 55 per cent, and CIN in 23 per cent of rats (Nanra and Kincaid-Smith 1973*b*). The ability of aspirin to induce RPN was confirmed by Molland (1976, 1978); RPN developed in 75 per cent of rats given 318 mg/kg/day of aspirin for 18–24 weeks, and in 100 per cent of uninephrectomized animals fed 325 mg/kg/day of aspirin for 12–15 weeks (Table 3.2). Simultaneous gavage feeding of sodium bicarbonate, 100 mg/kg/day, with aspirin, 500 mg/kg/day, over 20 weeks prevented the development of RPN; sodium bicarbonate given to rats in a lower dose, 50 mg/kg/day, afforded only partial protection with RPN developing in 20 per cent of animals (Nanra and Kincaid-Smith 1973*b*).

The Gunn rat also readily develops RPN with aspirin, the lesion developing in 45 per cent of rats given 250 mg/kg/day over 4 weeks (Axelsen 1975). Axelsen (1976) also demonstrated a dose–response effect; increasing single doses of aspirin from 175 to 280, 450, 720 and 1150 mg/kg resulted in RPN in 17, 33, 33, 50 and 100 per cent of animals, respectively. A single dose of sodium salicylate, 3 mmol/kg, also induced RPN in 50 per cent of animals

(Harper and Axelsen 1982). The effects of aspirin in Gunn rats were magnified by subjecting the animals to uninephrectomy; a single dose of aspirin, 1.25 mmol/kg induced RPN in 90 per cent of rats and CIN in 20 per cent of rats (Henry and Tange 1984) (Table 3.3). Briggs *et al.* (1982) had noted that the RPN induced by aspirin was more severe than that seen with paracetamol.

3.1.4 Caffeine

Data relating to caffeine nephrotoxicity has been conflicting. Caffeine had been shown to induce haematuria and renal tubular epithelial celluria in clinical studies (Prescott 1965), and impaired renal concentrating capacity and dose-related acute tubular necrosis in laboratory animals (Vinci 1914; Boyd 1959*b*; Boyd *et al.* 1965; Steele and Edwards 1970). However, feeding rats with caffeine alone, 150 mg/kg/day for 20 weeks, failed to induce RPN (Nanra *et al.* 1971; Nanra and Kincaid-Smith 1972) or uroepithelial changes suggestive of malignancy (Takayama and Kuwabara 1982). In fact, it had been suggested that caffeine may reduce the nephrotoxicity of analgesics (Nanra and Kincaid-Smith 1970), and this was supported by functional studies in animals (Steele and Edwards 1970; Steele *et al.* 1971). De Crespigny *et al.* (1990) have found that 23 per cent of rats given 100 mg/kg/day of caffeine over 16 weeks developed weight loss, haematuria and mild RPN (Tables 3.1, 3.2).

3.1.5 Pyrazolon derivatives

Antipyrine (phenazone), aminopyrine and isopropylantipyrine, all commonly used in analgesic mixtures, especially in Europe, have been shown to be nephrotoxic.

In studies in animals over 7 weeks, antipyrine caused renal tubular epithelial celluria, proteinuria, impaired concentrating capacity and a reduction in glomerular filtration rate (GFR) (Aosima 1940*a*,*b*; Brown and Hardy 1968). Aosima (1940*a*,*b*) had noted minor histological changes in rabbits given 30 mg/kg/day of antipyrine. However, 13 per cent of rats fed antipyrine, 1000 mg/kg/day, for 12–30 weeks developed RPN (Nanra *et al.* 1971; Nanra and Kincaid-Smith 1973*a*, 1986). More recently, Gunn rats with uninephrectomy were given a single intravenous dose of antipyrine, 2.5 mmol/kg, and the kidneys were examined after 1 month; 80 per cent developed moderate RPN and 40 per cent had significant CIN (Henry and Tange 1984).

Aminopyrine was also found to be nephrotoxic in a series of experiments in rabbits, Fazekas *et al.* (1960*a*,*b*, 1961) reporting oliguria or polyuria, proteinuria, glycosuria, and elevation of blood urea concentration. RPN was noted in 83 per cent of rats given 500–1200 mg/kg/day of aminopyrine for 7 weeks (Brown and Hardy 1968).

Phenylbutazone is nephrotoxic and induces RPN and calcification. Cats fed phenylbutazone, 44 mg/kg/day, and rats given oxyphenbutazone, developed acute tubular necrosis, cystic dilatation of tubules and nephrocalcinosis (Carlisle *et al.* 1968; Arnold *et al.* 1976). A single dose of phenylburazone, 400 mg/kg, induced RPN, in some rats within 1 h, and in the majority of animals within 54 h (Arnold *et al.* 1976); RPN was also seen with a single low dose of 50 mg/kg of phenylbutazone. In long-term studies over 8–20 weeks, RPN developed in 11 per cent, and nephrocalcinosis in 33 per cent, of rats gavage-fed 10 mg/kg/day of phenylbutazone (Nanra *et al.* 1971; Nanra and Kincaid-Smith 1973*a*, 1986).

3.1.6 Indomethacin

Indomethacin, a potent suppressor of prostaglandin (PG) synthesis, readily induces RPN in experimental studies. In 1971, Bokelman *et al.* reported that indeneacetic acid, a drug closely allied to indomethacin, caused haematuria, acute tubular necrosis, uroepithelial hyperplasia, and RPN. A single dose of indomethacin, 20–75 mg/kg, induced RPN in 60–80 per cent of rats; RPN developed within 1 hour with the higher dose (Arnold *et al.* 1974, 1976). RPN has been reported with chronic oral feeding of indomethacin in a dose of 12 mg/kg/day for 12–30 weeks in 29 per cent of animals, with papillary calcification in 43 per cent, and CIN in 14 per cent (Nanra and Kincaid-Smith 1973*a*, 1986).

3.1.7 Fenemates

In animal studies, mefenamic acid, flufenamic acid and meclofenamic acid, and glafenine, a related drug, readily induce tubular lesions (Kaump 1966; Gaetani *et al.* 1972; Lechat *et al.* 1974) and RPN (Kaump 1966). The papillotoxicity of the fenemates is confirmed by induction of RPN in animals by a single dose of flufenamic acid, 50–100 mg/kg, or an allied drug, *N*-phenylanthranilic acid (Hardy 1970*a*,*b*). Chronic feeding of rats over 8–20 weeks with 100 mg/kg/day of mefenamic acid also resulted in RPN in 67 per cent of animals; medullary calcification was noted in the lesions (Nanra *et al.* 1971; Nanra and Kincaid-Smith 1973*a*, 1986; de Crespigny *et al.* 1990).

3.1.8 Propionic acid derivatives

Adams *et al.* (1969) had reported the development of tubular lesions in animals given ibuprofen. Subsequent experiments in which animals were given naproxen, sudoxicam, 2 mg/kg/day, or fenoprofen, 40–305 mg/kg/day for 18 months resulted in the development of RPN and CIN (Hallesy *et al.* 1973; Wiseman and Reinert 1975; Ingram 1979; Curt *et al.* 1980).

3.1.9 Mixed analgesics

Renal functional studies in rats fed with a mixture of aspirin, phenacetin, and caffeine (APC), in doses of 500–2700 mg/kg/day for 6–39 weeks (Steele

Table 3.4 *Renal papillary necrosis with analgesic mixtures*

Drug	Dose	Duration of feeding	Renal papillary necrosis	
	mg/kg/day	weeks	per cent	grade
Aspirin, phenacetin, caffeine	900	8–30	46–70	++
Aspirin, paracetamol, caffeine	900	8–30	38–75	++
Aspirin, salicylamide, caffeine	900	12–30	54	++
Aspirin, phenacetin	750	8–20	40	++
Antipyrine, phenacetin, caffeine	840	12–30	17–36	+
Mefanamic acid, caffeine	200	16	62	++

and Edwards 1970; Edwards *et al.* 1971; Nanra *et al.* 1973), have shown defects in concentration, acidification and sodium conservation, and elevation of blood urea and serum creatinine concentrations. The concentrating capacity appears to recover upon cessation of analgesics, and the raised blood urea and serum creatinine levels to improve after separation of the necrotic papilla and healing of the papillary stump; the latter has been well demonstrated with lesions induced by *N*-phenylanthranilic acid (Hardy 1970*a*). Physiological studies performed in rats with RPN induced by analgesic mixtures containing combinations of aspirin, phenacetin, paracetamol, salicylamide, phenazone (antipyrine), and caffeine, have shown changes which are similar to those seen in clinical analgesic nephropathy (Nanra *et al.* 1981*a*). The significant abnormalities which are different from control animals are hypertension, reduced total body sodium, sodium excretion, renal vein PGE_2, and concentrating capacity, and increased renal vein plasma renin and hepatic salicylate esterase activity (Table 3.1).

In most studies, experimental RPN has been readily induced by APC mixtures (Table 3.4). In 1967, Abrahams and Levin reported RPN in 63 per cent of rats given A (27), P (20), and C (4 mg/kg/day) for 44 weeks. To shorten the time of feeding, rats were gavage-fed the A (380), P (380), and C (140 mg/kg/day) for 8–30 weeks and subjected to 18 hours dehydration daily; 46–70 per cent of animals developed RPN (Nanra and Kincaid-Smith 1970, 1973*a*; Nanra *et al.* 1971; Nanra *et al.* 1980). Replacement of phenacetin by paracetamol or salicylamide in, or removal of caffeine from, the analgesic mixture, did not alter the incidence or severity of RPN; 38–75 per cent of the rats developed RPN (Nanra and Kincaid-Smith 1970, 1973*a*; Nanra *et al.* 1971; Nanra *et al.* 1980). In a short-term study in rabbits given 5–7 g of APC over 6–36 h, electron microscopy revealed that the early renal changes were proximal tubular brush border calcification, mitochondrial calcification and peroxisomal changes (Hennis *et al.* 1982).

Early attempts to produce RPN with isopropylantipyrine (150) plus phenacetin (250) plus persidon (50) plus caffeine (50 mg/kg/day) in animals were unsuccessful (Studer and Zbinden 1955; Thölen *et al.* 1956). However, gavage feeding rats with a higher dose of phenacetin (300) plus antipyrine (300) plus caffeine (240 mg/kg/day) for 12–30 weeks resulted in RPN in 36 per cent of animals (Nanra *et al.* 1980); similarly, Johansson (1981) found RPN in 17 per cent of animals.

In a recent study, rats given mefenamic acid (100) plus caffeine (100 mg/kg/day) for 16 weeks developed total RPN in 62 per cent of animals (de Crespigny *et al.* 1990). Electron microscopic studies revealed increased interstitial tissue around bundles of vasa recta. The animals also developed weight loss and haematuria.

Studies in Gunn rats administered APC showed a high incidence of RPN with a dose–response (Table 3.3); all animals given 1190 mg/kg/day of the mixture for 5–18 days developed RPN, compared to 70 per cent of animals given 238 mg/kg/day for 25–34 days (Axelsen 1975). The predisposition of Gunn rats to RPN is also demonstrated in studies with analgesics delivered intravenously (Henry and Tange 1984) (Table 3.4). Homozygous Gunn rats with unilateral nephrectomy given a single intravenous dose of aspirin (1.25) plus paracetamol (3 mmol/kg) developed moderate RPN in all, and CIN in 70 per cent. Similar results were obtained with a single intravenous dose of antipyrine (2.5) plus paracetamol (3 mmol/kg), with RPN in 95 per cent and CIN in 75 per cent of rats. No renal lesions developed in uninephrectomized albino rats given the same analgesic mixtures.

3.2 Causation of renal papillary necrosis

3.2.1 Countercurrent concentration

The countercurrent concentration mechanism plays a central role in RPN, and numerous experimental studies with analgesics suggest that dehydration aggravates, and that diuresis ameliorates, RPN (reviewed by Bach and Bridges 1985); this is also seen with 2-bromoethanamine-induced RPN (Sabatini *et al.* 1983). Prior papillectomy in animals, which interferes with the long loops of Henle and the countercurrent arrangement, also protects against experimental RPN (Hardy 1970*b*; Molland 1978). It has been suggested that the renal countercurrent concentration mechanism is responsible for the specific concentration of toxicokinetic factors in target cells in the renal medulla (Mudge 1985). The earliest histological lesions in experimental RPN are toward the tip of the papilla, the site of maximal concentration of analgesics. In hydropenic animals the medullary-to-cortical concentration gradient of conjugated paracetamol is 10 : 1 and that of free paracetamol is 16 : 1 (Bluemle and Goldberg 1968; Duggin and Mudge 1975, 1976*a*,*b*; Duggin 1980). This cortico-medullary gradient is not seen with phenacetin (Duggin and Mudge 1976*b*). Studies with aspirin either do not show a concentration gradient, or show a mild gradient between medulla and cortex, 1.9–4.5 : 1; there is some evidence of accumulation of aspirin in the cortex in the pars recta of proximal tubules (Bluemle and Goldberg 1968; Gault 1971; Molland 1978; Duggin 1980). Aspirin and salicylate have an intracellular distribution which is augmented by maximal urinary acidification (Caterson and Duggin 1978; Duggin 1980); this explains the protective effect of sodium bicarbonate on experimental RPN with aspirin (Nanra and Kincaid-Smith 1973*b*). An additional effect of dehydration is the promotion of medullary ischaemia (Thurau 1964), an important mechanism in RPN (Nanra *et al.* 1973; Shimamura and Trojanowski 1976).

3.2.2 Medullary ischaemia

The renal medulla has low oxygen tension and is susceptible to anoxic injury. Thus RPN readily develops in experimental renal arterial or venous occlusion, or ureteric ligation (Muirhead *et al.* 1950; Sheehan and Davis 1959*a*,*b*; Beswick and Schatzki 1960; Davies 1968; Baum *et al.* 1969). Medullary ischaemia has been demonstrated in experimental analgesic nephropathy and correlates with evidence of medullary dysfunction, such as impaired concentrating capacity and sodium conservation (Nanra *et al.* 1973). The histological features of RPN are suggestive of an ischaemic infarction, and vasa recta lesions with endothelial necrosis, vascular obliteration and narrowing, platelet aggregation, increased interstitial fibrosis, and a more generalized microangiopathy or capillary sclerosis, have all been demonstrated early in RPN (Kincaid-Smith *et al.* 1968*a*,*b*; Abrahams and Levinson 1970; Nanra *et al.* 1973; Burry *et al.* 1977; Molland 1978; Mihatsch *et al.* 1983*a*; de Crespigny *et al.* 1990).

3.2.3 Disturbed arachidonic acid and prostaglandin metabolism

Most antipyretic-analgesics and non-steroidal anti-inflammatory drugs (NSAIDs) interfere with arachidonic acid metabolism resulting in reduced prostaglandin $(PG)E_2$ or increased thromboxane $(TX)A_2$ synthesis by suppression of cyclooxygenase, leading to vasoconstriction and medullary ischaemia (Shelley 1978; Nanra 1980; Dunn and Zambraski 1980; McGiff 1981; Frölich *et al.* 1981). Matsuda *et al.* (1983) have shown that the potency of suppression of PG synthesis by NSAIDs is flubiprofen > ketoprofen > naproxen > indomethacin > diclofenac > meclofenamic acid > mefenamic acid > aspirin; this ranking accords with their potency in inducing RPN (Hardy 1978, unpublished data). It has been suggested that altered PG metabolism may have a role in carcinogenesis (Honn *et al.* 1981).

3.2.4 Metabolic activation and changes in intermediary metabolism

Aspirin undergoes metabolic activation with formation of a reactive metabolite mediated by the microsomal cytochrome p450 dependent monooxygenase (Mitchell *et al.* 1977). Aspirin has a number of major effects on intermediary metabolism. It: (1) inhibits the hexose monophosphate shunt resulting in reduced tissue glutathione and a predisposition to covalent binding of electrophilic molecules (Goldberg *et al.* 1971; Duggin 1980); (2) irreversibly blocks fatty acid cyclooxygenase causing reduced lipogenesis in the renal medulla, and also leads to reduced levels of glutathione (Caterson *et al.* 1978; Zenser *et al.* 1978; Roth and Siok 1978; Humes *et al.* 1981; Beynen *et al.* 1982; von Bruchlausen and Baumann 1982; Tolman *et al.* 1983); (3) provides the acetyl group for transacetylating macromolecules, resulting in inhibition of PG synthetase in the renal cortex and medulla (Hawkins *et al.* 1969; Caterson *et al.* 1978; Shamsuddin *et al.* 1974; Roth and Majerus 1975); (4) uncouples cortical oxidative phosphorylation, resulting in reduced intracellular adenosine triphosphate (ATP) (Quintanilla and Kessler 1973; Dawson 1975); (5) inhibits amino acid incorporation into cellular proteins, an effect that is enhanced by paracetamol (Davidson *et al.* 1973*a,b*); and (6) may induce tissue hypoxia by reducing red cell 2,3-diphosphoglyceride (Kravath *et al.* 1972).

Other NSAIDs also undergo metabolic activation by PG-hydroperoxidase or other peroxidase-mediated metabolic pathways (Marnett 1981; Bakkenist *et al.* 1981; Egan *et al.* 1981; Eling *et al.* 1983; Wise *et al.* 1983). The reactive metabolites which result have effects similar to those of aspirin, including reduced medullary lipogenesis, reduced tissue levels of glutathione, and medullary ischaemia (Beynen *et al.* 1982).

Paracetamol, and its metabolite *p*-aminophenol, undergo p450 mediated activation to a reactive alkylating intermediate metabolite, probably *N*-acetyl-*p*-benzoquinoneimine, as well as peroxidative activation to reactive phenolic or aromatic metabolites (McMurtry *et al.* 1978; Crowe *et al.* 1979; Calder *et al.* 1979; Moldéus and Rahimtula 1980; Boyd and Eling 1981; Mohandas *et al.* 1981*a*; Carpenter and Mudge 1981; Gemborys and Mudge 1981; Nelson *et al.* 1981*a*; Newton *et al.* 1982; Zenser *et al.* 1983*a*; Hinson 1983). Like aspirin and other NSAIDs, paracetamol also has significant effects on intermediary metabolism: (1) markedly depleting serum sulphate and sulphate clearance thus limiting sulphate availability for medullary synthesis of proteoglycans (PoGs) and glycosaminoglycans (GAGs), essential constituents of medullary matrix (Lin and Levy 1983); and (2) generating reactive metabolites which covalently bind to cellular proteins and nuclei leading to intracellular depletion of glutathione in renal cortex and medulla (Mudge *et al.* 1978), an effect which is augmented during antidiuresis (McMurtry *et al.* 1978; Mudge *et al.* 1978).

The major deacetylated metabolite of phenacetin, *p*-phenitidine, also produces biologically reactive species with toxic effects similar to those of paracetamol (Kadlubar *et al.* 1982; Andersson *et al.* 1983).

3.3 Pathogenesis of experimental renal papillary necrosis and chronic interstitial nephritis

The renal functional changes induced by analgesics have been fully reviewed by Nanra and Kincaid-Smith (1972, 1986) and Prescott (1982*a*) (Table 3.1). The reduction in renal oxygen consumption and phenol red uptake are considered non-specific effects. Most of the urinary abnormalities reflect tubular epithelial toxicity and mimic the changes seen with model proximal tubular nephrotoxins (Kennedy and Saluga 1970). However, medullary toxicity is manifest by defects in concentration, acidification, sodium conservation, medullary ischaemia, and increased urinary excretion of PoGs and GAGs.

Metabolic activation of analgesics and NSAIDs generates free radicals, strongly electrophilic intermediates or unstable metabolites which are normally removed by intracellular nucleophiles, such as glutathione, and antioxidants; failure of this protective mechanism, also caused by analgesics and NSAIDs, results in the binding or arylation of intracellular proteins by toxic metabolites, leading to cell dysfunction and death in the renal medulla (Nelson 1982). In RPN, the medullary interstitial cells, which are active metabolically, are damaged and reduced in number (Molland 1976, 1978; Henry and Tange 1983). The interstitial cells contain lipooxygenase and peroxidase enzymes, and fatty acids, and are involved in glycolysis, gluconeogenesis, PoG and GAG synthesis, and lipogenesis; the low oxygen tension in the medulla facilitates the lipooxygenase reaction and makes these cells extremely vulnerable to papillotoxins (Bojesen 1974; Moldéus and Rahimtula 1980; Mohandas *et al.* 1981*a*; Nelson *et al.* 1981*a*; reviewed by Bach and Bridges 1985). The earliest lesions in experimental RPN occur in the loops of Henle, vasa recta bundles and interstitial cells (Kincaid-Smith *et al.* 1968*a*,*b*; Molland 1976,1978; Axelsen 1978), especially at the papillary tip, the site of maximal concentration of papillotoxins and maximal tissue ischaemia, due to suppression of vasodilator medullary PGs and lipids, and to vasa recta lesions. The combination of cytonecrosis and medullary ischaemia leads to the development of RPN, with features of ischaemic infarction. Obstruction of tubules in the necrotic medulla leads to the changes of CIN in the cortex. The presence of mononuclear cells in CIN may represent interference to the normal trafficking of these cells through the interstitium as well as the effect of chemotactic metabolites in the lipooxygenase pathway (Bach and Bridges 1985). However, CIN may develop without RPN, especially with aspirin (Molland 1978; Nanra 1983); aspirin may achieve a six-fold cortical concentration in hydropenic animals (Duggin 1980), and has significant cortical cytotoxic effects.

In analgesic- and NSAID-induced RPN, the medullary matrix is also damaged and shows altered staining characteristics (Molland 1976; Bach and Bridges 1985). There is reduced medullary synthesis of PoG and GAG by interstitial cells due to inhibition of sulphate incorporation, decreased glycosamine turnover in renal mitochondria and microsomes, depolymerization of GAG by reactive metabolites, extensive loss of medullary mucopolysaccharides and increased urine excretion of GAG (Näntö *et al.* 1964; Molland 1976, 1978; Bach and Bridges 1985). The possible effects of medullary loss of PoG–GAGs include loss of concentrating capacity, loss of Tamm–Horsfall mucoprotein, tendency to microcrystallization and stone formation, susceptibility to urinary tract infections, and basement membrane thickening of loops of Henle and vasa recta (Angervall *et al.* 1964; Hardy 1970*a*; Nanra and Kincaid-Smith 1972; Burry *et al.* 1977; Molland 1978; Nanra 1980; Macklin and Szot 1980; Mihatsch *et al.* 1983*a*); uroepithelial hyperplasia and carcinoma may also be secondary to loss of PoG and GAG (Kennedy 1979). The loss of vasodilator medullary PG and antihypertensive lipids may also contribute to the development of hypertension in RPN (Nanra *et al.* 1981*a*).

Thus, the histopathological features of RPN and CIN, and the functional abnormalities in experimental analgesic nephropathy, are similar to those in man. On the basis of available data, the following stages in the pathogenesis of experimental analgesic nephropathy are proposed (modified from Nanra 1976*a*; Nanra and Kincaid-Smith 1986):

Stage I. The concentration of analgesics or NSAIDs in the renal medulla by the countercurrent mechanism leads to reversible medullary ischaemia due to suppression of PG synthesis.

Stage II. Damage to medullary interstitial cells and medullary matrix by reactive metabolites with loss of PoG and GAG. This stage may be associated with impaired concentrating ability, hypertension, papillary calcification, and thickening of basement membrane of loops of Henle and vasa recta.

Stage III. Necrobiosis of loop of Henle cells and vasa recta endothelial cells leading to occlusive changes and irreversible medullary ischaemia.

Stage IV. The extreme vulnerability of the renal medulla to ischaemic damage results in necrosis of the papilla with histological features of an ischaemic infarct caused by irreversible medullary ischaemia, cytotoxic cell necrosis, and medullary matrix damage.

Stage V. Obstruction of renal tubules in the necrotic medulla leads to secondary atrophy of the overlying cortex with histological changes of CIN.

3.4 The aetiological agent

All analgesics and NSAIDs which cause RPN produce large quantities of toxicokinetic molecules, and both the parent drug and the metabolites are excreted via the kidney (Prescott 1982*a*). Thus most analgesics and NSAIDs are able to induce RPN, and their potency in the induction of the medullary lesion is partly consequent upon their degree of suppression of PG synthesis (Hardy 1978, quoted by Bach and Bridges 1985). The nephrotoxicity of these drugs is time–dose dependent and dose–response effects have been demonstrated.

In the APC mixture, aspirin appears to be the most potent nephrotoxin. The papillotoxicity of phenacetin is largely related to paracetamol, its major immediate metabolite; the possible role of *p*-phenitidine, its major de-acetylated metabolite should also be considered. However, the papillotoxic potential of aspirin and phenacetin or paracetamol is greatly enhanced in combination, and this synergistic nephrotoxicity is readily explained by their effects on intermediary metabolism (Duggin 1980; Nanra and Kincaid-Smith 1970, 1973*a*).

4
The implication of analgesics in human kidney disease

M.M. Elseviers and Marc E. De Broe

The abuse of analgesics was described for the first time in 1907 in Australia in a local newspaper article entitled 'What the drink habit is among men, the headache powder is among women' (Nanra *et al.* 1978*a*). During and after the Second World War, the consumption of analgesics increased. In 1952, an investigation was started in Sweden into the cause of high mortality due to end stage renal failure observed in an area where a locally produced analgesic powder had widespread use (Grimlund 1963), and in 1953, Spühler and Zollinger published the first report of a possible association between the increased incidence of chronic interstitial nephritis observed by autopsy and a history of excessive use of analgesics.

The initial reports, observing that phenacetin was present in most of the abused analgesic mixtures, generated the oversimplified conclusion that phenacetin was the nephrotoxic agent. Consequently the associated renal disease received the name 'phenacetin nephritis', and restrictive measures on the sale of analgesics were focused on this ingredient (Scandinavia, Canada, United Kingdom). The success of these measures in decreasing new cases of analgesic nephropathy, especially in Scandinavia, supported the phenacetin misconception. However, experimental work showed that the analgesics usually taken in combination with phenacetin (salicylates, antipyrine, aminopyrine) are also nephrotoxic in animals, and Australian data indicated that the withdrawal of phenacetin did not lead to the expected decrease in end stage renal failure due to analgesic nephropathy (Disney and Roy 1988). However, these data must be interpreted with caution because incidence rates were confounded by the steady rise in the average age of patients accepted into dialysis so that patients with analgesic-induced kidney disease, who would earlier have died without treatment, were now being recorded (McCredie *et al.* 1989; Disney 1991). In the 1970s and 1980s, it became accepted that excessive use of different kinds of analgesic mixtures, whether or not including phenacetin, may cause renal damage. The more appropriate term, analgesic nephropathy (AN), was introduced and progressively the phenacetin misconception was abandoned.

In most populations studied, abuse was found to be more common in females and consequently the reported incidence of AN was higher in women than in men. End-stage renal failure due to analgesic abuse was observed after consumption for approximately 20 yr, and most patients with AN entered renal replacement therapy in their fifth decade. Headache has been the reason most often advanced for regular ingestion of analgesics. However, in the case of excessive use, headache is often a result, rather than a cause, of continuing analgesic consumption (Dichgans *et al.* 1984).

In this chapter, the implication of analgesics in human kidney disease will be discussed. Actual knowledge concerning the prevalence of AN, and the epidemiological evidence of the nephrotoxicity of analgesics, will be presented.

4.1 Quantification of the problem

Different methods have been used to measure the occurrence, and to follow the evolution, of AN in a given area. Autopsy incidence rates of renal papillary necrosis associated with a history of analgesic ingestion, showed a marked increase during the 1950s and 1960s, maximum incidences being between 1.75 per cent in Switzerland and 8.6 per cent in Australia (reviewed by Prescott 1982*a*). In Canada, the evolution of AN in relation to restrictive measures on the sales of phenacetin was investigated using numbers of newly diagnosed cases. A decrease of 50 per cent in less then a decade was observed after restriction of phenacetin and paracetamol (Gault and Wilson 1978; Wilson and Gault 1982). However, to quantify AN, measurement of incidence (number of new cases per year) and prevalence (number of current cases) of patients in renal replacement programmes are most reliable.

4.1.1 Prevalence of analgesic nephropathy

Although there is overwhelming clinical evidence linking analgesic abuse with a particular form of chronic renal damage evolving towards end-stage renal failure, and cases are reported from all over the world, structured information concerning the extent of the problem is limited (Fig. 4.1).

It is obvious that prevalence data are available only in countries providing renal replacement therapy on a broad scale. This is not the case in most third world countries, where a disease with an incidence rate no more than 20 per million of population does not constitute a pressing problem. Even in industrialized countries, differences in observed prevalences may be influenced by selection practices according to race, sex, age, or social class, and must be interpreted with caution. Furthermore, differences in clinical practice may result in underestimation of the diagnosis of AN in several countries. National rates are known only in Europe/North Africa and Australia/New Zealand. These data (1986) are derived from reports of the European Dialysis and Transplant Association (EDTA) and the Australian

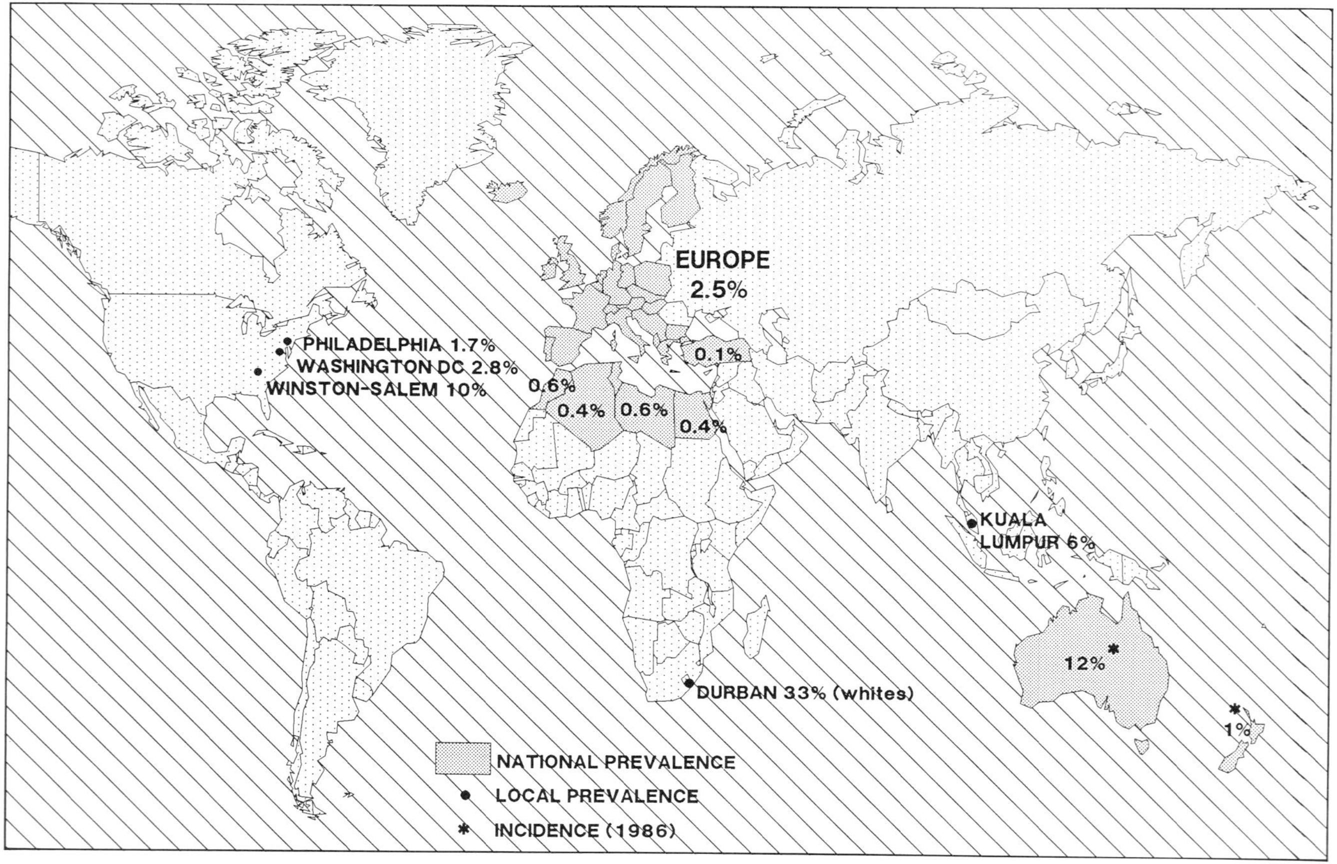

Fig. 4.1 Prevalences of analgesic nephropathy in patients on renal replacement therapy (1980–6).

and New Zealand Dialysis and Transplant Registry (ANZDATA) respectively (Wing *et al.* 1989; Disney and Roy 1988). Both organizations maintain an almost complete record of each individual patient commencing renal replacement therapy for end stage renal failure.

In Europe, more than 140 000 patients were on renal replacement therapy in 1986; 2.5 per cent had the diagnosis of AN. Prevalence was highest in Switzerland (18.1 per cent), Belgium (17.9 per cent), and West Germany (13 per cent), whereas in the United Kingdom, France, Italy, and Spain, the prevalence was less than 1 per cent (Wing *et al.* 1989; Elseviers and De Broe 1988; Pommer *et al.* 1986). In Scandinavia, a marked decrease in prevalence was observed, from more than 20 per cent in the 1960s to 1–5 per cent at present, due to restriction on the sales of phenacetin and paracetamol in compound analgesic preparations in 1961 resulting in an almost complete disappearance of mixtures containing more than one analgesic substance (Bengtsson 1989). In most Eastern European countries, reported prevalences are low. In several of these countries however, due to age limitation in acceptance on to renal replacement therapy, and perhaps to discrimination against self-inflicted disease, disproportionate numbers of patients with AN may have been refused entry to dialysis programmes (Kokot 1989; Taraba 1989). On the other hand, taking into account the high consumption of analgesic mixtures, mostly still containing phenacetin, an increase of recorded AN from Eastern Europe can be expected for the next decade (Kokot 1989; Taraba 1989; Prát 1989; Precht *et al.* 1989; Thieler and Sicker 1989; Thieler *et al.* 1990).

In contrast to all other prevalence data given in Figs 4.1 and 4.2, the Australian and New Zealand rates are incidences, i.e. new patients entering renal replacement therapy during 1986. Although, the Australian prevalence of AN was considered as being the highest in the world during the 1970s, a decrease was observed after restriction of the sales of over-the-counter analgesics in 1979 (Kincaid-Smith 1979, 1986*a*; McCredie *et al.* 1989).

The national prevalence of AN in the United States is unknown, local studies ranging from 1.7 per cent in Philadelphia and 2.8 per cent in Washington, DC, to 10 per cent in north-west North Carolina (Murray *et al.* 1983, McAnally *et al.* 1983; Gonwa *et al.* 1981). While Murray and Goldberg (1978) noted analgesic abuse in 7 per cent of new patients entering dialysis in 30 centres in the United States, the national prevalence in the 1980s is estimated to be 1–2 per cent. The controversy between those who consider AN to be a rare (Maher 1986), or a significant (Buckalew and Schey 1986*a*), cause of renal disease in the United States can only be resolved by careful registration of all cases (Goldberg 1986).

Few other national data are available. In Canada 2.5 per cent of patients on dialysis in 1976 had AN; current prevalence is likely to be lower (Gault and Wilson 1978). In South Africa, 33 per cent of the white patients accepted on to renal replacement therapy between 1974 and 1980 in Durban had this diagnosis, and the disease was more common in males than in females; AN was rare in the Black, Indian, and Coloured populations (Seedat *et al.* 1984). Among 180 Malaysian dialysis patients, 14 (8 per cent) had consumed excessive quantities of analgesics and 7 of them had renal papillary necrosis (Segasothy *et al.* 1988).

4.1.2 Geographical variation in the prevalence of analgesic nephropathy

Investigators have been intrigued by the strikingly different occurrence of AN observed between areas in the same country. In Australia, the proportion of AN in patients entering renal replacement therapy in the period 1971–7 varied from approximately 30 per cent in Queensland and New South Wales, to 5 per cent in the four southern states (Stewart 1978; Kincaid-Smith 1979). In Europe, local pockets of high prevalence of AN could be observed, even in countries with a low national prevalence (Fig. 4.2) (Vanherweghem and Even-Adin 1982; Pommer *et al.* 1986; Tepavčevic *et al.* 1986; Lusvarghi *et al.* 1987; Elseviers and De Broe 1988; Stummvoll and Breitenfellner 1989; Wing *et al.* 1989; Thieler *et al.* 1990).

It has been suggested that climatic conditions causing dehydration play a role in the geographic distribution of AN in Australia (Kincaid-Smith 1979), and drinking habits may be one of the factors explaining the north–south decline in observed prevalence in Germany, consumption of alcohol being higher in southern Germany than in the north (Pommer *et al.* 1986).

Nevertheless, it is generally accepted that the degree of analgesic use or abuse in a given population is the most important factor to explain the striking geographical variation in prevalence. Many investigators have correctly emphasized the correlation between regular analgesic use or the per capita consumption of analgesics and the prevalence of AN (Stewart 1978; Prescott 1982*a*; Buckalew and Schey 1986*b*; Elseviers and De Broe 1988). However, the question arises why people tend to abuse analgesics more in some countries than in others. The over-the-counter availability of analgesic mixtures and the practice of adding habituation components (caffeine, codeine, barbiturates) may play an important role in the development of addictive behaviour (Murray 1978; Stewart 1978). The existence of pockets of higher prevalence can also be related to psychological and social factors such as addiction within families, availability of analgesics in the workplace, and stress in the living environment (e.g. Durban and Berlin), and to marketing strategies.

4.1.3 Is the prevalence of analgesic nephropathy underestimated?

The prevalence of AN is unknown in most parts of the world (Fig. 4.1). However, there is evidence to suggest that the disease is overlooked and

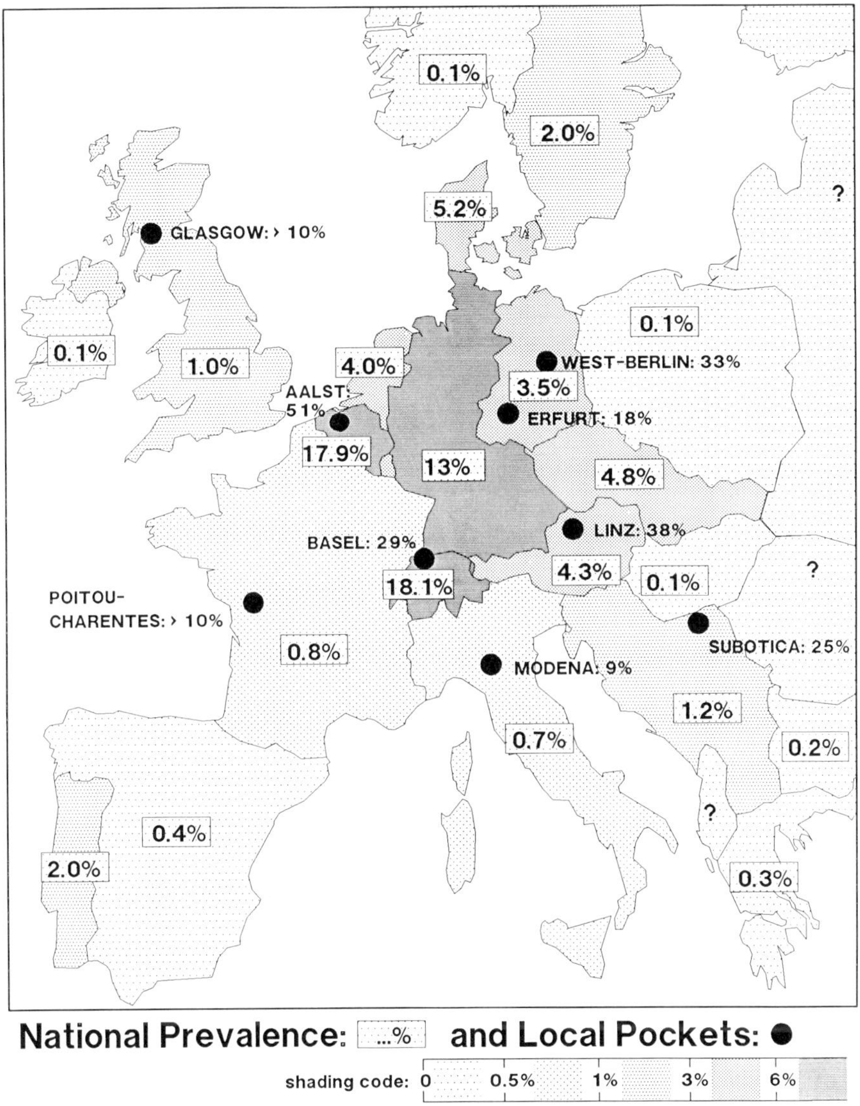

Fig. 4.2 Prevalences of analgesic nephropathy in Europe (1986).

underestimated in some countries. Indeed, the diagnosis is not always easy. AN is associated with mainly non-specific clinical manifestations, particularly at the onset of the disease when renal function is nearly normal. Support for the diagnosis has been to a large degree provided by a history of analgesic abuse. However, it has repeatedly been documented that abusers tend to deny their analgesic abuse and that anamnestic information concerning previous analgesic consumption is unreliable (Joubert *et al.* 1977; Murray 1978; Schwarz *et al.* 1984).

In Europe, several lines of reasoning indicate that AN is underestimated. First, there was a discrepancy between the data collected yearly by the EDTA, and national studies investigating the prevalence of this disease. In a German study, a prevalence of 13 per cent was found while the corresponding EDTA rate was never more than 6 per cent (Pommer *et al.* 1986). Secondly, an inverse correlation between the prevalence of AN and renal failure of unknown aetiology was shown (Fig. 4.3; Buccianti 1989). Wing *et al.* (1989), analysing the EDTA data, found additional information in favour of an underestimation from comparison of the age distribution of primary renal diseases, the demography of urothelial malignancies, an evaluation of diagnostic criteria, a market survey of analgesic usage, and a search for local pockets of AN.

4.2 The relation between analgesic abuse and kidney disease

Although, the existence of analgesic-associated nephropathy is generally accepted, the causality of excessive analgesic consumption in chronic renal failure is not clearly established, nor is it known whether analgesics are a direct causative, or a predisposing, factor. Arguments against the existence of AN are partly based on contradictory results of experimental studies; also many clinical and epidemiological investigations have failed to demonstrate a relation between abuse of analgesics and the development of renal failure (reviewed by Schwarz 1987). On the other hand, several well-controlled epidemiological studies of the 1980s were in support (Table 4.1).

4.2.1 Clinical observations

The weight of clinical evidence linking analgesic abuse with chronic renal disease is overwhelming. There are numerous reports demonstrating a high incidence of heavy analgesic consumption in patients with renal failure or papillary necrosis (reviewed by Prescott 1982*a*). Also the observed deterioration of renal function in patients with AN who continued their abuse, and in contrast the stabilization of renal failure after discontinuation of the abuse, is in favour of this association (Murray 1972; Nanra *et al.* 1978*a*; Schwarz *et al.* 1989). Further evidence came from the declining incidence of AN in countries where the sales of phenacetin and paracetamol, or the over-the-counter sales of analgesic mixtures, were legislatively restricted (Wilson and Gault 1982; Bengtsson 1989; McCredie *et al.* 1989; Disney 1991).

4.2.2 Epidemiological studies

Analytical epidemiology involves studies which may be prospective, proceeding from cause to effect (cohort study), or retrospective, proceeding from

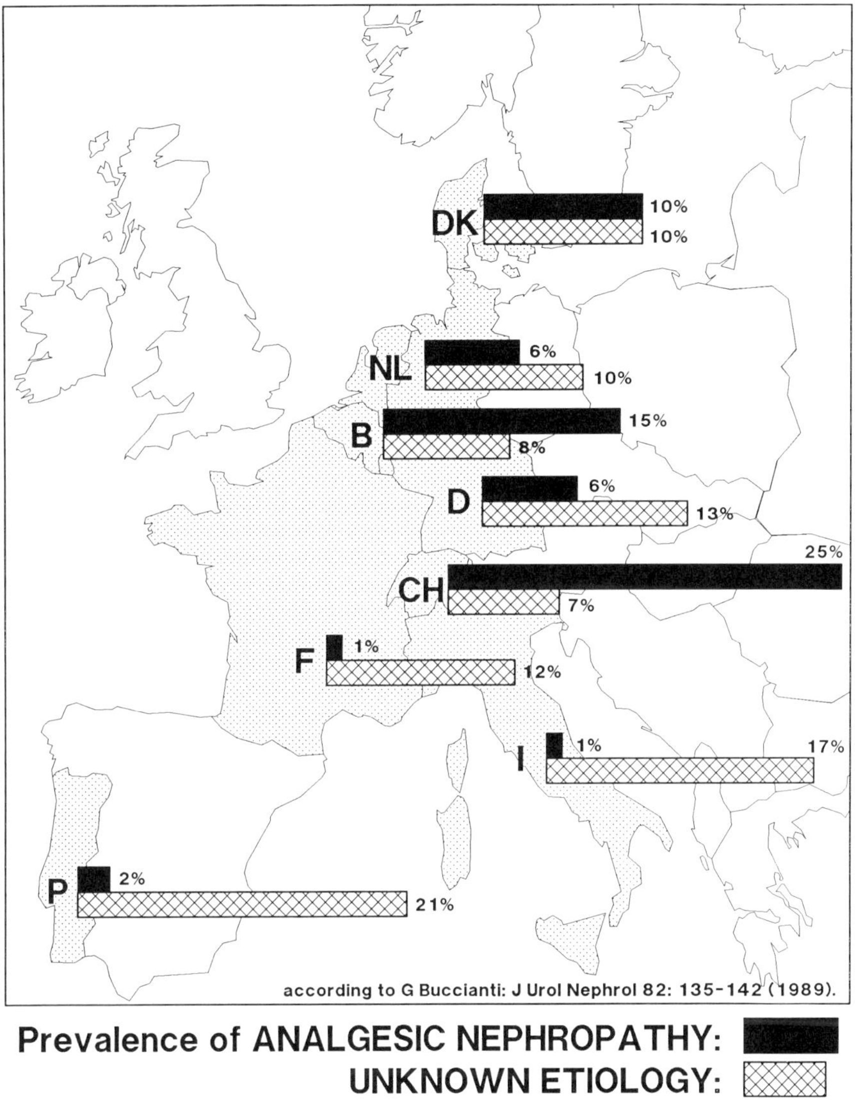

Fig. 4.3 The prevalence of analgesic nephropathy in relation to renal disease of unknown aetiology in European patients on renal replacement therapy (1980–4).

effect to cause and attempting to identify antecedents that led to the disease (case–control study). Within the limited number of epidemiological studies in the field of AN, most have been of the case–control type (Table 4.1) which has the advantages of rapidity of execution, requiring smaller groups, and relatively low cost. Case–control studies are especially useful for studying diseases which are rare or of long latency, both true for AN. The max-

Table 4.1 *Formal epidemiological studies measuring the risk of renal disease from analgesic consumption*

	Case	Controls	Definition of minimal abuse	Principal results as odds ratios (95% confidence interval)
Retrospective studies				
McCredie (1982) Australia	n = 80; prevalent women with RPN	n = 80; women with kidney disease of other aetiology	total consumption ≥ 0.1 kg	17.2 (8.5–34.7)
Murray (1983) United States	n = 527; prevalent patients with ESRF	n = 1047 hospitalized patients	almost daily for 30 days	1.08 (0.8–1.5)
Sandler (1989) United States	n = 554; incident patients with CRF	n = 516 population based	daily for 1 yr	2.79 (1.85–4.21)
Pommer (1989) Germany	n = 517; prevalent patients with ESRF	n = 517 clinic out-patients	15 units/month for 1 yr	2.44 (1.77–3.39)
Prospective studies				
Dubach (1983) Switzerland	n = 623; healthy working women 30–49 yr with regular analgesic intake	n = 621; healthy working women 30–49 yr with no regular analgesic intake	NAPAP in 2 consecutive specimens of urine	impaired concentration— 4.2 (2.54–6.98)[1] elevated serum creatinine— 8.08 (2.82–23.18)[1] death from renal disease— 4.8 (1.05–22.17)[1]

Abbreviations: RPN = renal papillary necrosis, ESRF = end stage renal failure, CRF = chronic renal failure. [1] Recalculation of results of Dubach according to Buckalew and Schey (1986*b*).

imum annual incidence is 20 per million of population, and the absolute risk of developing end stage renal failure is estimated to be 0.2–1 per cent of analgesic abusers (Schwarz *et al.* 1986; Elseviers and De Broe 1989). In AN, end stage renal failure is preceded by daily analgesic consumption for periods of 5–45 yr.

4.2.2.1 Cohort study

The only cohort study reported is that of Dubach *et al.* (1983, 1991) who followed a group of healthy working women with objective evidence of intake of phenacetin containing mixtures, and a group of matched controls, from 1968 to 1979, investigating the incidence of renal disorders (raised serum creatinine, low specific gravity of urine, bacteriuria, proteinuria, and haematuria) and mortality occurring during the study period. Because of the difficulty of obtaining a reliable drug history, which compromises most epidemiological research in this field, Dubach used objective measures of analgesic consumption for his cohort study. Urine specimens of the investigated women were analysed for the presence of *N*-acetyl-*p*-aminophenol (NAPAP), the main metabolite of phenacetin. Subjects with at least one out of three urine specimens positive for NAPAP during each of the two screenings, were enrolled in the study group. Subjects with either negative results during the first screening, or no additional positive specimens at the second screening, were used as controls (Dubach 1967).

Compared to the controls, cases with objective evidence of intake of phenacetin-containing analgesics showed more frequently a raised serum creatinine (6.7 per cent vs 0.9 per cent) and a low specific gravity of urine (23 per cent vs 7 per cent). The two groups did not differ in development of bacteriuria, haematuria, or proteinuria. Adjusted analyses of mortality over 11 years showed significant differences overall (39 vs 13 deaths), and in mortality due to urinary tract disorders (10 vs 2 deaths) or cardiovascular diseases (15 vs 3 deaths). Odds ratios shown in Table 4.1 were calculated from these original results by Buckalew and Schey (1986*b*).

The strongest proof of causality in the field of AN came from this study, although the absolute incidences remain small. This is not surprising knowing that AN is characterized by silent progression and that early symptoms are non-specific or minimal.

4.2.2.2 Case–control studies

Four case–control studies have been reported, from Australia (McCredie *et al.* 1982*b*), West Berlin (Pommer *et al.* 1989), and from a low, and a high, prevalence area respectively of the United States (Murray *et al.* 1983; Sandler *et al.* 1989). Methodological details are summarized in Table 4.1. In all, controls were matched to cases at least according to sex and age, and randomly selected except in the study of McCredie. Enrolling either hospitalized (McCredie, Pommer) or population-based (Sandler) controls can influence the results of the study, since analgesic consumption is found to be higher in a hospital, than in the general, population (reviewed by Prescott 1982*a*; Schwarz 1987). A history of analgesic consumption was obtained by direct interview of the subject, except for the study of Sandler where telephone interviews were used and where, for 55 per cent of the cases and 10 per cent of the controls, these interviews were conducted with proxies.

The results shown in Table 4.1 are odds ratios, estimating the relative risk for developing the disease under study when analgesics of any kind were taken regularly according to the minimum doses defined. Only Murray *et al.* (1983) failed to find a significant odds ratio. One of the factors leading to that result could be the definition of analgesic abuse, which was low compared to what is considered to be a minimum amount needed to develop end stage renal failure. Furthermore, the low prevalence in the area investigated would necessitate a larger number of subjects to obtain significant results. McCredie *et al.* (1982*b*) showed the highest odds ratio, due to the fact that the disease under study was renal papillary necrosis, which could be considered as the hallmark of AN, and which is more specific than newly diagnosed chronic renal failure or end stage renal failure, used in the other studies. Sandler *et al.* (1989) and Pommer *et al.* (1989) found comparable odds ratios, of a 2–3-fold increased risk for developing end stage renal failure after regular analgesic consumption.

4.3 Nephrotoxicity of different kinds of analgesics

4.3.1 Phenacetin misconception

In the majority of early reports of AN, phenacetin was singled out as the culprit on the basis of association and circumstantial evidence. Indeed, nearly all patients initially reported had taken large amounts of analgesics containing phenacetin. However, the potential nephrotoxicity of other products invariably taken with phenacetin was largely overlooked. This misconception burdened the research of AN which was almost totally focused on phenacetin for many years. It was only in the 1970s and 1980s that the nephrotoxicity of other analgesic products became more apparent. Prescott (1982*a*), in his review concerning the nephrotoxic role of phenacetin and other analgesics, argued that numerous chronic toxicity studies in animals with phenacetin have failed to produce renal papillary necrosis, that the removal of phenacetin in some countries has not been followed by the expected fall in mortality from AN (but see above), and that AN has a poor prognosis if phenacetin is discontinued but other analgesics are allowed.

4.3.2 The nephrotoxicity of single analgesics

It is clearly demonstrated that abusers prefer analgesic mixtures, and although experimental evidence of the nephrotoxicity of single analgesics exists, abuse of these products is rare and associated renal disease is reported only exceptionally (reviewed by Prescott 1982*a*). Pommer *et al.* (1989) investigated the relative risk of regular consumption of single analgesics and did not find a significantly increased risk (Table 4.2).

The nephrotoxicity of aspirin has been investigated in patients with rheumatoid arthritis for which high dose salicylate therapy was once the mainstay of treatment. Ferguson *et al.* (1977) and Emkey and Mills (1982) concluded that long-term salicylate ingestion did not cause renal damage. Other studies reviewed by Prescott (1982*a*) failed to given conclusive results because most investigators were not able to control rigorously the abuse of other analgesics taken in addition to the high doses of aspirin consumed. Additional information came from Sandler *et al.* (1989) (Table 4.2) in which the regular use of aspirin alone did not increase the risk.

In contrast, Sandler found an estimated risk ratio of 3.21 for the regular consumption of paracetamol used as a single analgesic. This result received much attention and controversial reaction (Gates and Temple 1989; McCredie 1989; Mandel 1989). Her results are supported by the clinical observation of Segasothy *et al.* (1984; 1988) who found 15 cases of renal papillary necrosis attributable to paracetamol consumption, mostly in patients believed to have consumed the drug alone. However, their findings should be considered as preliminary.

4.3.3 The nephrotoxicity of analgesic mixtures

Pommer *et al.* (1989) estimated that the relative risk of developing end stage renal failure after regular analgesic intake of at least 15 doses per month was 2.69, increasing to 4.83 when more than 60 doses per month were consumed over a period of at least 5 years. There is no doubt that epidemiological studies have supported the view that analgesic mixtures containing phenacetin are nephrotoxic (Table 4.2). Moreover, an increasing odds ratio with increasing consumption of phenacetin was demonstrated in all studies (Table 4.3).

However, the results for analgesic drugs other than phenacetin (Table 4.2) must be interpreted with caution. Most abusers had consumed different kinds of analgesics, and it is not easy to estimate the risk for one type of analgesic while controlling for all others. Additionally, the majority had consumed analgesics during a long period during which the pharmaceutical industry was replacing phenacetin by other analgesic substances (frequently paracetamol), usually without changing the name of the product.

McCredie and Stewart (1988) did not find an increased risk for paracetamol abuse, but virtually all their kidney disease patients who had taken paracetamol, had earlier taken phenacetin. Pommer *et al.* (1989), controlling for the additional abuse of phenacetin, found an increased risk of 6.09 in subjects who had consumed more than 1 kg of paracetamol, a tentative, but not conclusive, result because the number of subjects was small.

Table 4.2 *Epidemiological evidence of the nephrotoxicity of different kinds of analgesics*

	Any analgesics	Single analgesics			Analgesic mixtures			
		Any	Aspirin	Paracetamol	Any	Phenacetin-containing	Paracetamol-containing	Phenazone-containing
McCredie (1982)	17.2	..	..	..	..	18.1	NS	..
Sandler (1989)	2.79	..	NS	3.21	..	7.59	6.90	..
Pommer (1989)	2.44	NS	..	..	2.69	4.76	4.06	2.73

Results given as odds ratios for development of renal disease following consumption at or above threshold levels (definitions as in Table 4.1). .. = Not reported, NS = not significant.

Table 4.3 *Relation of risk to exposure dose reported in epidemiological studies*

	Amount of phenacetin consumed	Odds ratio
McCredie (1982)	< 2 kg	4.4
	2–4.9 kg	15.7
	5–9.9 kg	44.6
	≥ 10 kg	65.6
Sandler (1989)	weekly	2.33
	daily	7.59
Pommer (1989)	< 2 kg	2.94
	2–4.9 kg	4.76
	≥ 5 kg	9.20
Dubach (1989)		
increased serum creatinine	low NAPAP	8.10
	high NAPAP	15.25
impaired concentration	low NAPAP	4.2
	high NAPAP	7.6

NAPAP = *N*-acetyl-*p*-aminophenol.

Thus the nephrotoxicity of analgesic mixtures not containing phenacetin is not yet clearly established in humans. However the number of cases with a history of analgesic abuse, who had never consumed phenacetin, is increasing and clinical observations indicate the nephrotoxicity of these drugs (e.g. Elseviers and De Broe 1987). It can be expected that this issue will be resolved in the coming decade.

4.3.4 Effects of legislative measures

Apart from studies previously cited, the effect of legislative measures on the sales of analgesics provides additional information concerning nephrotoxicity. There seems to be a contradiction between the effects observed. In Scandinavia, a significant decline in the incidence of AN was demonstrated after restriction of phenacetin and paracetamol in 1961. But in Australia during the 1970s, when phenacetin was withdrawn from most analgesic mixtures, no clear decline in incidence rates was observed until after restriction of the over-the-counter sales of all analgesic mixtures (McCredie *et al.* 1989). In Belgium, the total sales of analgesics containing phenacetin dropped from more than 30 per cent to less than 1 per cent in two decades, but there was no decline in the incidence of AN (Elseviers and De Broe 1988).

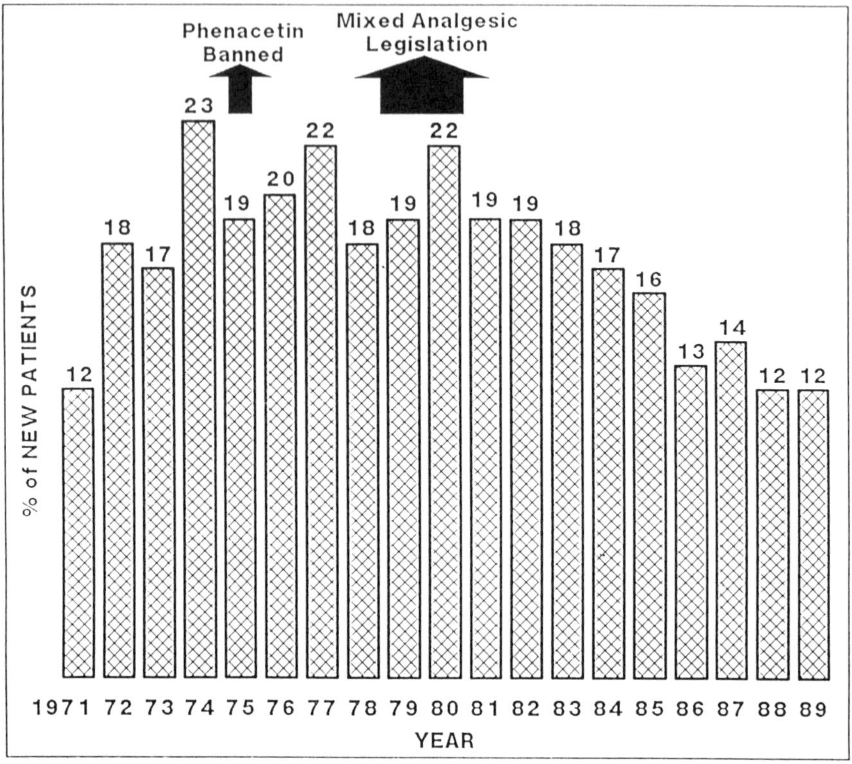

Fig. 4.4 Annual incidences of analgesic nephropathy in patients entering renal replacement therapy in Australia (1971–89).

How can such different effects be explained? Sweden still has high over-the-counter sales of analgesics, of which 40 per cent are products still containing caffeine or codeine. However, all the most popular products contain one analgesic substance only (Wessling 1987). In Australia, Belgium, West Germany, and Switzerland, phenacetin was removed from the market spontaneously by the pharmaceutical industry, but replaced by another analgesic substance (usually paracetamol), resulting in continuing high volume sales of analgesic mixtures containing two or more analgesic substances. These observations strongly suggest that the nephrotoxicity of analgesic mixtures is largely influenced by the additional or synergistic effect of several analgesic substances present in those mixtures.

4.4 Conclusion

Analgesic-induced kidney disease constitutes a serious health problem in several countries, while in others the prevalence of this disease is unknown or is underestimated. In some countries, a decrease in the prevalence was observed following appropriate legislative measures.

AN is caused by excessive consumption of analgesic mixtures containing adjuvants (caffeine, codeine, barbiturates) which are considered the principal causative agents in creating a psychic dependence leading to addictive behaviour. Abuse of single analgesics is rare, and associated renal disease is exceptional.

Further investigations are needed to establish the prevalence of AN in most countries, using validated diagnostic criteria, and to study the nephrotoxicity of analgesics not containing phenacetin. The additional information so derived will be helpful for the development of preventive action in countries still confronted with a high prevalence.

5
The abuse of non-narcotic analgesics

D. Ladewig

After reports had first been published from Switzerland referring to the abuse of antipyretic–analgesics containing phenacetin (Kielholz 1954; Horisberger *et al.* 1958; Battegay 1958*b*), and to the possibility of a causal connection between such abuse and chronic renal disease (Spühler and Zollinger 1953), numerous authors drew attention to the problem of abuse of non-narcotic analgesics (see Gsell *et al.* 1968). Such abuse may lead to genuine dependence (Eddy *et al.* 1965; Jaffe 1970), which on theoretical grounds might be assigned to the barbiturate type of drug dependence.

Most of the antipyretic–analgesics abusively used consisted of mixed preparations (Woodbury 1970) which contained substances such as: salicylates; *p*-aminophenol derivatives, e.g. phenacetin, paracetamol, acetanilide; pyrazolone derivatives, e.g. antipyrine (phenazone), aminopyrine, phenylbutazone; caffeine; hypnotics; and codeine.

Phenacetin was withdrawn in many countries during the 1970s due to renal damage, and in the 1980s barbiturates or other hypnotics were withdrawn step-wise from combination due to their toxicity and potential for psychotropic dependence.

5.1 Symptomatology and aetiology of the abuse of non-narcotic analgesics

Distinctive features exhibited by analgesic habitués were their dirty greyish-brown complexion and cyanotic lips. During the stage of intoxication, they are befuddled, dysarthric, and ataxic, their psychomotor status being characterized either by disinhibition and enhanced drive, or by retardation and apathy. They bump into objects and may fall, thus sustaining typical injuries. Haematomas may be seen on the face, shoulders, or pelvis. The basic mood in such cases was anxious, sub-depressive, dysphoric, or less often, irritable and hypomanic. Following years of such drug abuse, memory is impaired.

5.1.1 Reasons given for analgesic consumption

The reasons given for consuming excessive quantities of non-narcotic analgesics were painful syndromes of predominantly psychosomatic origin, such as headaches, pains in the neck, limb or back, gastrointestinal spasms, cardiac oppression, dysmenorrhoea, or feelings of pressure which assume various forms.

5.1.1.1 Headache

When the chronic consumer of analgesics describes the type of headache to which he is subject, he confines himself to generalities, the description usually being vague, long-winded, and depending on the degree and duration of the intoxication, either verbose or monosyllabic. Such descriptions frequently contain references to changes in the intensity and location of the pain or to alterations in the symptomatology. The picture presented by the patient must also be interpreted to some extent in terms of his or her reaction to the type of interrogation used, to the manner in which the interview is conducted, and to the attitude of the physician.

The headache as described may be unilateral or bilateral. Though rather difficult to classify accurately, the headache has been identified as migraine, or more often as vasomotor cephalalgia or due to muscular tension (tension headache), as chronic post-traumatic neuralgic headache, or as headache due to diseases of the nose, sinuses, teeth, ears, temperomandibular joint, or pharynx. Patients most commonly complain of a feeling of pressure over the eyes or forehead, or of a sensation such as would be produced by a helmet pressing on their head. Less often they report pain in the nuchal or occipital region. In patients of this type headache is usually not the only painful symptom encountered.

5.1.1.2 Other symptoms

Pain may occur in any of the muscles, in the limbs, neck, shoulder, or back. Occasionally an abdominal syndrome consisting of pain or discomfort, of loss of appetite amounting sometimes to frank anorexia (an increase in appetite is less common), or of nausea, the sensation of a lump in, or dryness of, the throat or of choking, vomiting, heartburn, epigastric tenderness, gastrointestinal spasms, constipation (possibly alternating with diarrhoea), and tenesmus is seen. In certain instances the condition becomes such that even surgery is performed; following the operation, the patient obtains temporary relief from the symptoms which later recur and are associated with increased headaches.

More frequent than these abdominal symptoms is the occurrence of headaches associated with a variety of complaints which include tiredness, impairment of performance, sleep disorders, hypoaesthesia or hyperaesthesia, pruritus, tremor, jitteriness, mental unrest, sweating, shivering, impotence, frigidity, and frequency of urination. In the general symptomatology of these syndromes, sleep disorders such as difficulty in getting to sleep, light sleep, and early awakening constitute cardinal signs. Less often encountered are cardiopulmonary syndromes marked by a sensation of pressure or stabbing pains in the region of the heart, precordial anxiety, pseudoangina, tachycardia, extrasystoles, a tendency to syncope, dizziness, feelings of pressure and constriction in the chest and dyspnoea, as well as endocrine symptoms such as disturbances in the water balance, hypoglycaemia, loss of weight, and menstrual disorders.

5.1.2 Psychosomatic basis for analgesic abuse

In female patients, headache, in conjunction with the above-mentioned categories of symptoms, is an early manifestation of systemic psychosomatic disease. These women tend to have personalities that are predominantly of the asthenic, sensitive type, i.e. they take life very seriously and feel uncertain of themselves. Owing to their emotional weakness and sensitivity, they are afraid of injury to their feelings, which they therefore strive to bottle up. This tendency to introversion is often further intensified by the attitude which others adopt towards them. When they do voice their intuitive opinions, anxieties, and apprehensions, they are not adequately understood. Consequently, they become increasingly withdrawn and isolated.

The personalities of the male patients are likewise largely of the asthenic, sensitive, egocentric type which, though passive, is characterized by the desire to assert itself. Ambition and the urge toward self-assertion induce such men to aim at high goals, but the discrepancy between their goals and actual performance results in feelings of failure, in resignation and dysphoria, in overcompensating pompousness, and in increasing emotional encapsulation coupled with the feeling of not being understood by others.

Though in such cases we may suspect various conflict situations, we learn little about these at first. It is often not until after weeks of intensive interviewing that the patients begin to thaw out. As they are progressively weaned from the drug, they show less tendency to suppress their feelings, to deny their difficulties, and to explain away their unpleasant experiences. We are then informed by the patients that the headaches had the habit of worsening after they had suffered losses or disappointments, and that a change of environment, a pleasant experience, or success at work caused the pains to disappear temporarily.

Underlying the psychosomatic disturbances as described above are longstanding emotional tensions. In women these take the form of presistent tensions due to thwarted yearnings for love, sexual satisfaction, or recognition. Such tensions are usually attributable to lack of affection, tenderness, appreciation, and sexual fulfilment, to chronic emotional upsets, or to the husband's infidelity or alcoholism. Alternatively, they may arise from emotional overstrain, from inability to cope with the household chores and with the upbringing of the children, from dissatisfaction with employment, or from financial worries. The strain of having to perform work which taxes the patient's inner resistance rapidly leads to autonomic nervous disturbances and to organic manifestations of functional disorders.

In men, on the other hand, the main causative factors are conflicts occuring in connection with their occupations—ambitions, rivalries, the fear of failure at work, or simply anticipatory, competitive, or existential anxiety as such.

5.1.3 The onset of drug habituation

It is quite understandable that to combat their psychosomatic symptoms these patients resort to analgesics and hypnotics which are on sale everywhere and are claimed to be safe and harmless. The persons who take them certainly have no desire to become dependent on drugs, nor do they consciously wish to escape from reality; they are merely trying to treat themselves so that they can keep going and live free of the symptoms that afflict them. In much the same way as hypnotics are taken in order to combat insomnia, so drugs are consumed by these individuals in response to anticipatory anxiety, in the hope that they will ward off pain and discomfort.

Very gradually the patient becomes habituated to the drug and slowly has to increase the dose so as to obtain the desired analgesic affect. The interval between doses becomes shorter and the dosage progressively higher. Often only after prolonged habituation does the patient suddenly find that, in addition to its analgesic properties, the drug also relieves tiredness, exerts a reviving and stimulant effect, and apparently helps to improve performance. This effect—which serves to combat weariness, apathy, and general listlessness and which as a rule makes itself felt only secondarily—is the one that the patient can no longer do without. The insidious feature of the phenacetin- and caffeine-containing combinations is that, when taken in high dosage, they themselves give rise to headache and so prompt further consumption. Such patients thus become caught up in a vicious circle, which leads to intoxication and may ultimately result in genuine dependence.

Analgesics do not only influence pain receptors, but also the subjective experience of pain, thus exhibiting a latent psychotropism, as when a patient states that a certain analgesic 'does him good'. The experience of the effects of a medicament as 'pain-killing' or as calming, relaxing, pleasant or stimulating, is a very personal one in which the substance has become psychotropic. In the development of psychotropism it is essential that an analgesic reacts continuously in the way mentioned and that the consumer has developed the ability to perceive this effect. The more a patient tends to recognize and utilize this new effect in a medicament, the more he runs the risk of misusing it.

5.2 Drug withdrawal

When antipyretic analgesics are discontinued, withdrawal symptoms set in within 12–48 h, and persist for 10 days in the acute phase of abstinence and for 2–4 months in the protracted withdrawal period. Among the chief symptoms encountered are headache, excessive wakefulness, mental unrest, sleep disturbances, fine tremor, muscular twitching, rheumatic pains in the limbs, mood disorders marked by anxiety and depression, pre-collapse, diarrhoea alternating with constipation, vomiting and, finally, withdrawal deliria, hallucinations, and grand mal seizures. As in the case of barbiturates, the severity of the withdrawal symptoms—including especially the occurrence of epileptic seizures and deliria—seems to be dose-dependent.

Immediately after the withdrawal, non-specific generalized abnormalities, which are usually of mild–moderate severity and are rarely of an episodic character, can be detected in the electroencephalogram (EEG). The EEG pattern generally shows a tendency towards normalization, as evidenced by stabilization of the α-frequency and a decrease in θ-, δ- and β-waves. In one-third of the patients, however, the electrical activity of the brain showed only mild abnormalities in the first EEG recordings made after withdrawal of the drug, but underwent a deterioration during the following 7–10 days—a deterioration marked by an increase in slow waves, asymmetry, localized focal abnormalities, or even paroxysmal electrical manifestations. Recurrences of abnormalities are observed seldom. These phenomena are probably attributable to the withdrawal of a preparation which the patient has been taking for years resulting in disruption of the equilibrium which the electrophysiologic functions of the brain have gradually established, the disruption persisting until such time as a new balance is attained.

5.3 Psychological aspects of drug use patterns

What are the mutual effects of personality and abuse of non-narcotic analgesics? In the field of epidemiological studies, psychometric methods such as multidimensional personality inventories are particularly valuable. In English-speaking countries such inventories are well known in the form of the Minnesota Multiphasic Personality Inventory (MMPI) and the Maudsley Personality Inventory (MPI). In German-speaking countries one newly developed has been the Freiburg Personality Inventory (FPI) (Fahrenberg *et al.* 1973).

We focused our interest on the relationship between chronic use and abuse of non-narcotic analgesics and personality features as tested by inventories such as the FPI. In 1968, Dubach started a prospective study to determine whether phenacetin-containing non-narcotic analgesics are detrimental to kidney function. The study group was chosen from a total of 1258 women, from 87 factories in the north-western part of Switzerland, who had volunteered to be screened for renal disease and diabetes mellitus. Those women, in whose urine phenacetin metabolites were found on two occasions in 1968, were chosen. A control group was matched by age, number of pregnancies, nationality, marital status, and type of work. The two cohorts were

Table 5.1 *Mean Freiburg Personality Inventory values in persons who did and did not consume analgesics over the years 1972, 1975, and 1978*

Scale	Permanent consumers	Permanent non-consumers
	n = 112	*n* = 160
Nervousness	3.75	2.71
Depressiveness	3.48	2.41
Excitability	4.06	3.07
Equanimity	3.03	3.68
Emotional Lability	3.44	2.46
Masculinity/Femininity	2.62	3.29

psychologically investigated in 1972, 1975 and 1978 (Ladewig *et al.* 1978, 1979; Ladewig 1979; Meier-Hirschi 1980). As the consumption changed over the years, other groups could be differentiated according to the time course ('starters' and 'stoppers'), and the frequency and intensity of use from metabolites detected in urine samples ('high intakers' and 'low intakers').

5.3.1 Do consumers differ from non-consumers with regard to personality?

When comparing consumers and control subjects we noted significant differences in the following FPI scales (Tables 5.1, 5.2):

Scale 1—Nervousness
The consumers mention physical symptoms involving various functions: autonomic complaints (circulation, respiration, digestion), sensitivity to pain, synaesthesia, general psychosomatic disturbances (insomnia, weakness, easy fatiguability, sensitivity to changes in the weather, susceptibility to stimuli, and restlessness), intense physical affect resonance, e.g. intense autonomic and muscular phenomena accompanying affective stimulation.

Scale 3—Depressiveness
Besides ill-humour and lability of mood tinged with general depression, the consumers exhibit anxiety, a feeling of apathy and inner emptiness, lack of concentration, and guilty feelings extending to a general feeling of insufficiency. This gives a picture of an ill-humoured, depressed and unself-reliant person.

Scale 6—Equanimity
The consumers are easily irritated and disappointed, tend to take things hardly, are solicitous and disinclined to quick or spontaneous decisions. They are further characterized by their expectant attitude.

Table 5.2 *Probabilities of equality of means (inter-group differences) obtained by paired* t*-tests*

Factor	1972						1975					
	I	II	III	IV	V	VI	I	II	III	IV	V	VI
1 Nervousness	0.00[c]	0.04[a]	0.25	0.26	0.54	0.17	0.01[b]	0.15	0.16	0.65	0.94	0.44
2 Aggressiveness	0.32	0.57	0.09	0.04[a]	0.97	0.01[b]	0.40	0.35	0.49	0.18	0.56	0.13
3 Depressiveness	0.00[c]	0.07	0.01[b]	0.86	0.79	0.91	0.01[b]	0.60	0.67	0.46	0.31	0.98
4 Excitability	0.06	0.43	0.79	0.60	0.84	0.23	0.03[a]	0.52	0.15	0.72	0.66	0.99
5 Sociability	0.99	0.64	0.83	0.50	0.57	0.80	0.71	0.98	0.65	0.71	0.81	0.80
6 Equanimity	0.03[a]	0.57	0.58	0.44	0.67	0.05[a]	0.31	0.18	0.87	0.24	0.43	0.33
7 Dominance	0.38	0.47	0.33	0.99	0.74	0.61	0.26	0.94	0.56	0.78	0.61	0.84
8 Inhibition	0.98	0.34	0.75	0.30	0.26	0.70	0.42	0.19	0.76	0.34	0.31	0.80
9 Openness	0.32	0.81	0.20	0.55	0.80	0.48	0.58	0.66	0.33	0.26	0.44	0.44
E Extraversion	0.63	0.33	0.16	0.05[a]	0.22	0.25	0.33	0.81	0.09	0.14	0.44	0.23
N Emotional Lability	0.00[c]	0.11	0.02[a]	0.85	0.49	0.54	0.02[b]	0.91	0.16	0.31	0.15	0.89
M Masculinity	0.03[a]	0.06	0.65	0.24	0.37	0.26	0.06	0.36	0.34	0.84	0.99	0.71

[a] $2p \leq 0.05$; [b] $2p \leq 0.01$; [c] $2p \leq 0.001$. I Consumers vs controls; II consumers vs starters; III consumers vs stoppers; IV starters vs stoppers; V starters vs controls; VI stoppers vs controls. With kind permission of Elsevier Sequoia SA, Lausanne.

Scale N—Emotional Lability
The consumers see themselves as emotionally labile, oppressed, readily injured, quick-tempered, tormented by guilty feelings, and unjustly treated.

Scale M—Masculinity/Femininity
The consumers show components of the somewhat problematic concept of 'typical female self-portrayal'. They appear as restrained and shy, show little self-reliance and complain of multiple psychosomatic symptoms.

Considering the inter-group differences at the point of investigation, it is clearly shown that permanent consumers were distinct from non-consumers in 1972 as well as in 1975 and 1978. In their self description they differed from the control group in 1972 in Scales Nervousness, Depressiveness, Equanimity, Emotional Lability and Masculinity.

5.3.2 Do groups of consumers with varying patterns of use differ?

In addition, it was shown (Tables 5.2, 5.3) that different groups of consumers could be distinguished according to their intensity of use measured by the optical density (od) in the spectrophotometric determination of *N*-acetyl-*p*-aminopherol (NAPAP) in urine samples. When comparing, for example, 'high-intakers' (NAPAP values of over 0.47 od) with 'low-intakers' (NAPAP values 0.047–0.199 od), there were differences in a range of additional scales. Whereas the 'high-intakers' could be distinguished very clearly from 'low-intakers', it was not possible to differentiate in the same clear way between 'low-intakers' and non-consumers. It could be summarized that the 'high-intakers' stand out from the non-consumers as well as the 'low-intakers', particularly as regards psychosomatic and contact disturbances, lack of self-reliance tinged with depression, and emotional immaturity.

Comparing the control group, the 'starters', the 'stoppers', and the consumers in 1972 and in 1975, again differences could be found, partly to be interpreted as a sort of maturation due to the ageing process. The steady consumers did not share this development; they were more likely to remain depressive and emotionally unstable. Whereas the group of 'stoppers' showed a psychological improvement over the period from 1972 to 1975 in terms of less excitability, less emotional lability, and a tendency to a more 'masculine' self-portrayal, the 'starters' did not change significantly.

Summarizing these results, it can be said that permanent consumers or 'high-intakers' differ clearly from non-consumers. The abuse of a drug over a period of years can hamper the psychologically normal process of maturation, but a certain normalization of the process of personality disturbation is possible too. The results of our first study in 1972 have been confirmed by reinvestigation in 1975 and 1978. It is not clear if the personality structure of the consumers, as measured by this multidimensional personality inventory,

Table 5.3 *Means, standard deviations and probabilities of equality of means (intra-group differences) obtained by* t-*tests*

Factor		Consumers, n = 40					Starters, n = 10					Stoppers, n = 24					Controls, n = 216				
		1972		1975			1972		1975			1972		1975			1972		1975		
		$\bar{x}$	s	$\bar{x}$	s	$2p$	$\bar{x}$	s	$\bar{x}$	s	$2p$	$\bar{x}$	s	$\bar{x}$	s	$2p$	$\bar{x}$	s	$\bar{x}$	s	$2p$
1	Nervousness	4.28	2.12	4.03	2.27	0.35	2.60	2.72	2.80	2.74	0.51	3.63	2.20	3.21	2.21	0.20	3.01	2.05	2.86	2.11	0.03[a]
2	Aggressiveness	1.00	1.04	0.80	1.22	0.14	1.20	0.79	1.20	1.14	1.00	0.58	0.78	0.58	1.21	0.55	1.19	1.43	0.97	1.19	0.01[b]
3	Depressiveness	4.48	2.01	3.63	2.24	0.01[b]	3.10	2.47	3.20	2.44	0.88	2.96	2.61	2.50	2.50	0.11	2.90	2.26	2.49	2.14	0.00[c]
4	Excitability	4.28	2.06	3.95	1.87	0.29	3.70	1.83	3.50	2.27	0.78	4.13	2.21	3.21	2.11	0.01[b]	3.55	2.23	3.20	2.05	0.01[b]
5	Sociability	3.33	2.24	3.53	2.43	0.16	3.70	2.16	3.50	2.51	0.74	3.21	1.82	3.79	1.84	0.08	3.32	2.08	3.67	2.22	0.00[c]
6	Equanimity	2.88	1.54	3.25	1.77	0.19	3.20	1.87	4.10	1.66	0.11	2.63	2.00	3.17	2.18	0.21	3.49	2.06	3.59	1.99	0.32
7	Dominance	2.25	1.82	2.05	1.62	0.47	1.80	1.32	2.00	2.16	0.73	1.79	1.74	1.79	1.89	1.00	1.99	1.74	1.72	1.71	0.03[a]
8	Inhibition	3.93	2.36	3.83	2.46	0.67	3.10	2.56	2.70	2.00	0.59	4.13	2.63	3.63	2.70	0.11	3.94	2.29	3.49	2.40	0.00[c]
9	Openness	2.85	1.70	2.43	1.82	0.09	2.70	2.16	2.70	1.42	1.00	2.29	1.65	1.96	1.83	0.20	2.56	1.73	2.26	1.78	0.00[c]
E	Extraversion	3.03	1.95	3.33	2.14	0.29	3.70	1.83	3.50	1.78	0.62	2.33	1.79	2.42	1.93	0.73	2.85	2.14	2.96	2.15	0.41
N	Emotional Lability	4.60	2.01	3.40	2.37	0.00[c]	3.40	2.46	3.50	2.72	0.91	3.21	2.73	2.54	2.34	0.05[a]	2.91	2.20	2.48	2.15	0.01[b]
M	Masculinity	2.18	1.81	2.53	2.06	0.21	3.50	2.55	3.20	1.99	0.68	2.42	2.34	3.04	2.12	0.02[a]	2.91	2.02	3.21	2.11	0.00[c]

[a] $2p \leq 0.05$; [b] $2p \leq 0.01$; [c] $2p \leq 0.001$.

is the cause or the result of drug use, but it is obvious that this group of people tend to manipulate their mental and physical condition by means of drugs.

5.4 Treatment and prevention

Treatment has to be conducted within a specialized context with adequate medical and psychosocial conditions. Results are favourable if the original psychosomatic disturbances are not ingrained. Cognitive psychotherapy, physical training and pharmacotherapy, are the modalities within a frame of a long-term out-patient treatment which help patients to cope with their disabilities.

Prevention may be achieved in two ways. The reduction or exclusion of dependence-producing ingredients of analgesics in favour of the development of monosubstances is the most important. The other is in the form of general information and education to promote a sense of healthy behaviour.

6

The analgesic syndrome

J.H. Stewart

As only antipyretic–analgesic preparations containing at least two pharmacologically active ingredients have caused chronic kidney disease (Chapter 4), and then only when taken in large amounts, it follows that patients with analgesic nephropathy will be at risk of toxic effects in other organs and tissues of the individual drugs present in these preparations. The 'analgesic syndrome', as the composite clinical pattern of these toxic effects is known, will vary between countries, depending upon the constituents of the commonly abused analgesics (Table 6.1). Thus there are syndromes characteristic of aspirin, phenacetin, and caffeine (APC) ingestion, the most common; aspirin, phenacetin, and codeine; aspirin, paracetamol, and caffeine; phenazone and phenacetin with or without caffeine, etc.

Unlike the aetiology of renal papillary necrosis, in which there appears to be contributions from two drugs (e.g. aspirin and phenacetin), the non-renal toxicity of the antipyretic-analgesics on the whole is due to the individual drugs acting alone. Thus to aspirin may be attributed gastric ulcer, iron deficiency anaemia, and perinatal morbidity; to phenacetin, cyanosis, splenomegaly, and pigmentation; to caffeine, headaches and perhaps alterations in mood or behaviour; and to codeine, constipation.

Nevertheless, it must not be overlooked that it is the presence of more than one ingredient that potentiates habituation to analgesics, and thus the persistent and heavy consumption of the drugs which individually cause the elements of the analgesic syndrome. Moreover, accelerated atherogenesis and premature ageing, claimed but not yet proven to be consequences of analgesic abuse, may be multifactorial in their aetiology; and in the case of central nervous system toxicity, it is not possible to separate the particular effects of the components of the analgesic mixtures taken. It follows that the analgesic syndrome is essentially a consequence of compound analgesic consumption.

For the sake of clarity, the individual elements of the analgesic syndrome will be described, grouped according to aetiology.

However, the composite picture created by joining the several vignettes with the manifestations of analgesic nephropathy itself, does not describe fully the clinical picture of the patient who has consumed large amounts of

Table 6.1 *The elements of the various analgesic syndromes seen in different parts of the world*

Components of analgesic preparations	Countries where syndrome is prevalent	Clinical manifestations
Phenazone, phenacetin[1] (with or without caffeine)	Switzerland Sweden	haemolytic anaemia, cyanosis, splenomegaly pigmentation headache, psychiatric abnormalities urothelial cancer
Aspirin, phenacetin,[1] caffeine	Australia Canada Iceland Scotland	as above plus peptic ulcer bleeding, bruising, iron deficiency anaemia perinatal morbidity acute organic brain syndrome accelerated atherogenesis premature ageing
Aspirin, phenacetin,[1] codeine	England Canada Australia	as above plus constipation

[1] When paracetamol is substituted for phenacetin, haemolytic anaemia, cyanosis, and splenomegaly are not seen, and there is no proven association with urothelial cancer.

compound analgesics. The traits that have drawn that person towards analgesic dependency must be added. As these form the subject matter of Chapter 5, they will not be described again here, except insofar as these people are inclined to turn to self medication or the use of prescribed sedatives and the like for relief of the side-effects of their primary drug habituation. The clinical effects of what might be called secondary abuse of drugs—aperients, antacids, tranquillizers, sedatives—also may be considered as part of the analgesic syndrome.

6.1 Caffeine

Caffeine is a drug of dependence (Griffiths and Woodson 1988), partly as a result of its directly generated psychotropic action and its indirect effects mediated through catecholamine release, but also because of the headache which occurs as its pharmacological effect wears off (van Dusseldorp and Katan 1990). Consequently, the combination of analgesic with caffeine is masterfully designed to ensure continuing consumption, each repeated dose being taken to ward off the effects of withdrawal from previous self medication. It is not surprising therefore, that it is caffeine-containing analgesics, often in powder form which promote rapid absorption, that are associated predominantly with chronic analgesic toxicity (Gault *et al.* 1968*a*; Murray 1978; Stewart 1978).

6.1.1 Withdrawal headache

The analgesic habitué generally can avoid headache by regular spacing of intake, but the overnight break from analgesic ingestion characteristically is marked by headache, or at least a 'thick head', on wakening. This headache may be caused by adenosine-mediated cerebral vasodilatation; other components of compound analgesic preparations, aspirin, paracetamol, and (presumably) phenacetin, also contribute to rebound headache, in these instances tension being the chief mechanism identified (Kudrow 1982; Michultka *et al.* 1989).

6.1.2 Direct caffeine toxicity

Caffeine is used, on the whole innocently, as a cerebral and physical stimulant by most people from time to time, but its effects are difficult to demonstrate by objective testing. Most clear-cut is its stimulation of certain psychomotor functions when impaired by fatigue. This, together with its ergogenic action, which is used to enhance competitiveness in endurance sports (Flinn *et al.* 1990), gives substance to the frequent claim by analgesic habitués that they take APCs to 'give themselves a lift' or to improve performance at work.

The amount in an analgesic powder or tablet (20–150 mg) is about the same as in a cup of coffee (40–150 mg) or tea (25–100 mg), and caffeine is not as strong a stimulant as sympathomimetic drugs such as amphetamine. Moreover, repeated consumption may lessen its pharmocological activity, presumably through up-regulation of adenosine receptors, its primary site of action (Benowitz 1990). Nevertheless, taking an APC may do more than to 'give a lift'; in some analgesic habitués it causes restlessness by day or sleeplessness by night, palpitations, frequency of urination, or lack of appetite.

Given the personality which predisposes to analgesic habituation, it is to be expected that tranquillizers or sedatives, not to mention tobacco or alcohol, are often used to ameliorate the physical symptoms of caffeine toxicity.

6.2 Codeine

Codeine, an opiate, may be addictive depending upon the quantity taken and the susceptibility of the subject. Indubitably it is responsible for some analgesic habituation. However, the amount in proprietary analgesics (usually 8 mg per tablet) is unlikely to cause overt withdrawal symptoms, although this may not be true for the larger doses in those preparations generally available only by prescription (usually 32 mg per tablet).

The chief side-effect of regular proprietary codeine-containing analgesic consumption is constipation, to which unsatisfactory eating habits may contribute. This is likely to account for the frequency of purgative abuse in patients with analgesic nephropathy; it has been suggested that laxatives may potentiate the toxicity of analgesics (Wainscoat and Finn, 1974). If aperients are taken, irregularity of bowel evacuation and abdominal discomfort may ensue.

6.3 Aspirin and salicylates

Aspirin frequently is a component of compound analgesics, but other salicylates only rarely. The gastric sequelae of aspirin and other non-steroidal anti-inflammatory drugs are the same, but only aspirin suppresses platelet cyclooxygenase irreversibly at very low dosage (0.45 mg/kg body weight/day) (Chapters 2, 12 and 13). As platelets survive for about 8 days in the circulation, a single dose of aspirin will have an effect on haemostasis, albeit steadily diminishing, for about a week. Thus, while gastric ulcer will occur with any of these drugs, iron deficiency anaemia is common only with aspirin.

6.3.1 Gastric ulcer

Billington (1960, 1963) was able to show that, starting about 1943, chronic gastric ulcer once again became prevalent in young, later in older, women in the Australian states of New South Wales and Queensland. The time and place of this change in incidence of gastric ulcer is the same as that of the appearance of the habit of taking of APC powders by women who were joining the work-force in large numbers for the first time because of the Second World War. No increase in gastric ulcer was seen in other parts of Australia or in several countries, including England and Wales, New Zealand and the United States, where analgesic abuse has not been common. Astute clinical observation (Douglas and Johnston 1961), confirmed by formal epidemiological study (Gillies and Skyring 1968, 1969), has implicated regular and prolonged consumption of APC powders with chronic gastric, rather than duodenal, ulceration, whereas acute haemorrhagic gastric erosion may be a consequence of taking even a single aspirin tablet (Douthwaite and Lintott 1938).

Although it was in New South Wales and Queensland that gastric ulcer was shown to be a consequence of APC abuse, the association of peptic (predominantly chronic gastric) ulcer with analgesic nephropathy has also been noted in another Australian state, Victoria (Dawborn *et al.* 1966), and in many parts of the world where aspirin is a constituent of the commonly taken analgesics, but not in Sweden or Switzerland, where proprietary compound analgesics usually contain no salicylate (listed by Gault *et al.* 1968*a*).

6.3.1.1 Pathogenesis of peptic ulcer

Aspirin-related peptic ulcer has dual pathogenesis, salicylate toxicity within the gastric epithelium and inhibition of mucosal cyclooxygenase (Kauffman 1989; Schoen and Vender 1989).

Aspirin, like most non-steroidal anti-inflammatory drugs, is a weak acid which is undissociated in the acid environment of the gastric lumen; accordingly it readily enters the epithelial cell, becomes ionized at neutral pH, and consequently trapped at high concentration which is toxic to enzyme and transport proteins. The resultant untoward effects include uncoupling of oxidative phosphorylation, loss of transepithelial potential gradient, and influx of hydrogen ions.

Local production of prostaglandins, dependent on cyclooxygenase, sustains the gastric mucosal protective barrier by promoting secretion of bicarbonate and the glycoproteins of mucus, the hydrophobicity of the epithelial surface, mucosal blood flow, and epithelial proliferation in response to injury. Each of these is adversely affected by aspirin and most non-steroidal anti-inflammatory drugs. Aspirin toxicity is most pronounced in the stomach, but the intestine, especially the first part of the duodenum, is also susceptible.

Despite the data presented above, the link between gastric ulcer and analgesic abuse may be partly indirect, due to the frequency with which consumption of other gastric irritants, particularly alcohol and tobacco, is found in analgesic habitués (Chapter 5).

6.3.1.2 Milk–alkali syndrome

In societies such as New South Wales where APC consumption has been common, the milk–alkali syndrome (alkalosis, hypercalcaemia, transient renal failure) is rare except in association with analgesic nephropathy (Posen, personal communication). Impaired kidney function, which compromises the excretion of excess calcium and bicarbonate, increases susceptility to the syndrome.

6.3.2 Bleeding tendency

Since a single tablet of aspirin can prolong bleeding time for some days, a tendency to bleed or bruise is a frequent finding in analgesic habitués. This may manifest as iron deficiency anaemia with or without occult or frank gastrointestinal haemorrhage (Dawborn *et al.* 1966; Gault *et al.* 1968*a*; Duggan 1970*a*, 1974; Murray *et al.* 1971*a*), easy bruising or prolonged bleeding after minor injury (Frick 1956), menorrhagia (no direct references, but several to gynaecological complaints, e.g. Murray 1973*a*; Bailey *et al.* 1974; Duggan 1974), or ante- or post-partum haemorrhage (Lewis and Schulman 1973; Collins and Turner 1975).

Moreover, aspirin readily crosses the placenta (Levy *et al.* 1975) and may affect platelet function in the new-born infant (Bleyer and Breckenridge 1970). Thus, infants born before 34 weeks of gestation appear to be at greater risk of intracranial haemorrhage if their mothers had taken aspirin during the week before delivery (Rumack *et al.* 1981*b*).

6.3.3 Perinatal morbidity and mortality

Aspirin increases the likelihood not only of perinatal haemorrhage, but also of delayed, prolonged or obstructed labour, presumably due to suppression of uterine contractile prostaglandins (Lewis and Schulman 1973; Collins and Turner 1975). More contentious are assertions that aspirin is teratogenic, which is unlikely (Collins 1981), or causes retardation of fetal growth, a claim made only in relation to heavy and prolonged ingestion of APC powders in which the effect of phenacetin or caffeine cannot be discounted (Turner and Collins 1975; Shapiro *et al.* 1976). Cyclooxygenase inhibitors, including high-dose aspirin, may result in neonatal pulmonary hypertension if taken before delivery to close the ductus arteriosus (Rudolf 1981). However, low-dose aspirin is widely and safely used now to prevent the placental microangiopathy of idiopathic fetal growth retardation (Beaufils *et al.* 1985; Wallenburg and Rotmans 1987) and pregnancy-induced hypertension (Benigni *et al.* 1989).

6.4 Phenacetin and paracetamol

Although paracetamol in large amounts is acutely toxic to hepatic and renal tubular cells (Chapter 15), chronic toxicity is not certain. For instance, paracetamol rarely, if ever, causes chronic active hepatitis or cirrhosis (Seeff 1981).

6.4.1 Cyanosis, haemolysis, and splenomegaly

Acetic-4-chloranilide, a contaminant found in preparations of phenacetin, and *p*-phenetidin, a minor metabolite of phenacetin but not of paracetamol (Chapter 2), are oxidants which cause methaemoglobinaemia and sulphaemoglobinaemia (Schnitzer *et al.* 1965; Schnitzer and Smith 1966), the latter an irreversible reaction resulting in Heinz body formation, sequestration of erythrocytes in the spleen, and haemolysis (Lorenzen and Schwartz 1960; Forsström 1968; Millar *et al.* 1972; Gault *et al.* 1974). The result is central cyanosis (Harvald 1963; Gault *et al.* 1968*a*; Duggan 1974), which however may be less readily discerned in the presence of anaemia. When phenacetin consumption is especially heavy and prolonged, the spleen may be modestly enlarged (Fordham and Huffines 1967; Duggan 1970*b*).

6.4.2 Pigmentation

Haemosiderin, presumably emanating from intravascular haemolysis Reynolds and Edmondson 1963), or lipofuschin (Murray *et al.* 1971*b*; Lee *et al.* 1974) granules in tubular epithelial cytoplasm, and a pigmented cholesterol ester resembling lipofuschin in and around capillary basement membranes (Munck *et al.* 1970; Mihatsch *et al.* 1983*a*), cause pigmentation of the kidneys and urinary mucosa. Hyperpigmentation of the skin (Berneis and Studer 1969; Clarkson and Lawrence 1970; Nanra *et al.* 1978*a*) and other tissues is due to the same lipofuschin-like material (Mihatsch *et al.* 1983*a*). Brown urine, due to the presence of a chemical derivative of paracetamol or *p*-phenetidin (Miller *et al.* 1970), is characteristic of phenacetin intoxication (Gault 1975).

6.5 Pyrazolon derivatives

Aminopyrine (amidopyrine, pyramidon) had to be withdrawn from therapeutic use because it caused aplastic anaemia, but phenazone (antipyrine) and other closely related drugs are innocent of this ill effect, and indeed, of any other serious extra-renal human toxicity.

6.6 Disorders of mixed or uncertain aetiology

6.6.1 Central nervous system toxicity

Hallucinations, convulsions, confusion, coma, ataxia, tinnitus, and deafness, in some cases ascribed to salicylate intoxication, have been observed in analgesic abusers (Greer *et al.* 1965; Murray 1973*b*), and an electroencephalographic pattern indicating metabolic encephalopathy, or with a focal abnormality, is present in some of these patients (Kasanen and Valleala 1963; Murray 1973*b*; Chapter 5). Phenacetin abuse (together with aspirin, but not aspirin alone) has been associated with dementia in which there are cerebral lesions, including lipofuscin deposition, resembling Alzheimer's disease (Murray *et al.* 1971*b*). As aspirin, phenacetin (Prescott *et al.* 1970), caffeine (Curatolo and Robertson 1983; Benowitz 1990) and codeine all have pharmacological effects in the central nervous system, any or all may contribute to these elements of the analgesic syndrome.

6.6.2 Accelerated atherogenesis

That ischaemic heart disease is unduly common in this syndrome (Fellner and Tuttle 1969; Duggan 1974; Mahony *et al.* 1974; Kaladelfos and Edwards 1976) has been corroborated in objective studies (Krishnaswamy *et al.* 1974; Nanra *et al.* 1978*a*; Dubach *et al.* 1983, 1991). However, the coincidental presence of other risk factors for coronary atheroma, particularly hypertension, smoking, and uraemic dyslipoproteinaemia, may have confounded these observations.

Caffeine probably increases the risk of myocardial infarction and death from coronary artery disease, either by its effect on cholesterol (which is questioned by van Dusseldorp *et al.* 1990), or by causing arrhythmias (Curatolo and Robertson 1983; Benowitz 1990). Other analgesic drugs are not known to worsen serum lipids.

6.6.3 Premature ageing

That analgesic habitués appear older than their chronological age, a necessarily subjective observation, has been remarked upon (Gault *et al.* 1968*a*; Nanra *et al.* 1978*a*); if true, accelerated atherogenesis or Alzheimer-like cerebral lesions (see above) could be responsible, as conceivably could longstanding depletion of prostglandin-dependent inflammatory mediators in the connective tissues.

6.7 A typical analgesic habitué

It must be kept in mind that the analgesic syndrome varies between countries or regions, not only because of differences in the composition of proprietary compound analgesics, but also because the type of person who is susceptible to analgesic habituation may differ, depending upon such things as its social acceptability, the pressure and type of advertising, and the availability and seemliness of alternatives such as tobacco, alcohol, or tranquillizers.

In Australia, Canada, Iceland (Ólafsson *et al.* 1966), and Britain (Prescott,

1966), headache, gastric ulcer, and anaemia have been more common than cyanosis and splenomegaly. Psychiatric abnormalities and abuse of other drugs (including alcohol and tobacco) have occurred not much more frequently than in the general population in communities where analgesic nephropathy is prevalent, but have been characteristic of analgesic habitués in Britain (Murray 1973*a*,*b*), North America (Gault *et al.* 1968*a*; Fellner and Tuttle 1969) and the southern states of Australia where regular consumption of analgesics is not common (Dawborn *et al.* 1966; Clarkson and Lawrence 1970).

Few of the published associations have been subjected to statistical validation, but the descriptions are for the most part consistent with each other and the patterns of disease accord with the known side-effects of analgesic components. Least reliance can be placed on those associations for which there is not a known aetiological link with analgesic drugs (accelerated atherogenesis, premature ageing) and those based upon subjective criteria (personality, psychiatric abnormalities).

It is easy, perhaps too easy, to generalize in representing the personality and physical condition characteristic of the patient with renal disease caused by analgesics, and many have done so. It is true that the recognition of these characteristics may alert the clinician to the possibility of analgesic abuse or of renal papillary necrosis, but there is a danger in placing too much reliance upon such subjective criteria. The certain diagnosis of drug abuse depends upon history, if necessary supported by information obtained from relatives or friends, and by detection of drug in urine; and that of analgesic nephropathy is based upon organ imaging, perhaps supplemented by tests of renal function or histopathology.

7
The pathology of analgesic nephropathy

Michael J. Mihatsch and H.U. Zollinger

In 1953, Spühler and Zollinger described chronic interstitial nephritis (CIN) in patients with an excess intake of phenacetin-containing analgesics. Renal papillary necrosis (RPN) was present in the majority. This syndrome, characterized by (RPN), CIN, cortical atrophy, and brown pigmentation of the papillae and urothelium, is known now as analgesic nephropathy (AN).

AN results from the abuse of not only phenacetin, but of analgesic mixtures in general (Prescott 1982*a*), but is rare with non-steroidal anti-inflammatory drugs (Clive and Stoff 1984). Morphologically, it is not a uniform syndrome, the only well-characterized variant being that described below, induced by phenacetin- or paracetamol-containing analgesic mixtures. More detailed work is required on the morphology of the nephropathy associated with other analgesics.

7.1 The lesions of analgesic-induced renal disease

The history of AN as a syndrome in its own right can be divided into three phases. In the first, it was deemed to be characterized primarily by interstitial nephritis (Spühler and Zollinger 1953), and in the second, primarily by papillary necrosis. In the final and current phase, it has come to be recognized that capillary sclerosis and analogous changes in the tubular basement membrane play the decisive role in the development of RPN. The evolution of AN from the earliest detectable lesion in the urinary tract to the terminal stage of bilaterally contracted kidneys will be traced below. Three stages can be identified: capillary sclerosis of the lower urinary tract; RPN; and cortical changes (Fig. 7.1).

7.1.1 Capillary sclerosis

The earliest detectable change in analgesic abuse is capillary sclerosis of the urinary mucosa (Torhorst 1976; Mihatsch *et al.* 1978, 1979, 1983*a*, Gloor 1982), found in 80–90 per cent of cases. Basement membrane thickening is seen in the capillaries immediately underlying the urothelium, which itself is unaltered (Fig. 7.2), and in severe cases also in the muscle layer (Palvio *et al.* 1985). With increasing severity the basement membrane thickens causing constriction of the lumen and eventually complete occlusion. Basement

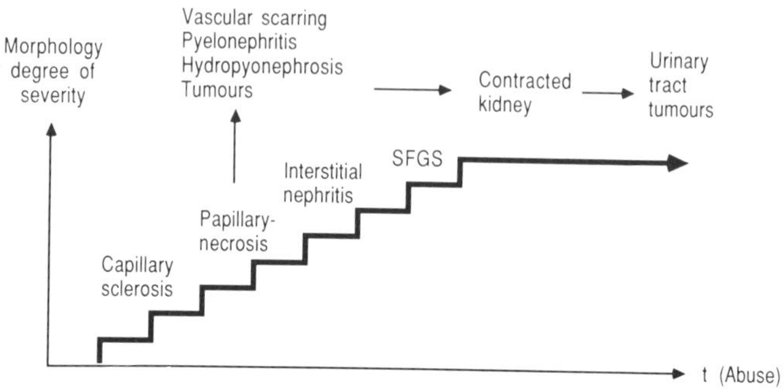

Fig. 7.1 Stages in the development of analgesic nephropathy. SFGS = segmental focal glomerulosclerosis.

membrane thickening has been shown by electron microscopy to result from the concentric deposition of thin basement membrane lamellae in an onion- or tree-ring structure. Massively constricted or occluded capillaries may exhibit over twenty such lamellae entrapping polymorphous cell debris and a dense concentration of lipids, visible on Sudan staining (Fig. 7.3). In particularly severe cases the lipid deposition causes a brownish pigmentation of the urinary tract mucosa, visible to the naked eye (Gloor 1982; Berneis *et al.* 1983). Such pigmentation is a particular feature of the abuse of phenacetin-containing analgesics, and is thought not to occur with phenacetin-free analgesics (Nanra, personal communication). Capillary sclerosis increases in severity from the calyces to the pelvi–ureteric junction, is most marked in the proximal ureter, and gradually decreases to the bladder where it may be found especially around the ureteric ostia in severe cases (Fig. 7.4).

In mild capillary sclerosis evidence of nephropathy is absent in some half of patients and RPN is detectable macroscopically in only 15 per cent; in moderate or severe capillary sclerosis, 40 per cent have macroscopically evident RPN, but in 15 per cent no RPN is detectable even by microscopy (Mihatsch *et al.* 1983*a*).

7.1.2 Development of papillary necrosis

The morphology of RPN is well-documented since the fundamental studies by Burry (1967; Burry *et al.* 1966, 1977) and Gloor (1960, 1961, 1974, 1978*a*,*b*) and can be divided into three stages: early, intermediate, and late or full-blown, RPN.

In the early stage, the macroscopic appearance of the kidney is virtually normal; however, in abuse of phenacetin-containing analgesics, the medullary pyramids show yellow-brown streaks converging on the papillary tips (Fig. 7.5). Histologically, the lesion is confined to the central part of the inner medulla, the outer medulla and cortex being unaffected. Transverse

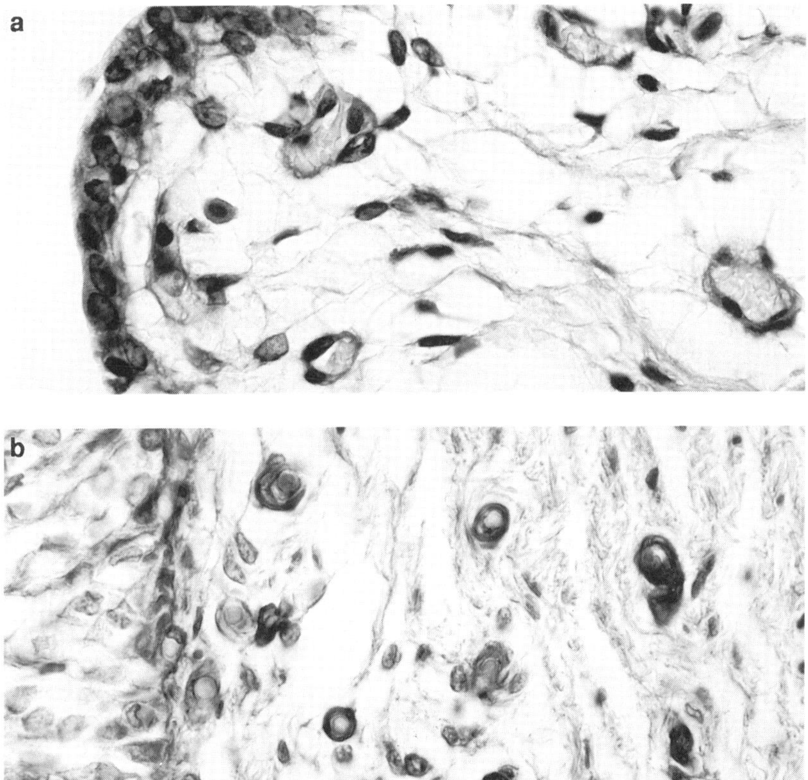

Fig. 7.2 Different degrees of severity of capillary sclerosis in the urothelial mucosa. (a) Normal mucosa with hardly visible capillary basement membranes. (b) Slight capillary sclerosis with thickened basement membranes. (c) Severe capillary sclerosis with narrowing or complete occlusion of the lumen.

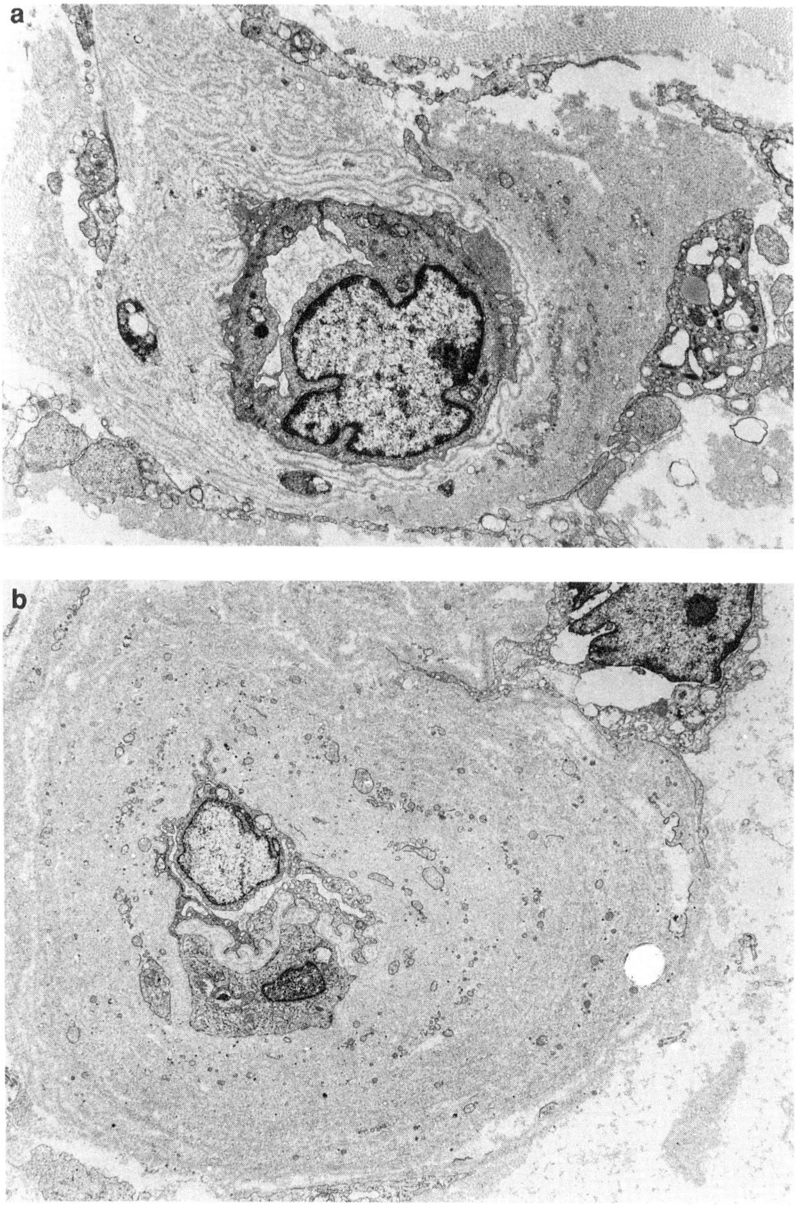

Fig. 7.3 Capillary sclerosis seen by electron microscopy. (1) Slight capillary sclerosis: the basement membrane is thickened and consists of a few thin membrane lamellae. (b) Severe capillary sclerosis with numerous densely-packed thin basement lamellae. The vascular lumen is very narrowed. The endothelial cell is still preserved. Between the basement membrane lamellae polymorphous, partly lipid-containing, debris is present.

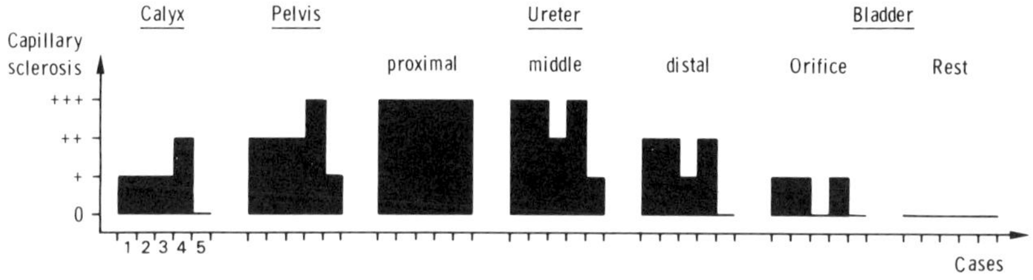

Fig. 7.4 Different degrees of capillary sclerosis in the urinary tract from the calyx to the bladder. The most severe form is always present in the proximal and middle third of the ureter.

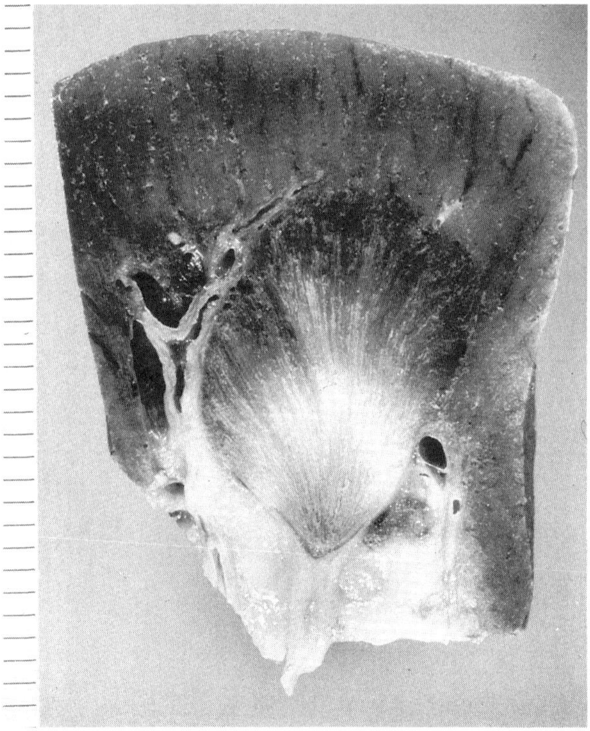

Fig. 7.5 Early stage of papillary necrosis with streaks converging to the papillary tip.

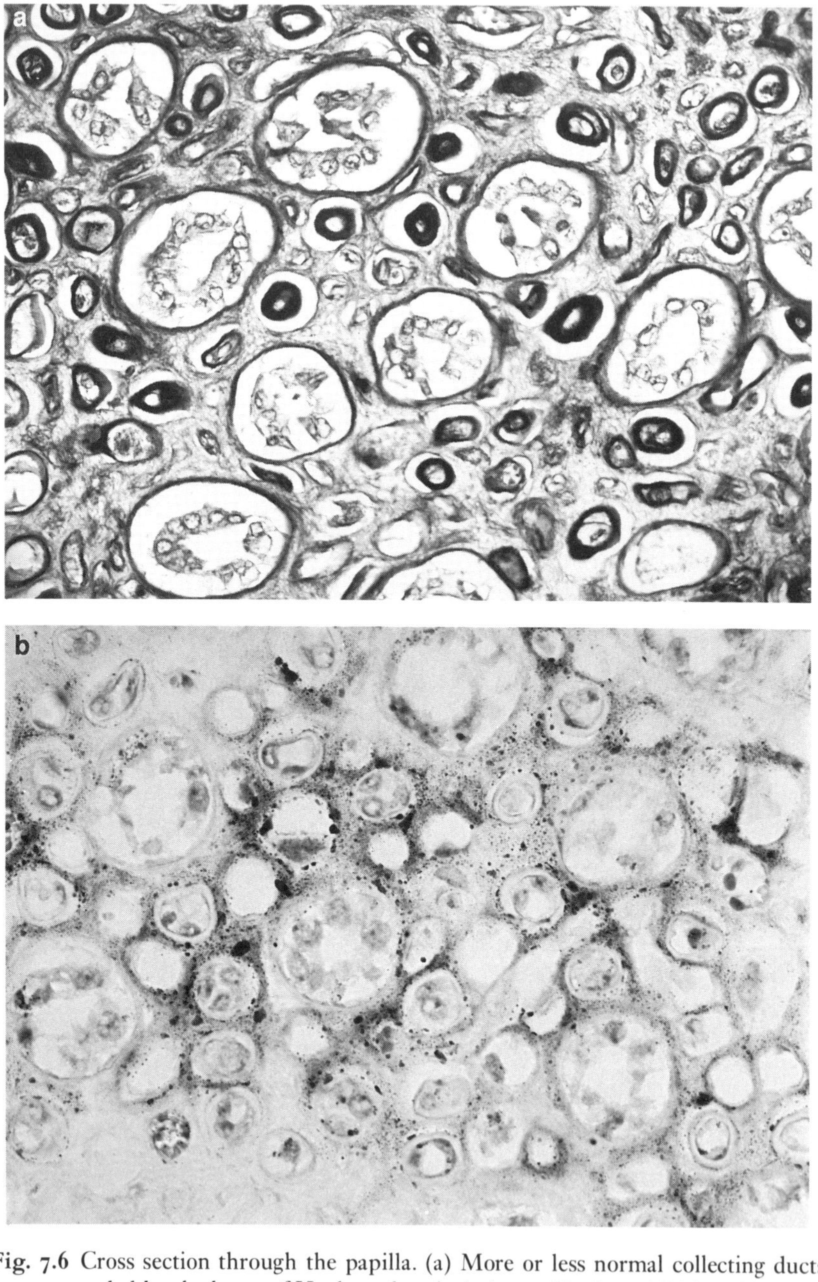

Fig. 7.6 Cross section through the papilla. (a) More or less normal collecting ducts are surrounded by the loops of Henle and peritubular capillaries exhibiting thickened basement membranes. (b) The thickened basement membranes contain lipid deposits (black).

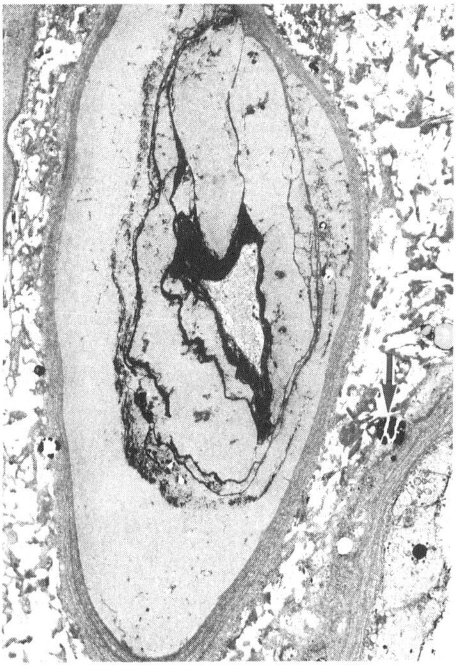

Fig. 7.7 Henle's loop and peritubular capillaries exhibit thickened basement membranes consisting of thin lamellae which also contain calcium deposits (arrow). The endothelial cell is necrotic and artificially detatched from the underlying basement membrane.

sections through the papillary tips show patchy lesions distributed around the collecting duct bundles. The interstitium is widened by an increase in ground substance and contains markedly altered peritubular capillaries and ascending limbs of Henle's loops; adjacent descending limbs, collecting ducts, and vasa recta show little or no abnormality (Fig. 7.6(a)). The basement membranes of the ascending limbs and peritubular capillaries are thickened by layers of newly formed basement membrane lamellae (Fig. 7.7) (Mihatsch *et al.* 1983*a*). The tubular epithelium of the ascending limbs and the peritubular capillary endothelial cells show degenerative changes or are fully necrosed. Interstitial cells likewise die (Burry *et al.* 1977; Gloor 1978*a*; Mihatsch *et al.* 1983*a*). Sudan-stained sections from abusers of phenacetin-containing analgesics show lipid infiltration of the thickened basement membranes and surrounding interstitium (Fig. 7.6(b)). Focal deposits of calcium salts are seen also in the basement membranes (Burry *et al.* 1977) (Fig. 7.7).

In the intermediate stage of RPN, foci become confluent in the papillae

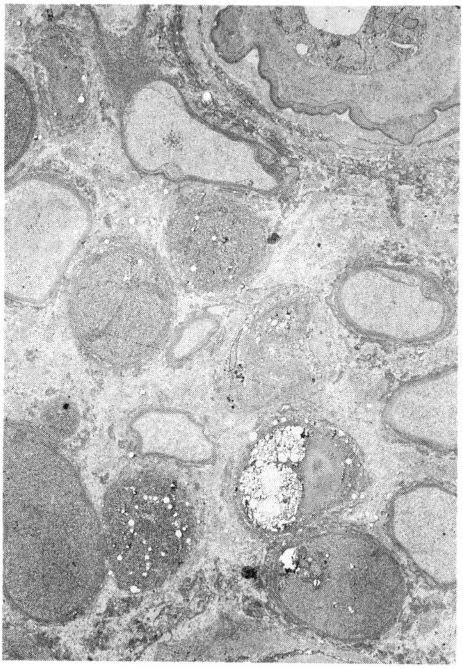

Fig. 7.8 Intermediate stage of papillary necrosis with preserved collecting ducts and complete necrosis of Henle's loops and capillaries. Massive lipid deposition (vacuoles), calcium deposits (black), and lamellar thickening of the basement membranes.

and extend up to the border of the outer medulla. The lateral parts of the inner medulla, which receive the collecting ducts of the columns of Bertin, remain well preserved as do the collecting ducts themselves and the vasa recta (Fig. 7.8).

In late, full-blown, necrosis the collecting ducts and vasa recta are also destroyed. Clefts develop within the necrotic areas, especially bordering viable renal parenchyma and, among other features, become lined with collecting duct epithelium. RPN is a non-reactive, granulocyte-free necrosis. Granulocytes are also virtually absent from adjacent viable tissue. Lymphocytes and histiocytes are common in the area surrounding the vascular bundles in the outer medulla.

7.1.3 The relationship of cortical change to papillary necrosis

RPN gives rise to a variety of scenarios (Fig. 7.9): rapid demarcation and sloughing of necrotic papillae, protracted sloughing, and persistence *in situ* of necrotic papillae (Gloor 1961, 1978*a*, Burry *et al.* 1977).

If a necrotic papilla sloughs partially or totally, the papillary cavity can re-

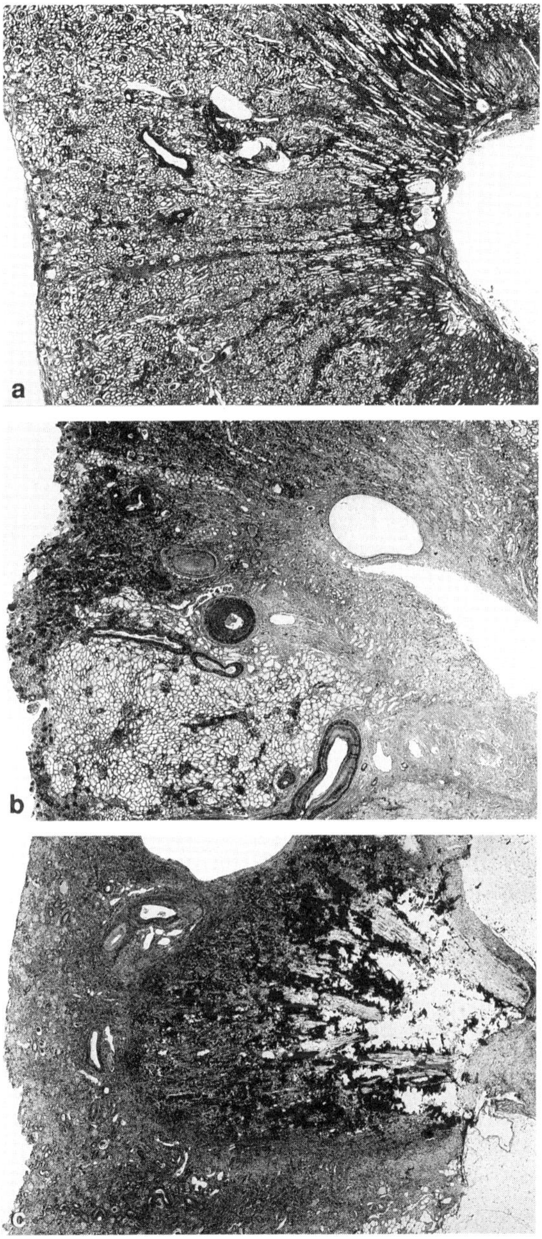

Fig. 7.9 (a) Renal cortex without significant abnormalities after rapid sloughing of the papilla. (b) Renal cortex after protracted sloughing of the necrotic papilla. The suprapapillary cortex is shrunken and atrophic. The column of Bertin, to the left, is hypertrophic and slightly elevated. (c) Necrotic, completely calcified and ossified papillary necrosis in a case of contracted kidney.

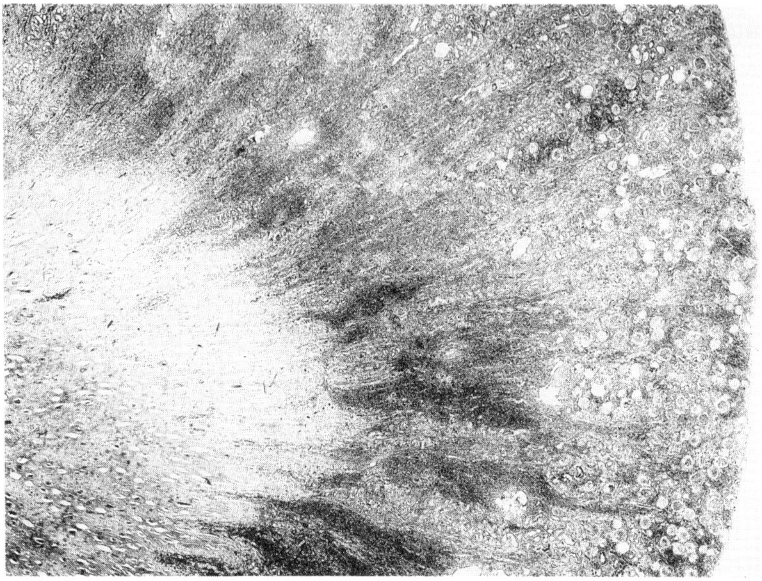

Fig. 7.10 Severe interstitial non-destructive nephritis: massive infiltrates are crowded along the cortico–medullary junction and extend into the cortex. Severe atrophy of the renal cortex (note densely-packed glomeruli).

epithelialize. Necrotic papillae remaining *in situ* can calcify and later ossify. For a long time a ghost outline of the original structure can be detected in the necrotic papilla, as shown by histological examination of papillary fragments spontaneously voided in urine.

What happens to the necrotic papillae is decisive for the renal cortex. If papillary sloughing is rapid, cortical changes may be absent. However, this rarely occurs.

On the other hand, if sloughing is delayed or incomplete, and particularly if the necrotic papillae remain *in situ*, progressive cortical atrophy ensues, with interstitial fibrosis and streaky infiltration by lymphocytes and histiocytes (chronic, non-destructive, interstitial nephritis—CIN) (Fig. 7.10). If some necrotic papillae slough rapidly, while others remain *in situ*, CIN and cortical atrophy develop only in relation to the unseparated papillae. The conclusion to be drawn is that CIN is the consequence, not the cause, of RPN (Kincaid-Smith 1967; Burry 1967; Burry *et al.* 1977; Gloor 1974). Thus obstruction of the intrarenal urine flow due to RPN leads to CIN as does urinary obstruction from other causes (Davies 1968).

Since RPN affects primarily the central papillary area, and spares the lateral area until much later, hypertrophy can occur of the cortical tissue of the columns of Bertin that drain urine mainly via the collecting ducts open-

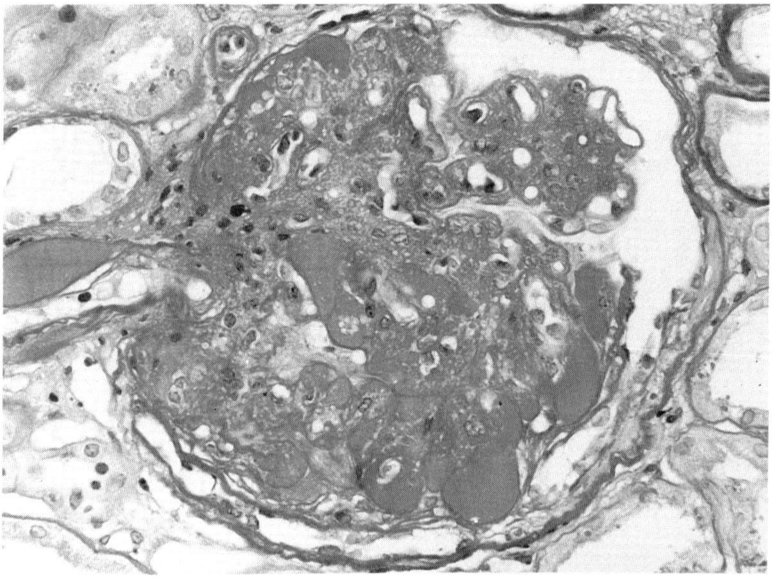

Fig. 7.11 Segmental focal glomerulosclerosis, as seen in the hypertrophied cortex of the column of Bertin (compare Fig. 7.9(b)).

ing laterally into the papillae (Burry *et al.* 1977). Compensatory hypertrophy of the columns of Bertin offsets the suprapapillary loss of parenchyma for a long while, and explains why glomeruli there particularly show focal segmental glomerulosclerosis and hyalinosis (Zollinger's (1966) overload glomerulitis) (Schmidt *et al.* 1983; Bürgin *et al.* 1984) (Fig. 7.11). In the atrophic suprapapillary cortex, however, non-specific glomerular changes, periglomerular fibrosis, collapse, or global sclerosis, predominate (Burry *et al.* 1977).

7.1.4 Fully developed analgesic nephropathy

The full-blown disease is the result of a complex series of events in which primary analgesic-induced lesions overlap with secondary pathology (Fig. 7.12). The kidneys are bilaterally contracted and in part ridged, with the contracted areas corresponding to RPN, and the ridges to the hypertrophied columns of Bertin. On the cut surface the cortico–medullary junction is poorly demarcated. Some papillae have sloughed, while others remain *in situ*. The renal pelvis is of normal or slightly increased width and may contain sloughed fragments of necrotic papillae. Brown pigmentation may be present in the urinary mucosa. RPN becomes difficult to identify in more severely contracted kidneys. Horizontal sections no longer suffice, and transverse sections across the calyces are required. In the terminal stage, even the

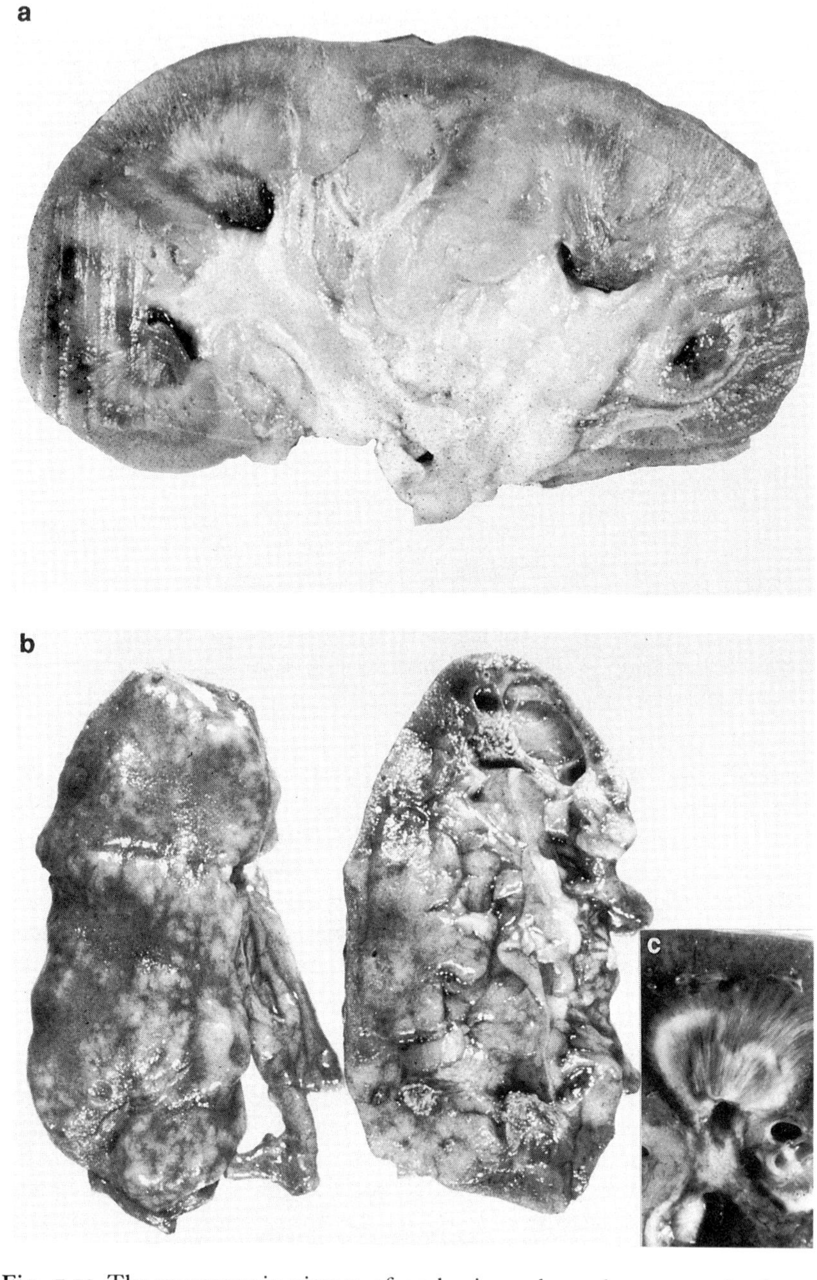

Fig. 7.12 The macroscopic picture of analgesic nephropathy as seen in the past and today. (a) Large pale kidney with numerous necrotic papillae and brownish discolouration, seen thirty years ago. (b) Small contracted kidney with numerous sloughed and retained papillae and a few areas of preserved renal tissue, usually seen today. (c) Inset: papillary necrosis (bright yellow) in acute pyelonephritis.

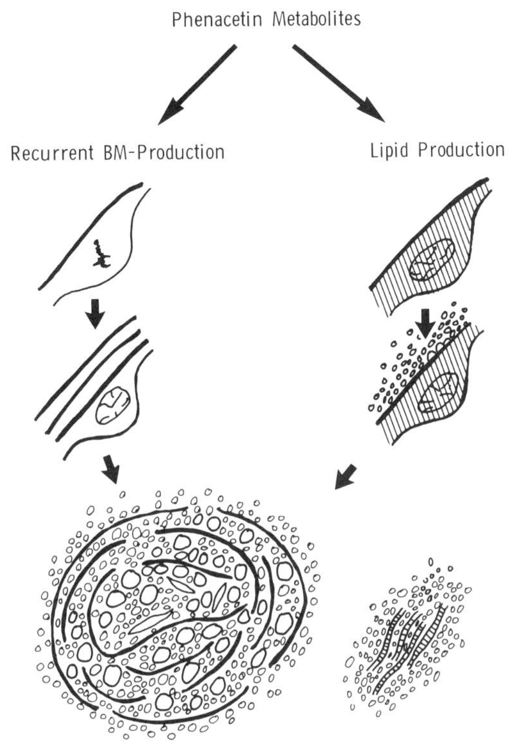

Fig. 7.13 Schematic presentation of the morphogenesis of capillary sclerosis.

previously hypertrophic tissue of the columns of Bertin becomes atrophic, resulting in small smooth kidneys.

7.2 Pathogenesis of analgesic-induced lesions

Capillary sclerosis of the urinary tract serves as a model for understanding AN, since the anatomical and functional conditions in urinary mucosa are essentially less complex than in the kidney.

Of the factors deemed to be involved in the pathogenesis of AN —ischaemia, inhibition of prostaglandin synthesis, immunological or toxic injury (Prescott 1982*a*)—only toxic damage is believed to cause capillary sclerosis (Fig. 7.13). The tree-ring morphology of the concentric layers of basement membrane suggests repeated toxic-induced endothelial necrosis (Mihatsch *et al.* 1978, 1979, 1983*a*). Each generation of cells develops its own basement membrane if it does not lie directly on the old basement membrane, as is the case with capillary sclerosis caused by deposition of cell debris (Vracko 1974). The frequency and variable severity of capillary sclerosis in the different segments of the urinary tract is best explained by the fact that strongly lipophilic analgesic metabolites diffuse out of urine and cause capillary damage. Thus capillary sclerosis is most marked at the points of maximum metabolite concentration and mucosal contact, i.e. distal renal pelvis, pelvi–ureteric junction and proximal ureter (Gloor 1982). The significant correlation between severity of capillary sclerosis on the one hand, and maximum daily dose of phenacetin on the other, emphasizes the importance of direct toxicity in its pathogenesis, as does its regression in the absence of exposure to toxic analgesic metabolites (Mihatsch *et al.* 1983*a*). Ischaemia, inhibition of prostaglandin synthesis, and immunological factors play no essential role in the pathogenesis of capillary sclerosis.

Similarly, toxicity is the common denominator of theories regarding the pathogenesis of AN. The topographical distribution of early changes in the inner medulla, with involvement of the loops of Henle, peritubular capillaries and interstitial cells in the presence of well-preserved collecting ducts, supports the hypothesis that the concentration of the toxic agent increases with that of the urine and exerts a direct effect at the points of maximum concentration (Kriz and Lever 1969). This assumption has been experimentally confirmed. Thus toxic compounds, e.g. paracetamol, aspirin, and others, can reach concentrations in the renal medulla which are many times higher than in blood (Duggin 1980). The relationship between the total intake of phenacetin and the severity of the analgesic-induced renal lesion supports the hypothesis of toxic injury (Burry *et al.* 1966). Stabilization or improvement of renal function after cessation of abuse also is an argument in favour of the toxic origin of AN (Nitzsche and Bock 1970), while further support is provided by biochemical evidence. It is probable that reactive metabolites, formed from aspirin and paracetamol under the influence of p450 monooxygenase, bind covalently to cell proteins causing cell damage (Nanra 1983). Ischaemic necrosis (Nanra *et al.* 1973; Molland 1978) is definitely not present, since the vasa recta running next to the necrotic papillae are unaffected. Furthermore, the selective occurrence of necrosis in the vicinity of the collecting duct bundle argues against the involvement of ischaemic necrosis. Immune processes (Raaflaub and Dubach 1969) likewise play no role in the development of RPN. Despite many experimental studies in animals, the primary target of analgesic-induced toxicity—tubular, endothelial, or interstitial cell—remains undeterminded (Shelley 1978; Prescott 1982*a*; Bach *et al.* 1983). The probability is that all three are equally susceptible.

7.3 Specificity of the analgesic-induced lesion

So far as we know, capillary sclerosis is specific to abuse of analgesics containing phenacetin and paracetamol (Mihatsch *et al.* 1983*a*). Other conditions associated with microangiopathy, e.g. diabetes mellitus and hypertension, do not produce changes which could be confused with capillary sclerosis, nor is it related to age, renal insufficiency, or malignancy.

Early papillary changes similarly are specific to AN (Gloor 1961; Burry *et al.* 1977). Increase in interstitial ground substance and calcification also can occur with advancing age, but not in association with changes in peritubular capillaries or loops of Henle. Basement membrane thickening in the loops of Henle and peritubular capillaries is seen in diabetes mellitus and cirrhosis of the liver, but does not lead to selective necrosis in the vicinity of the collecting duct bundle (Burry *et al.* 1977). It is hardly possible to mistake the non-reactive RPN in analgesic abuse with that of acute pyelonephritis (Gloor 1960). The latter is yellow, friable, and massively infiltrated with polymorphonuclear leukocytes (Fig. 7.12(c)).

The brown pigmentation of the urinary mucosa is also specific although it probably occurs only with abuse of phenacetin-containing analgesics. It is severe enough to be of diagnostic significance in only one third of cases (Gloor 1982).

7.4 Complications of analgesic nephropathy

Complications frequently overlay and blur the typical picture of AN and occasionally prevent the correct diagnosis being made. There are five principal complications: hypertension, pyelonephritis, hydronephrosis or pyonephrosis, urolithiasis, and urothelial tumours.

7.4.1 Hypertension

There is a direct correlation between frequency of hypertension and severity of renal failure (Mihatsch *et al.* 1982*b*). Thus hypertension is observed in approximately 80 per cent of patients with a serum creatinine of 885 μmol/l, but in only 30 per cent with a serum creatinine of 177 μmol/l. Additional lesions are found in the renal cortex in hypertension: arteriosclerosis, arteriolosclerosis (rarely), hypertensive glomerulosclerosis, and renovascular scarring, the last aggravating renal contraction. Hypertension-induced lesions often are more readily recognized in the columns of Bertin than in the markedly contracted suprapapillary cortical tissue. A rare complication is the central arterial contracted kidney, which may occasionally be bilateral, due to arteriosclerotic stenosis of the renal artery.

7.4.2 Pyelonephritis

Acute and chronic pyelonephritis occur in approximately 75 per cent of cases of AN. The necrotic renal papillae are an ideal culture medium for bacterial infection, but it is open to question whether scarring in interstitial destructive nephritis is due to bacterial infection (Gloor 1978*a*). Acute pyelonephritis with RPN is a red herring, which can result in failure to recognize analgesic-induced RPN (Gloor 1978*b*).

7.4.3 Obstruction

Similarly the typical picture can be obscured completely by hydronephrosis and pyonephrosis resulting from blockage of the lower urinary tract by sloughed necrotic papillae. A correct diagnosis is only reached in advanced renal destruction, particularly in nephrectomy specimens, if capillary sclerosis is deliberately looked for or if typical analgesic-induced sloughed papillae can be identified in the ureteral lumen. Capillary sclerosis can occasionally be destroyed by necrotizing mucosal inflammation, making it impossible to diagnose analgesic abuse on morphological grounds alone (Mihatsch *et al.* 1983*a*).

7.4.4 Cysts

After long-term haemodialysis, secondary cyst formation may also obscure the typical picture of AN. Once the whole kidney is permeated by cysts of variable size, the necrotic papillae are easily overlooked.

7.4.5 Urothelioma

About 10 per cent of abusers of phenacetin-containing analgesics develop malignant tumours of the urinary tract. One third of these tumours are located in the renal pelvis and/or ureter, the remaining in the bladder (Mihatsch and Knüsli 1982). In patients with renal pelvic tumours, the kidney may be completely destroyed, so that capillary sclerosis remains the only hint to previous analgesic abuse.

7.5 Correlation between clinical presentation and morphology

No functional disturbance is caused by capillary sclerosis in the urinary tract. However, once the inner renal medulla is involved—peritubular capillaries, loops of Henle, interstitial cells—then typical distal tubular disturbances occur: reduced urinary concentration, acidosis, and electrolyte losses (Dubach *et al.* 1983) (Fig. 7.14). Renal excretory function remains intact for a long time since the collecting ducts become recruited into the disease process only at a late stage, remaining patent even in complete necrosis and therefore still able to conduct urine. Once the necrotic papillae have sloughed, the collecting ducts flow into what remains of the medullary cone. Excretory function only begins to fall when cortical changes appear. Significant proteinuria is an unfavourable late symptom (Mehta *et al.* 1977). It is observed when excretory function is markedly reduced and in the pres-

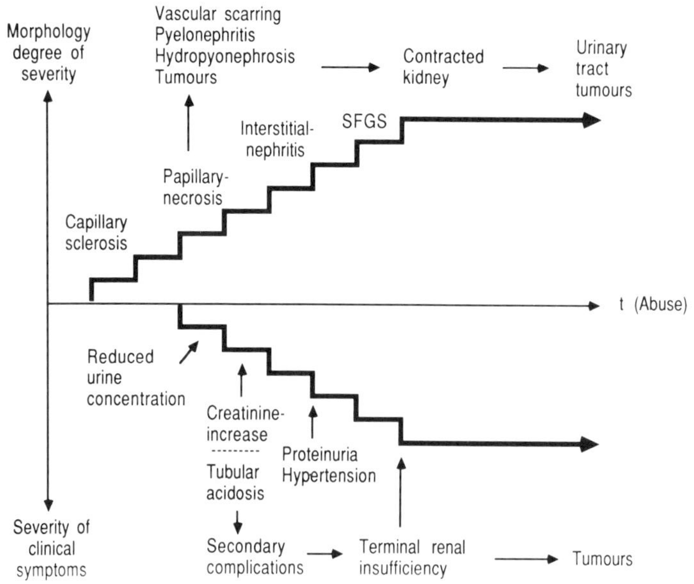

Fig. 7.14 Correlation between the morphologic stages of analgesic nephropathy and the clinical symptoms.

ence of segmental focal glomerulosclerosis (Schmidt *et al.* 1983; Bürgin *et al.* 1984).

7.6 Cessation of analgesic abuse

There have been few clinical and morphological investigations into what happens after analgesic abuse is discontinued (Mihatsch *et al.* 1983*a*). Analysis of individual cases suggests that capillary sclerosis halts and that partial regression of the basement membrane changes can occur as a result of continuous turnover. Thus, ureters which have been excluded from urine flow for some years show no further capillary sclerosis (Fig. 7.15). Remains of basement membrane can be detected in the stroma only by electron microscopy. That capillary sclerosis regresses would explain why this lesion may be absent from patients dying 10 or more years after cessation of analgesics. The hypothesis would also explain why renal function remains stable, or even improves, when analgesic abuse is abandoned in the early stages (Nitzsche and Bock 1970). This favourable outcome is assisted by compensatory hypertrophy of the columns of Bertin. Conversely, the morphogenesis of AN explains why cessation of abuse in advanced renal disease has no significant effect on the progression of renal impairment. The residual renal parenchyma of the columns of Bertin is progressively damaged

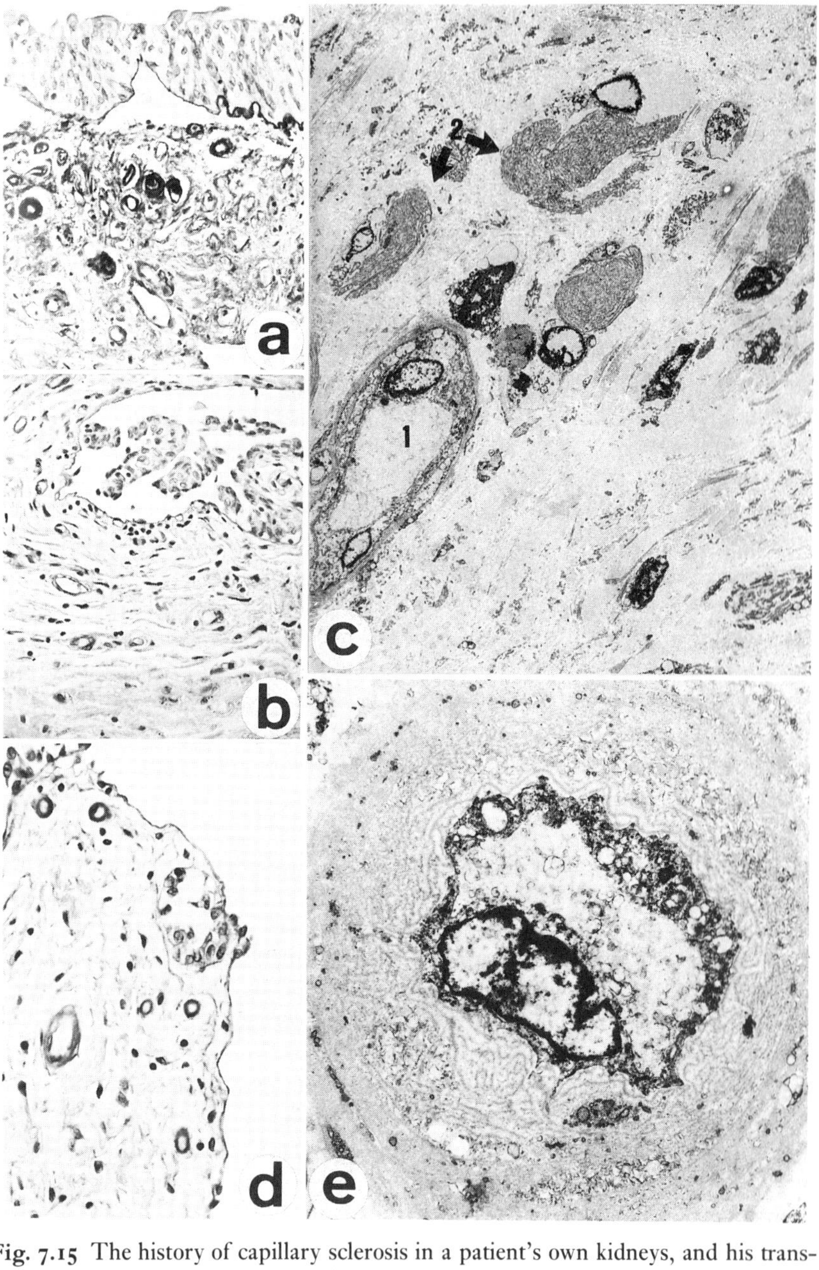

Fig. 7.15 The history of capillary sclerosis in a patient's own kidneys, and his transplant. (a) Moderate to severe capillary sclerosis in the host's ureter before transplantation. (b) No capillary sclerosis in the host's ureter at autopsy ten years later. (c) Electron microscopic finding of lumps of basement membranes representing remnants of completely occluded capillaries in the host's ureter at autopsy. Patent capillaries without significant capillary sclerosis. (d and e) Slight capillary sclerosis in the ureter of the kidney transplant.

by work hypertrophy and concomitant development of 'overload glomerulitis' so that loss of the still functioning nephrons continues.

7.7 Concluding remarks

AN is the most common completely avoidable renal disease. In all countries in which mixed analgesics containing aspirin, paracetamol, or phenacetin are on sale, the analgesic syndrome is reported (Chapter 6). In Switzerland, 18 per cent of patients with end stage renal disease still (in 1989) suffer from AN. In 1980, about 4 per cent of the autopsy cases had capillary sclerosis and/or a history of analgesic abuse (Mihatsch *et al.* 1982*a*).

These figures indicate that patients with end stage renal disease represent only the tip of the iceberg and that a large number of patients with minor renal disease and other symptoms of analgesic abuse must be expected. In all countries where compound analgesics are freely available, it is necessary to look for abuse using the classical tools of clinical history and determination of analgesic metabolites in urine (Dubach 1967).

For the pathologist, capillary sclerosis is a reliable morphologic feature of analgesic abuse and may be used for epidemiological studies. Such studies performed in Basel have shown that in 50 per cent of all patients with clear-cut morphologic evidence, analgesic abuse was unknown to the doctors attending the patients during their terminal illness (Mihatsch *et al.* 1982*a*).

8

The diagnosis of analgesic nephropathy by organ imaging

Hans Köhler, Elisabeth Zyzik, and Simin Schadmand

In analgesic nephropathy (AN) a variety of morphological changes can be demonstrated by imaging techniques. However, renal papillary necrosis (RPN) is the hallmark of AN (Table 8.1). RPN may occur less frequently in other conditions, such as diabetes mellitus (Günther 1937), obstructive uropathy (Friedreich 1877) or sickle cell disease (Harrow *et al.* 1963). The origin of RPN has been considered to be essentially ischaemic and common to the different aetiologies (Kincaid-Smith 1986*a*). In keeping with this, the radiographic changes of RPN are independent of aetiology.

8.1 Morphological features of analgesic nephropathy

8.1.1 Early signs

The detection of early changes is hampered by the fact that the normal renal papilla is invisible radiographically with the exception of the papillary blush, and can be imaged only indirectly by contrast in the adjacent calyx. Describing the radiographic changes of the papillary region, one has to keep in mind that in the normal kidney, about a dozen papillae drain into seven or eight calyces. The earliest changes of RPN are local papillary swelling, and decreased opacification in the adjacent calyx suggesting impaired renal function. Subsequently papillary atrophy occurs, causing irregularity of the papillary tip and widening of the fornix and the calyceal cup as a whole (Fig. 8.1). Thus the early features of analgesic nephropathy are large kidneys, diminished renal function and the signs of papillary atrophy (Table 8.2).

8.1.2 Partial papillary necrosis

Papillary necrosis and the associated development of cavities may start eccentrically at the fornix ('papillary' type), or centrally at the tip of the papilla ('medullary' type) (Fig. 8.1) (Poynter and Hare 1974). Partial papillary necrosis usually starts at the tip, forming a central cavity which may remain unaltered in size, or enlarge and progress to total papillary necrosis (Fig. 8.2). Eccentric partial papillary necrosis begins at the calyceal fornix,

Table 8.1 *Classification of renal papillary necrosis*

	Morphological signs	Diagnostic procedure
Total papillary necrosis	complete papillary sloughing	pyelography
Partial papillary necrosis	partial papillary sloughing	pyelography
(a) central (medullary)	cavity	
(b) eccentric (papillary)	cleft	
Necrosis *in situ*	no papillary sloughing	
(a) without calcification		histology
(b) with calcification		sonography, plain film, computed tomography

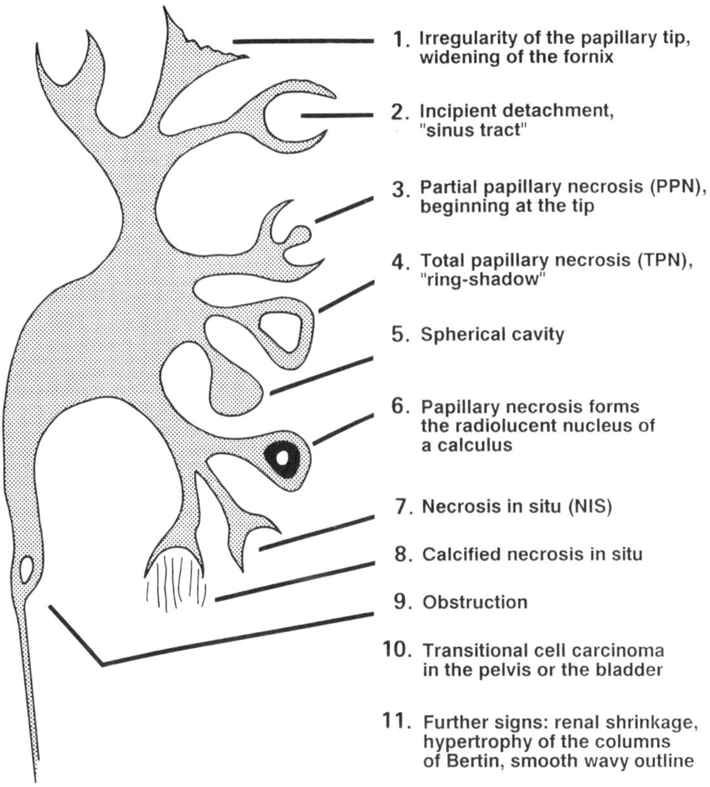

Fig. 8.1 Morphlogical features of analgesic nephropathy.

Table 8.2 *Incidence of radiological features in 57 patients with analgesic nephropathy.*[1]

	Per cent
Reduced renal function	85
Normal renal size	82
Medullary necrosis	65
Papillary atrophy	46
Papillary necrosis	46
Papillary cavity	39
Renal calcification	26
Ring shadows	14
Fistulae	11
Obstructive uropathy	3

[1] Mean creatinine clearance = 32 ml/min. From Adams and Murray (1975).

forming a cleft or 'sinus' into the papilla, and in most cases advances to total papillary necrosis (Fig. 8.2).

8.1.3 Total papillary necrosis

Total papillary necrosis may begin centrally or, more often, eccentrically, forming a cleft which results in papillary separation (Poynter and Hare 1974). After detachment, the papilla may remain in the calyx and be detected within a contrast-filled cavity (a 'ring shadow'). Sometimes the papilla appears triangular; if formed by 2–3 pyramids, its shape is irregular. However, ring shadows are rare because in most cases the sloughed papilla will be absorbed or pass into the urine, leaving a spherical cavity (Table 8.2). The characteristic feature of clubbed calyces is then demonstrable by pyelography (Fig. 8.1, 8.5, 8.6).

In some cases, especially with proteus infections, necrotic tissue forms the nucleus of a calculus. Then a radiolucent nucleus is surrounded by an opaque hull. Detached papillae passing into the urine may cause ureteric obstruction.

8.1.4 Necrosis *in situ*

The necrotic papilla may not separate, but remain attached as necrosis *in situ* (Poynter and Hare 1974). The more-or-less intact necrotic tissue may become calcified or even ossified. Non-calcified necrosis *in situ* may easily be missed, because the main radiological features of RPN depend on shrinking and, more importantly, separation of the papilla. A reported case illustrates this point: intravenous and retrograde pyelography showed a normal calyceal system without evidence of papillary necrosis, but RPN was demonstrated by renal biopsy, and 10 days later at autopsy extensive necrosis involved every papilla (Fairley and Kincaid-Smith 1968).

On the other hand, calcified necrotic papillae can be detected easily by sonography, plain film radiology or computed tomography (Köhler *et al.* 1987) (Fig. 8.3, 8.8). In a clinical study we demonstrated calcified papillae in 24 of 30 patients with AN and serum creatinine 142–841 μmol/l, and in 11 of 14 patients with AN undergoing regular haemodialysis.

However, calcification of papillae occurs late in AN. In a series of 57 patients with AN and a mean creatinine clearance of 32 ml/min, renal calcification was found in 26 per cent (Table 8.2), whereas in autopsy studies, calcified papillae have been demonstrated in more than 80 per cent of cases (Gloor 1978*a*).

8.1.5 The outcome of papillary sloughing

Detached papillae may remain in the calyceal cavity forming a ring shadow, or be absorbed, or calcify. However, usually they pass into the urine, either silently or causing renal colic and/or haematuria. To establish the diagnosis, the papillary tissue should be retrieved and examined histologically. Sloughed papillae may cause ureteral obstruction and require surgical intervention, for example by percutaneous nephrostomy to reduce intrapelvic pressure and provide an opportunity for antegrade pyelography, which yields optimal imaging of the renal collecting system (Fig. 8.5). This may also be achieved by conventional retrograde pyelography which, however, is accompanied by a higher incidence of infectious complications.

8.1.6 Parenchymal changes in analgesic nephropathy

Renal function and pyelographic density diminish early in the course of AN. Kidney size is variable, remaining nearly normal for a long time.

With progression of AN, the juxtamedullary nephrons atrophy and the peripheral cortex becomes thinner. This, and the loss of medullary tissue, leads to a shrinkage of the kidneys. The renal columns are spared, or may show hypertrophy. Although the renal outlines become slightly irregular, characteristically they appear smooth and wavy without focal scarring (Fig. 8.4). This may help to differentiate from reflux nephropathy in which there is focal loss of cortical tissue over clubbed calyces resulting in an irregular outline and disparity in size of the two kidneys (Fig. 8.11, 8.12). However, in AN some focal scarring may be superimposed, presumably due to intermittent bacterial infection.

8.1.7 Transitional cell carcinoma

In analgesic abuse, transitional cell carcinoma may develop after some 25 years, usually in the pelvis (Fig. 8.6), but also in the ureter and bladder (Fig. 8.7). It is seen most often in advanced kidney disease, including patients on

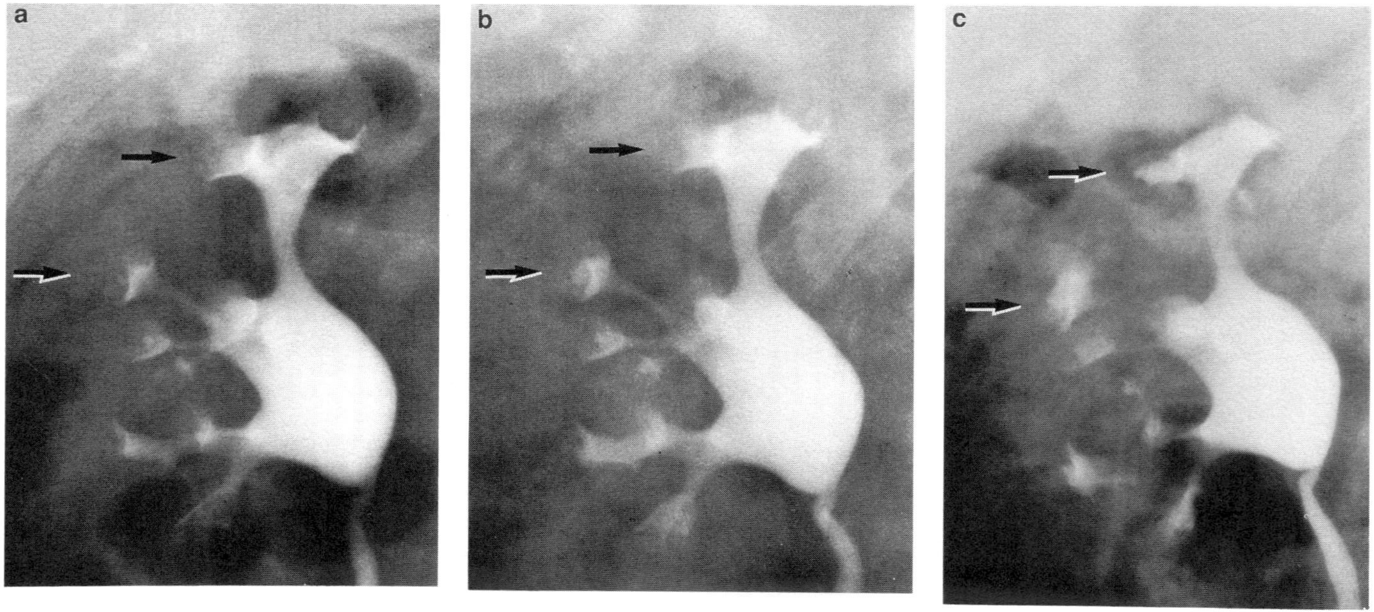
a
b
c

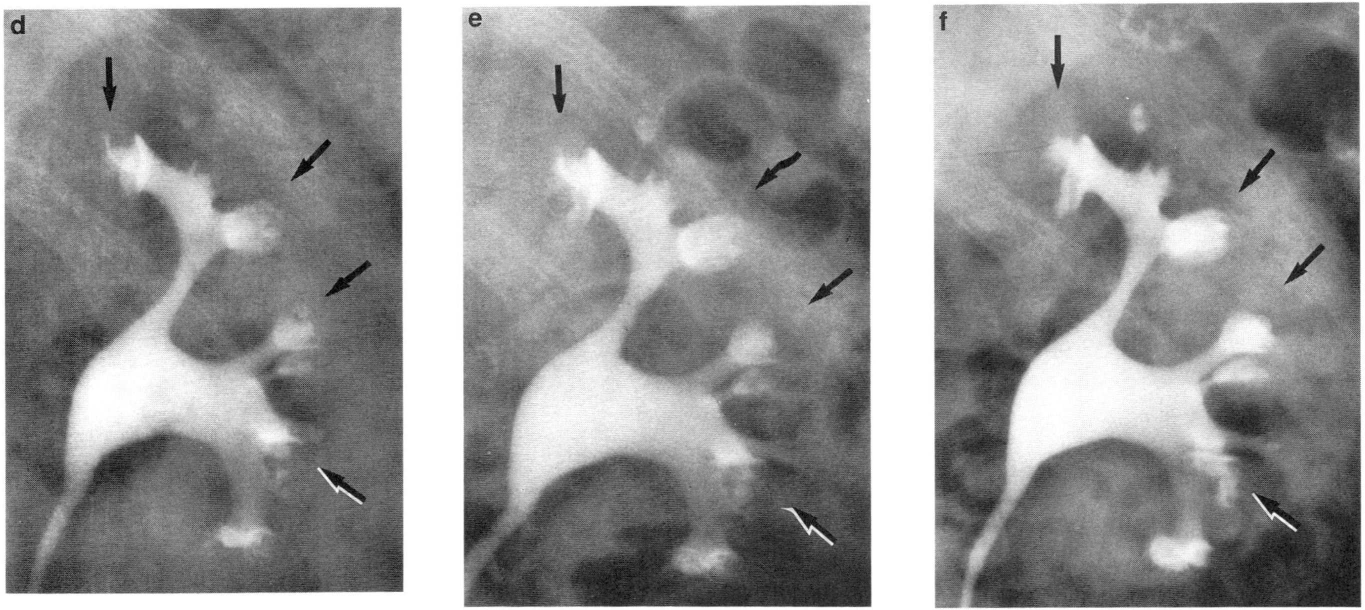

Fig. 8.2 Intravenous urograms at 2 yr intervals on a 73-yr old woman with a history of analgesic abuse (estimated at 8 kg over a period of 20 yr), recurrent haematuria, and renal colic; serum creatinine 60 μmol/l: (a–c) right kidney in 12/85, 3/87 and 5/89 respectively —multiple papillary necroses (upper arrow indicates progression from partial to total papillary necrosis; lower arrow shows that the papillary necrosis is of the central type); (d–f) left kidney at same dates—different stages of papillary necrosis in the one pyelogram, also showing progression; the top arrow shows central and cleft (eccentric) necrosis in one compound papilla.

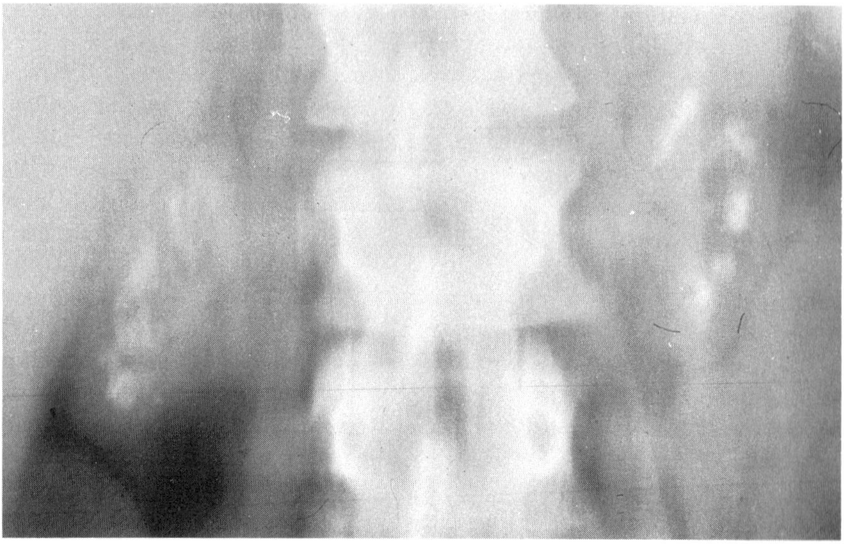

Fig. 8.3 Plain film from a dialysis patient with analgesic nephropathy shows shrunken kidneys with calcified papillary necrosis *in situ*.

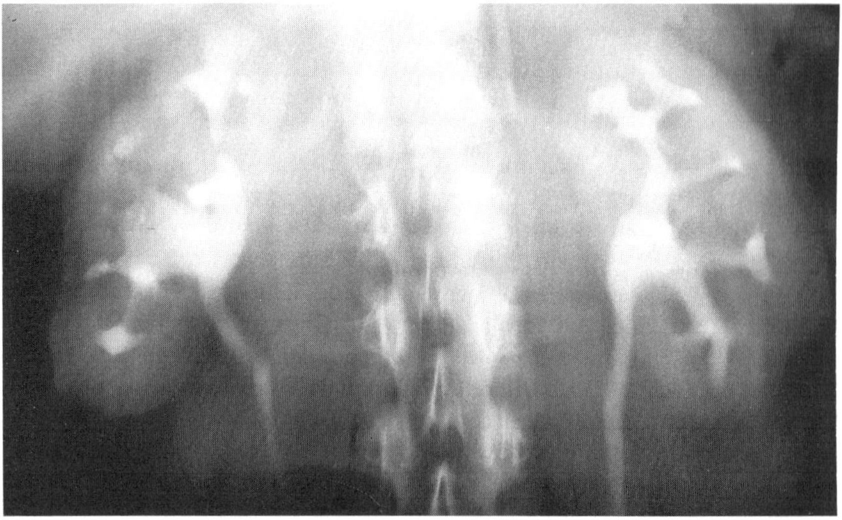

Fig. 8.4 Intravenous pyelography demonstrates the characteristic smooth wavy outlines of the kidneys in analgesic nephropathy.

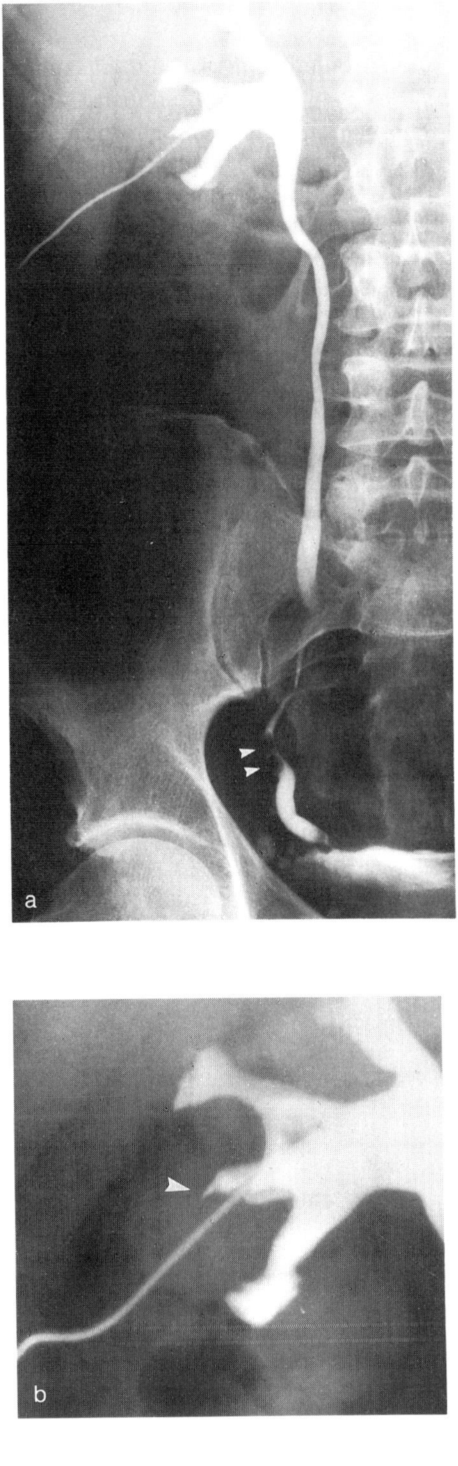

Fig. 8.5 Obstructive uropathy, in a 50-yr old patient with a serum creatinine 170 μmol/l and an analgesic consumption of 20 kg over a period of 30 yr, necessitated percutaneous nephrostomy. Antegrade pyelography demonstrated (a) in the ureter two filling defects, histologically identified as necrotic papillae, and (b) partial (arrow) and total papillary necrosis.

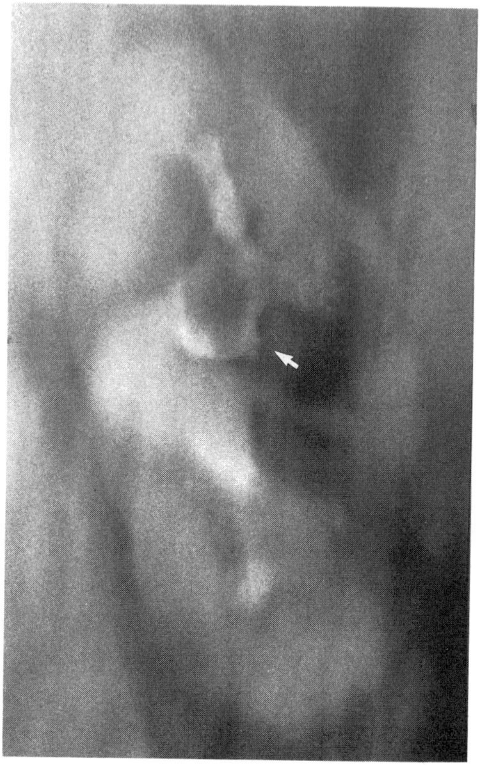

Fig. 8.6 Intravenous urogram, in a 69-yr old patient with analgesic abuse for 45 yr, demonstrates an irregular filling defect in the upper calyceal stem (a transitional cell carcinoma), total necrosis in the lower papilla, and eccentric partial necrosis in the upper papilla.

maintenance dialysis. Often concomitant calcified necrosis *in situ* can be detected. 'Displaced calcium', i.e. a displacement of calcified necrosis *in situ*, has been described as a sign of renal carcinoma (Marrocco *et al.* 1986).

8.2 Imaging techniques

8.2.1 Pyelography

Only pyelography (urography)—intravenous, antegrade, or retrograde—yields sufficient information about the early changes of analgesic nephropathy and about non-calcifying partial or total papillary necrosis. Non-calcifying necrosis *in situ* may not be detected with any imaging technique. In general, intravenous urography will be employed. One has to keep in mind that it is only reliable when ureteral compression, tomograms, and oblique films are performed (Fig. 8.10). Intravenous urography may demonstrate RPN and

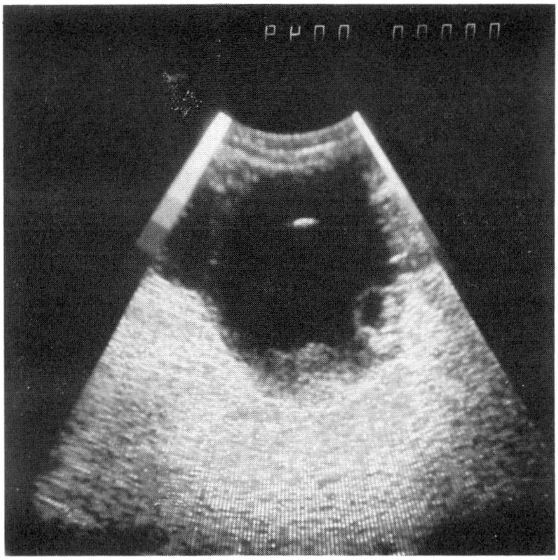

Fig. 8.7 Sonography shows a bladder cancer in a patient with analgesic nephropathy.

reveal the discrepancy between the diminished pyelographic density and normal kidney size.

With progressive loss of renal function, opacification becomes insufficient and either antegrade or retrograde pyelography, which usually provides optimal imaging of even subtle papillary changes (Fig. 8.5), is necessary. The additional definition obtainable with directly injected contrast may also be required in cases of suspected transitional cell carcinoma of the renal pelvis or ureter.

8.2.2 Ultrasonography

Calcified RPN, which occurs more frequently in advanced AN, may be diagnosed by ultrasonography, plain film tomography or computed tomography (Fig. 8.8). When compared, renal sonography is as sensitive and reliable as the other methods (Braun *et al.* 1983; Köhler *et al.* 1987; Weber *et al.* 1985). The normal human kidney shows low level echoes corresponding to renal pyramids, which form a typical garland pattern around the central sinus (Fig. 8.9(a)). In AN, the calcified papillae also surround the central sinus in a garland pattern (Fig. 8.9(b)), which in some cases is incomplete, suggesting either non-uniform calcification or papillary sloughing. Calcification usually starts at the tip of the papilla, often presenting a triangular shape. Distal shadowing is usually evident. In early cases the echolucent pattern of unchanged renal pyramids is usually present. However, necrosis

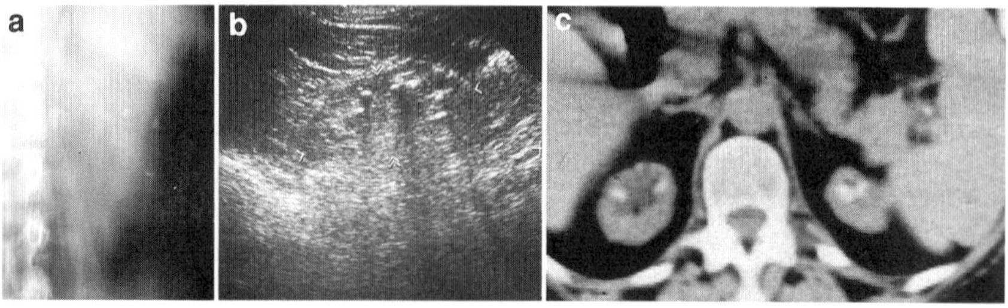

Fig. 8.8 Calcified papillary necrosis *in situ* can be demonstrated by (a) plain film radiography, (b) ultrasonography, and (c) computed tomography.

in situ may yield a comparable picture and may not be identified by any imaging technique.

A fluid-filled cavity, a sign of papillary detachment, is a rare finding with sonography.

8.2.3 Computed tomography and plain film radiology

Renal calcification can also be demonstrated by plain film or computed tomography (Fig. 8.3, 8.8). In patients with AN, papillary calcification was compared with all three imaging modalities (Weber *et al.* 1985). Calcified papillae were seen in 6 of the 16 patients only by computed tomography and sonography, and not by plain film radiology; in one patient only by computed tomography; and in another patient only by sonography. This underlines that plain film radiology is less sensitive than sonography or computed tomography, as is known for patients with nephrocalcinosis of other causation. Therefore, ultrasonography is the preferred procedure to detect calcified necrosis *in situ*.

8.3 Differential diagnosis

The radiological features may change during the course of the disease, varying from subtle changes with swollen papillae and widening of the calyceal cup, to incipient detachment starting centrally or eccentrically, complete sloughing leaving clubbed calyces, ureteral obstruction, or transitional cell carcinoma. These different manifestations of the disease may be seen together, or may change from one investigation to another. It should be stressed that besides renal papillary changes, the most important characteristics of AN are the relatively large or symmetrically shrunken kidneys with smooth, wavy outlines and early impairment of renal function.

RPN, the hallmark of AN, may also occur, but less frequently, in other pathological conditions such as diabetes mellitus, sickle cell haemoglobinopathy, and obstruction, which cannot be distinguished by imaging

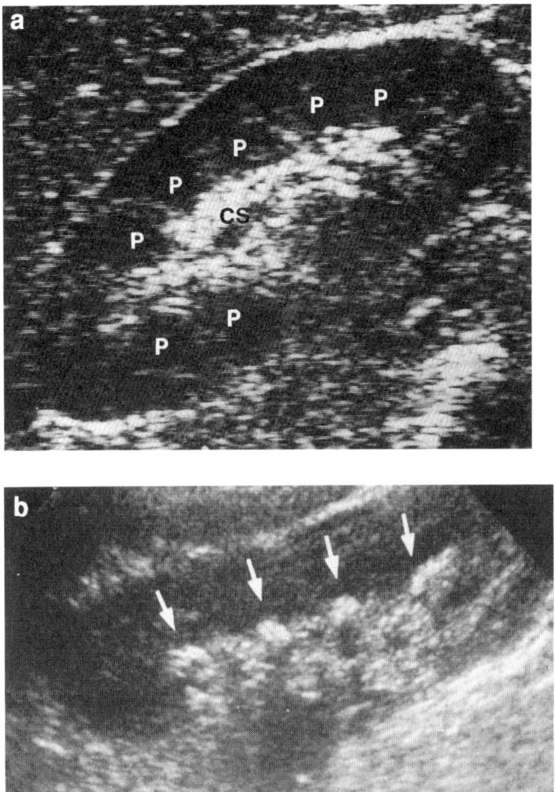

Fig. 8.9 The typical garland pattern of (a) low-level echoes corresponding to renal pyramids (P) around the central sinus (CS) in a normal human kidney, and (b and c) calcified papillary necrosis *in situ*; only some of the calcifications show distal shadowing (depending on the plane of the film).

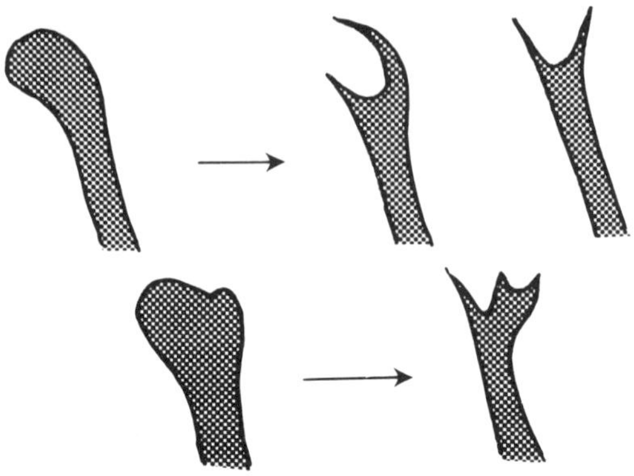

Fig. 8.10 Oblique films show calyces to be normal which otherwise would have been interpreted as papillary necrosis.

techniques. In a series of 32 patients with diabetic nephropathy and impaired renal function, for example, only one had calcified papillae (Weber *et al.* 1985).

8.3.1 Normal kidney

The early changes of AN may be subtle and hardly detectable by imaging techniques. A reduced contrast density due to an early impairment of renal function may be the only radiological feature suggesting the diagnosis. The wavy outlines of AN (Fig. 8.4) may resemble the normal multilobar structure, which is, however, more regular and built up of fewer lobes. Inadequate imaging techniques can give a false appearance which mimics papillary necrosis (Fig. 8.10).

8.3.2 Calyceal cysts

Calyceal cysts or diverticula may be confused with partial papillary necrosis. In contrast to partial papillary necrosis, calyceal cysts usually connect with the fornices, may contain calculi, and are solitary, whereas analgesic nephropathy is a generalized disease with a variety of morphological changes.

8.3.3 Reflux nephropathy (chronic pyelonephritis)

Reflux nephropathy is a focal disease, characterized by local but extreme cortical scarring overlying a clubbed calyx (Fig. 8.11, 8.12). Consequently, the outline is irregular and kidney size is asymmetrical. In contrast, AN involves the whole kidney, leading to a rather homogeneous and symmetrical shrinkage and relatively smooth, wavy outlines. Furthermore, reduction of renal function (reduced contrast density), occurs early in AN, when renal size may still be normal, whereas in reflux nephropathy the kidney can be

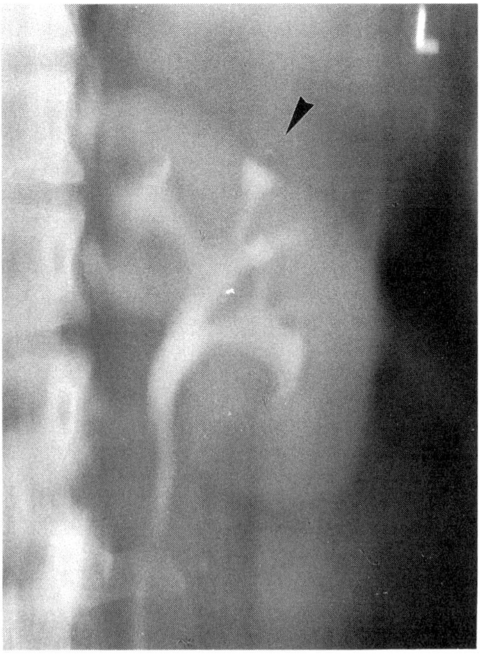

Fig. 8.11 Pyelographic appearances typical of reflux nephropathy (chronic bacterial pyelonephritis) with focal scarring over a clubbed calyx (arrow).

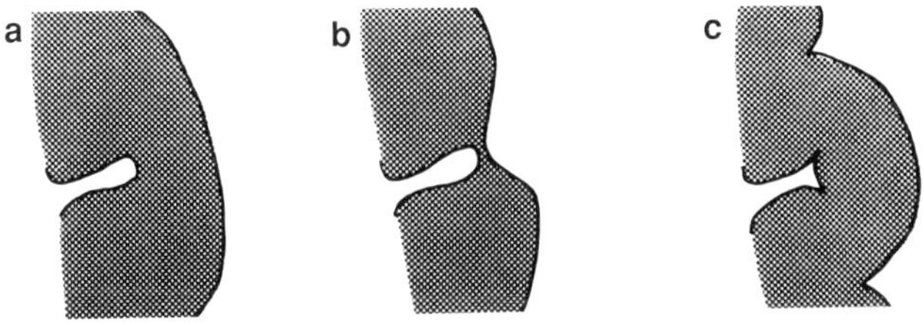

Fig. 8.12 Relationship between papilla and renal cortex in (a) total papillary necrosis, (b) reflux nephropathy, and (c) normally lobulated kidney.

quite shrunken yet produce good pyelographic concentration (Adams and Murray 1975).

8.3.4 Medullary sponge kidney

In medullary sponge kidney, intravenous urography shows cystic collections of contrast medium in the ectatic collecting ducts, which may resemble partial papillary necrosis of the central type (Fig. 8.13(a)). However, in AN there is rarely more than one cavity per papilla, whereas in medullary sponge

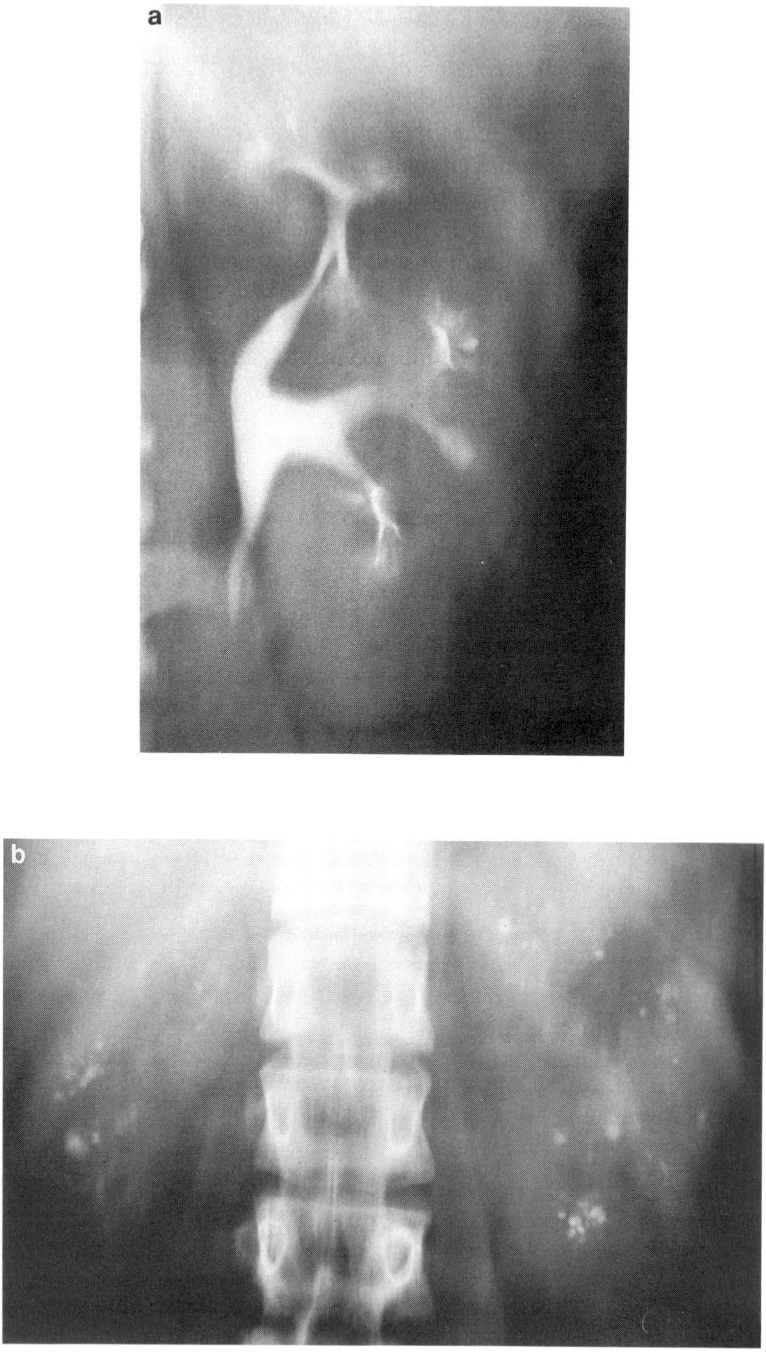

Fig. 8.13 Medullary sponge kidney: (a) intravenous urogram showing papillary blush and multiple cavities of different sizes; (b) plain film showing multiple calculi.

kidney multiple cavities of different sizes and shapes may be found in a single papilla; sometimes these contain calculi (Fig. 8.13(b)). Furthermore, a prominent papillary blush or characteristic radial linear striations may be seen.

8.3.5 Hydronephrotic atrophy

Longstanding urinary obstruction may cause loss of papillae and renal substance. The kidneys are shrunken but their outlines usually are relatively smooth. As these changes remain after the obstruction is relieved, previous bilateral obstruction may mimic AN with total papillary necrosis.

8.3.6 Tuberculosis

Early tuberculosis may resemble localized RPN, especially as sterile pyuria is characteristic of both diseases. However, in early tuberculosis, pyelographic density will be normal, and in advanced tuberculosis calcification may be irregular, involving structures beyond the papillae.

8.3.7 Metabolic nephrocalcinosis

In dialysis patients, cortical or medullary calcification may occur, whatever the underlying kidney disease, as a consequence of an elevated calcium–phosphorus product (Ibels *et al.* 1981). In most cases the kidneys are small. These metabolic changes may be superimposed upon calcified papillary necrosis *in situ* (Fig. 8.3).

In addition, nephrocalcinosis may be caused by diseases such as sarcoidosis, renal tubular acidosis, or primary hyperparathyroidism. In contrast to these conditions, calcification is a late event in AN, by which time the renal cortex usually is thin, and function poor.

9
Functional defects in analgesic nephropathy

Ranjit S. Nanra

The major renal pathological lesions in analgesic nephropathy (AN) are renal papillary necrosis (RPN), chronic interstitial nephritis (CIN) and the associated secondary glomerular lesions, transitional cell carcinoma, and atheromatous renal artery stenosis. The functional defects seen in AN are a reflection of these.

9.1 Urinary abnormalities

9.1.1 Microscopy

Visible or microscopic haematuria, which is seen in 40 per cent of patients with AN, is usually due to continuing abuse of aspirin-containing analgesics, recent acute RPN, a glomerular lesion, renal calculus, transitional cell carcinoma, pyelitis or cystitis, or malignant hypertension (Kincaid-Smith and Nanra 1988). Phase contrast microscopy of urine is helpful in differentiating dysmorphic red blood cells of glomerular origin from non-glomerular haematuria (Fairley and Birch 1982).

Sterile pyuria is common in AN and reflects covert urinary tract infection, active RPN or the presence of renal calculi. Other urinary abnormalities include renal tubular epithelial celluria, and a variety of casts including granular, broad, white blood cell, epithelial, and mixed casts (Kincaid-Smith and Nanra 1988). Urinary cytology is helpful in the detection of transitional cell carcinoma (Eriksson and Johansson 1976).

9.1.2 Proteinuria

Significant proteinuria, more than 0.3 g/day, may be seen in at least half of AN patients. The average protein loss is about 1 g/day; nephrotic syndrome is unusual. The proportion of patients with proteinuria increases with decline in glomerular filtration rate (GFR)—more than 90 per cent of patients with a creatinine clearance (C_{Cr}) less than 10 ml/min/1.73 m^2 have proteinuria. Unlike in glomerulonephritis, proteinuria tends to increase as GFR diminishes (Mehta *et al.* 1977).

Tubular proteinuria, indicated by elevation of urinary β_2-microglobulin concentrations, occurs in 56 per cent of AN patients; the proportion of patients with β_2-microglobulinuria, and its concentration in urine, increases as GFR declines. Urinary albumin concentrations follow a similar pattern to β_2-microglobulin, although its inverse relationship to GFR is less marked (Nanra, unpublished 1990). Data from Alt *et al.* (1979, 1983) and Nanra and Nanra (1988) suggest that in AN the proteinuria is mixed, glomerular and tubular, with large quantities of low and high molecular weight proteins, particularly β_2-microglobulin and albumin. However, it has been suggested that β_2-microglobulinuria may reflect not only proximal tubular damage but also the presence of transitional cell carcinoma (Russ *et al.* 1982).

In AN, persistent proteinuria usually indicates the presence of CIN with secondary glomerular lesions, but it may develop at an advanced stage of RPN; it is also a marker of adverse prognosis (Mehta *et al.* 1977; Kincaid-Smith and Nanra 1988).

9.1.3 Acute urinary response to analgesic ingestion

Acute urinary abnormalities occur with ingestion of aspirin and phenacetin (Prescott 1982*a*; Chapter 3); these include amino aciduria, changes in urinary acid mucopolysaccharides, transient haematuria and renal tubular epithelial celluria, decreased excretion of phenol red and increased urinary excretion of lactic dehydrogenase, β-glucuronidase, alkaline phosphatase, arylamidase and *N*-acetyl-β-glucosamidinase. The relevance of these acute tubular nephrotoxic changes to the chronic lesions of AN is not known.

9.2 Renal dysfunction

9.2.1 Glomerular filtration rate

Most patients with AN have reduced renal function; at initial presentation, 14 per cent have a C_{Cr} less than 5 ml/min/1.73 m^2 (Table 9.1) (Nanra 1989*a*). The mechanism of the reduced GFR is multifactorial. Possible hypotheses include: (1) blockage of renal tubules by atrophy and interstitial fibrosis; (2) destruction of postglomerular capillaries causing a fall in renal blood flow; (3) a modified Thurau hypothesis, in which impaired proximal sodium reabsorption leads to increased tubular flow rate, reduced local renin and angiotensin production, and a fall in GFR due to efferent arteriolar vasodilatation (REF); and (4) increased production of vasoconstrictor thomboxane A_2 by infiltrating mononuclear cells (Harris *et al.* 1989; Neilson 1989).

9.2.2 Tubular dysfunction

Patients with AN have disproportionately impaired tubular function including defects in urinary concentration, acidification, and sodium conservation (Bengtsson 1966; Steele *et al.* 1969; Cove-Smith and Knapp 1973; Krishnaswamy *et al.* 1976; Nanra *et al.* 1978*a*).

Table 9.1 *Renal functional abnormalities in analgesic nephropathy*

	1972–4	1984–6	
Number of patients	100	100	
Creatinine clearance			
< 5 (ml/min/1.73 m^2)	14	2	$p < 0.05$
5–19 (ml/min/1.73 m^2)	26	16	$p < 0.05$
20–89 (ml/min/1.73 m^2)	54	78	$p < 0.05$
> 90 (ml/min/1.73 m^2)	6	4	
Sterile pyuria	43	27	$p < 0.05$
Haematuria	41	20	$p < 0.05$
Proteinuria	58	45	
Hyperuricaemia or gout	23	23	
Renal osteodystrophy	34	31	
Hypertension			
benign	76	77	
malignant	8	0	$p < 0.05$

Table 9.2 summarizes the tubular functional defects in control subjects and patients with AN or glomerulonephritis (Krishnaswamy *et al.* 1976). AN is associated with a significant decrement in concentrating capacity (reduced maximum urinary osmolality and reabsorption of free water after pitressin), and excretion of titratable acid and ammonium (in the short oral acid load test). Ten per cent of AN patients had a partial renal tubular acidosis (minimum urinary pH values between 5.3 and 5.6). Complete distal renal tubular acidosis (urinary pH persistently greater than 5.7 and low ammonium excretion rates) was seen in AN only when C_{Cr} was less than 69 ml/min/1.73 m^2. Similar abnormalities in renal function had been reported by Steele *et al.* (1969) who also found reduced urinary citrate excretion in 9 of 15 patients, and noted a correlation between citrate excretion and the degree of systemic acidosis induced by ammonium chloride. Patients with AN and reduced GFR also had low fractional sodium excretion and urinary sodium/potassium ratios, indicating total body sodium depletion secondary to impaired sodium conservation. Cove-Smith and Knapp (1973) had found significantly defective sodium conservation in 7 of 10 patients with AN submitted to a diet of less than 20 mmol sodium/day for 3–5 days.

These tubular defects accord with the primary medullary lesion of RPN. The concentrating defect is a result of the disruption of the countercurrent mechanism and is the earliest clinical manifestation of AN (Nanra *et al.* 1978*a*; Nanra 1980). Impaired sodium conservation reflects damage to the deep juxtamedullary nephrons with their long loops of Henle, and to the

Table 9.2 *Renal tubular dysfunction in analgesic nephropathy and glomerulonephritis*

	Control	Analgesic nephropathy			Glomerulonephritis	
Number of patients	30	33	35	16	24	9
Creatinine clearance[1]	113 ± 21	98 ± 20	47 ± 11	22 ± 6	115 ± 28	54 ± 12
Phenol red excretion[2]	93 ± 27	82 ± 26	42 ± 16	28 ± 12	..	..
Maximum urinary osmolarity[3]	972 ± 133	655 ± 152[a]	558 ± 160[b]	410 ± 72	909 ± 110	695 ± 147
Tubular reabsorption of free water[4]	2.4 ± 0.9	1.6 ± 0.6[a]	0.9 ± 0.6[b]	0.5 ± 0.3	2.2 ± 0.7	1.4 ± 0.6
Minimum urinary pH						
5.3–5.6[5]	0	10%	28%	54%	4%	11%
> 5.7[5]	0	0	19%	8%	0	0
Urinary titratable acidity[6]	35.0 ± 8.7	26.1 ± 5.7[a]	18.3 ± 5.1	14.3 ± 5.1	31.6 ± 4.9	18.1 ± 8.3
Urinary ammonium[6]	53.1 ± 9.1	44.3 ± 11.2[a]	25.2 ± 8.4	18.7 ± 10.7	56.4 ± 19.5	24.3 ± 10.7

Values are means ± standard deviations. [1] ml/min/1.73 m^2; [2] % dose excreted at 15 min (per 100 ml creatinine clearance); [3] mosm/kg water; [4] ml/min; [5] per cent of all patients in category; [6] mmol/min/1.73 m^2; [a] significantly less than controls or group of glomerulonephritis with normal creatinine clearance, $p < 0.01$; [b] significantly less than group of glomerulonephritis with reduced creatinine clearance, $p < 0.05$.

collecting tubules. The renal tubular acidosis results from interference with ammoniagenesis and urinary acidification in the distal nephron.

9.3 Consequences of renal impairment

9.3.1 Hyperuricaemia

Secondary gout occurs in 22 per cent of patients with AN when the C_{Cr} falls below 60 ml/min/1.73 m^2. However, uric acid handling by the kidney appears to be similar in AN, glomerulonephritis, and control subjects (Nanra *et al.* 1978*b*).

9.3.2 Hypertension

Raised blood pressure, which increases in severity with declining renal function, is present in 15–70 per cent of patients with AN; up to 15 per cent have resistant hypertension, and 7 per cent develop malignant hypertension (Kincaid-Smith and Nanra 1988). It has been suggested that a proportion of patients who are diagnosed as having essential hypertension may have subclinical AN (Stewart and Gallery 1976).

As in other forms of hypertension secondary to renal parenchymal disease, the hypertension is related to fall in GFR, retention of sodium, elevation of angiotensin II, and a distorted relationship between intravascular volume and pressor agents (de Wardener and MacGregor 1988). In AN, angiotensin II levels are potentially higher, because of impaired sodium conservation and loss of medullary vasodilator substances due to RPN (Muirhead 1980). Thus some patients with acute RPN and intravascular volume depletion may have severe, or even malignant, hypertension (Nanra *et al.* 1978*a*).

Hypertension may be more common and severe in AN than in patients with other renal diseases. In analgesic abusers, 83 per cent of women, and 64 per cent of men, had hypertension, compared to 36 per cent and 33 per cent respectively in glomerulonephritis; all patients had a serum creatinine of less than 97 μmol/l (Küster and Ritz 1989). Our own unpublished data support these observations; in patients matched for age and renal function, 47 per cent of AN patients had a blood pressure greater than 150/90 mmHg, and 6 per cent had malignant hypertension, compared with 20 per cent and 1 per cent respectively of glomerulonephritics.

9.3.2.1 Renal artery stenosis

Atheromatous renal artery stenosis is a common cause of resistant hypertension in AN. Kincaid-Smith (1979) found this lesion in 38 per cent of 37 women with AN, and 14 per cent of 279 women without AN. In 148 consecutive patients with resistant hypertension, atheromatous renal artery stenosis was present in 64 per cent of 55 AN patients, and 40 per cent of the

93 who did not have AN; renal artery thrombosis occurred in 16 per cent and 7 per cent, respectively, in the two groups (Nanra, unpublished 1990).

9.3.3 Renal osteodystrophy

Metabolic bone disease is a common complication of chronic renal failure in AN (Ingham *et al.* 1974). More recently, it has been suggested that uraemic bone disease is worse in analgesic abusers with end stage renal failure than a comparable group of non-abusers; the patients with AN had higher osteoid volume, reduced calcification fronts, lower percentage of mineralization, and higher serum alkaline phosphatase and parathyroid hormone (Fassett *et al.* 1982). The mechanism for prominent renal osteodystrophy is unclear; it does not appear to relate to vitamin D metabolism, duration of renal failure, hypocalcaemia, systemic acidosis, or aluminium deposition.

9.4 Effect of cessation of analgesic abuse

Cessation of analgesic intake may be associated with stabilization or improvement in renal function (Prescott 1982*a*; Kincaid-Smith and Nanra 1988). Steele *et al.* (1971) had documented a significant improvement in maximum urinary concentration and ammonium excretion after an acid load in 16 patients with AN who had stopped analgesic abuse.

In Australia, the widespread availability of analgesic mixtures was restricted in 1979. The functional changes which were observed in patients during 1972–4, and those seen during 1984–6, are summarized in Table 9.1 (Nanra 1989*a*). The differences can be related to the cessation of analgesic abuse.

10

Clinical presentations of analgesic-induced nephropathy

Wolfgang Pommer

The term analgesic nephropathy (AN) covers a spectrum of disorders which are presumed to be associated with long- or short-term analgesic drug intake. Analgesic drugs in this sense include either the simple antipyretic–analgesics, such as salicylates, anilides, and pyrazolones, taken as single substances or compounds, or the group of non-steriodal anti-inflammatory drugs (NSAIDs), which have been more recently introduced to pain therapy. Within the spectrum of analgesic-associated kidney disease, classical AN is the best defined and most widespread (Gault and Wilson 1978; Murray and Goldberg 1978; Nanra *et al.* 1978*a*; Kincaid-Smith 1979; Fourie *et al.* 1982; McCredie *et al.* 1982*a*; Prescott 1982*a*; Maher 1984; Buckalew and Schey 1986*b*; Pommer *et al.* 1986; Buccianti *et al.* 1987; Elseviers and De Broe 1988; Mihatsch *et al.* 1980*a*). In contrast, renal diseases associated with NSAIDs are less well defined and regular intake of these drugs seems to be a minor problem as yet (Clive and Stoff 1984). The manifestations of analgesic-associated kidney diseases might be related to various factors such as individual susceptibility, type, duration and amount of coexisting drug usage, exposure to occupational and environmental hazards, as well as behavioural habits and life-styles.

The recognition of AN is subject to bias and, in many places the disease is under-reported, resulting in patients with regular analgesic intake and slow progression of renal insufficiency being designated as having chronic renal disease of unknown origin (Buccianti *et al.* 1987).

10.1 Approach to the evaluation of patients

10.1.1 Drug history

The exploration of drug intake is a crucial step in discovering the underlying cause of analgesic-induced renal disease. Because of the lack of standardized inventories for this purpose, there has been confusion about the role of denial, which is frequently attributed to patients with AN. It has been claimed that subjects with this disease deny previous regular intake in up to 80 per cent of cases (Purnell and Burry 1967; Finnigan *et al.* 1974;

Landmann-Suter and Dubach 1975; Murray 1978; Schwarz *et al.* 1984). None of these clinical studies has detailed the settings in which the interviews were conducted. Epidemiological studies based on structured inventories report a higher response to the exploration of analgesic history (Christie 1978; Murray *et al.* 1983; McCredie *et al.* 1988; Elseviers and De Broe 1988; Pommer *et al.* 1989; Sandler *et al.* 1989).

Nevertheless there is no doubt that regular analgesic intake, like other socially disapproved habits, tends to be under-reported by the consumers. In order to minimize this tendency, the interview should be performed empathetically and non-judgementally; additional visual auxiliaries or memory cards should be used. According to experience obtained in the West Berlin case-control study on analgesic intake and the risk of end stage renal failure (Pommer *et al.* 1989) the interview should focus on the life-long intake of all analgesics. The interview may start by evaluating knowledge of the most popular analgesic brands in the community, followed by questions about conditions associated with analgesic intake and the subject's own pattern of those complaints which might serve to justify analgesic intake. In this way type, amount, and duration of analgesic ingestion and the individually preferred brands can be explored with cross checking. The interview can be completed be recording coincidental habits, such as coffee and alcohol consumption, tobacco smoking, and the regular intake of diuretics and laxatives, as well as the family history of chronic drug intake. Drug–drug and drug–disease interactions should be also considered (Brater 1986). In our experience, interviews performed by staff not directly involved in the medical treatment result in better responses than those done by physicians or staff immediately involved in treatment.

The role of next-of-kin interviews, as used by some in this field (Sandler *et al.* 1989), has been less verified than in the evaluation of other types of drug ingestion or abuse (McLaughlin *et al.* 1991).

10.1.1.1 Analgesic intake in the family

The family background of patients with renal diseases associated with regular analgesic intake has been investigated rarely. Occasional reports focusing on this matter reveal a familial setting of broken homes and addiction to alcohol, barbiturates, and narcotic drugs (Fellner and Tuttle 1969; Murray 1973*a*; Duggan 1974; Cove-Smith and Knapp 1978; Basch 1980).

Traditional family analgesic intake plays an important role in the inception of regular analgesic use (Grimlund 1963; Gsell 1974; Murray and Goldberg 1975; Carro-Ciampi 1978; Murray 1978). In the West Berlin study (Pommer *et al.* 1989) the relatives of the study sample were found to have taken analgesic drugs to various extents (Fig. 10.1). Females outnumbered males in all the generations which have been investigated. The percentage of analgesic-induced renal diseases in the families of patients treated with end stage

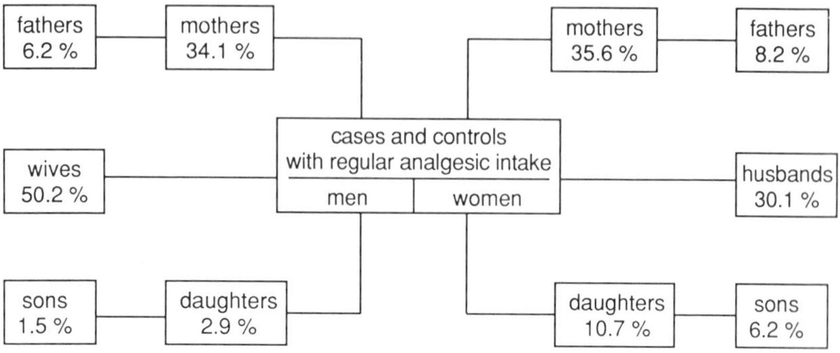

Fig. 10.1 History of regular analgesic consumption by close relatives of male and female renal patients known to have taken analgesics regularly. Unpublished data from the West Berlin case–control study on analgesic intake and the risk of end stage renal failure.

renal failure due to any cause yield about 1 per cent in this study area. The more frequent prevalence of HLA-B12 in patients with analgesic nephropathy may suggest a genetic predisposition (Kincaid-Smith and Nanra 1988).

10.1.1.2 Reasons for taking analgesics regularly

In most studies dealing with the pattern of complaints which serve to justify long-term analgesic intake, headache is the principal symptom given by both sexes (Gault *et al.* 1968*a*; Murray 1973*a*; Christie 1978; Cove-Smith and Knapp 1978; Sandler *et al.* 1989). Despite that and other medical symptoms, such as migraine, arthritis, and backache, statements of regular analgesic consumers indicate that analgesics are taken mostly for non-medical reasons (Table 10.1). It must be emphasized that the reasons and indications presented in the evaluation of a drug history depend on the setting. Responses obtained in a medical setting are usually covered by medical phrases whilst a more private setting allows a truer description of the motivation for analgesic intake.

10.1.2 Clinical examination

The clinical features have been described extensively for the group of patients with classical AN. In these the picture is varied and corresponds to that of a multi-system disease. The main features have been summarized under the term 'analgesic syndrome' (Duggan 1974; Carro-Ciampi 1978; Nanra 1983; Chapter 6) of which the extrarenal manifestations include anaemia, chronic gastrointestinal complaints, liver damage especially in conjunction with alcohol consumption (Kaysen *et al.* 1985), accelerated atherosclerosis (Kaladelfos and Edwards 1976; Kincaid-Smith 1979; Nanra 1980), and metabolic bone disease (Fellner and Tuttle 1969; Jaeger *et al.*

Table 10.1 *Frequently reported reasons for analgesic ingestion*

Specific indications	Non-specific reasons
Headache	Dimness
Backache	Tension
Osteoarthritis	To feel well
Sinus trouble	To prevent headache
Depression	Help to sleep
Hangover	To get through the day
Toothache	Cannot function without it
Menstrual pain	Sensitive to changes in the weather

1982; Fasset *et al.* 1982). A history of these conditions in patients with renal disease may indicate underlying analgesic use. Gastrointestinal lesions and other distinctive extrarenal disorders such as pulmonary and skin alterations due to the NSAIDs have been less often described (Carson *et al.* 1990; Velo and Milanino 1990).

10.1.3 Specific diagnosis of analgesic nephropathy

Although, a large number of signs are associated with AN, the sensitivity and specifity of the different diagnostic features are established for only three. Renal papillary necrosis (RPN) and irregular shrinking of both kidneys as detected by imaging techniques indicate AN with a high sensitivity and specificity (Weber *et al.* 1985; Puvaneswary and Segasothy 1988; Elseviers *et al.* 1992). The differential diagnosis of RPN includes obstructive uropathy and sickle cell haemoglobinpathy, but it seems to be a rare finding in chronic alcoholism, diabetes mellitus and intake of NSAIDs (Weber *et al.* 1985; Kincaid-Smith 1986*b*). Secondly, thickening of the capillary basement membrane (capillarosclerosis) in the mucous membranes of the urinary tract has been demonstrated with high specifity in nephrectomies of patients with long-term intake of phenacetin (Gloor 1978*a*; Mihatsch *et al.* 1978). Finally, repeated testing of blood or urine samples for analgesic substances, such as salicylates and paracetamol, is helpful when clinical findings are inconclusive.

10.2 Major clinical presentations

10.2.1 Renal insufficiency

Chronic renal failure is the common fatal complication in AN. The functional defects and the clinical course of renal deterioration depend on the types of substances ingested.

Table 10.2 *Synopsis of clinical findings in analgesic-associated kidney diseases*

Clinical finding	Analgesic mixtures[1]	Single analgesics[2]	Non-steroidal anti-inflammatory drugs
Renal insufficiency			
acute	–	occ	++
chronic	++	?	+
Urinalysis			
haematuria	++	occ	occ
leucocyturia	+/++	occ	occ
proteinuria	nil-moderate	occ	nil-heavy
Urinary infections	++	–	–/+
Obstructive uropathy	++	occ	–
Hypertension	++	–	+
Renal morphology			
papillary necrosis	++	occ	++
interstitial nephritis	++	occ	+/++
glomerular changes	secondary to interstitial disease	–	+/++
vasculitis	–	occ	occ
Neoplasia			
urothelial	++	–/+	–
renal	occ	–/+	–

[1] Containing salicylates, phenacetin or paracetamol, and/or pyrazolons; [2] salicylates or paracetamol. Symbols: – = not reported; –/+ = controversial; occ = occasionally reported; + = common; ++ = very common.

The long-term intake of analgesic mixtures containing salicylates, anilides such as paracetamol and phenacetin, and/or pyrazolons in combination with caffeine or codeine is the basis for the development of renal insufficiency in classical AN. Because AN comprises structural damage of the renal medulla with capillarosclerosis, papillary necrosis, interstitial nephritis and subsequent shrinking of the renal cortex (Burry *et al.* 1966; Gloor 1978*a*; Mihatsch *et al.* 1978), the earliest clinical findings are the loss of concentration capacity and decreased glomerular filtration rate as described in clinical (Larsen and Møller 1959; Bengtsson 1966 Krishnaswamy *et al.* 1976; Nanra *et al.* 1978*a*) and epidemiological studies (Dubach *et al.* 1983). About 25 per cent of patients with advanced renal impairment have an acidification defect; in 10 per cent there is frank tubular acidosis (Kincaid-Smith and Nanra 1988; Chapter 9).

The dose-related effect of analgesic intake in the development of renal deterioration, confirmed in autopsy, clinical, and retrospective epidemiological studies (Larsen and Møller 1959; Burry *et al.* 1966; Dubach *et al.* 1983; Pommer *et al.* 1989) suggests that intake of more than 1 kg analgesic mixtures over a period of 5 years results in significantly increased risks of severe renal insufficiency. But the fraction of patients with regular analgesic intake progressing to end stage renal disease is not known.

Cessation of regular analgesic intake has been said to improve or stabilize renal function in the absence of coincidental risk factors such as hypertension, upper urinary tract infections, or dietary habits (Bell *et al.* 1969; Nitzsche and Bock 1970; Gsell 1974; Porpáczy 1979; Schreiner *et al.* 1981).

10.2.2 Abnormal urinary findings

The findings in the urine vary depending on the type and severity of renal pathology, incidental urinary infections, and the presence of calculi or renal or uroepithelial tumours. They include macroscopic or microscopic haematuria, pyuria which frequently is sterile, and proteinuria which may be absent or of any grade but virtually never in the nephrotic range (Chapter 9).

10.2.2.1 Urinary infection

Recurrent overt or asymptomatic urinary tract infections are reported in 10–80 per cent of patients with classical AN (Gault *et al.* 1968*a*; Gsell 1974; Cove-Smith and Knapp 1978; Kincaid-Smith and Nanra 1988). It has been suggested that the incidence of urinary infections depends on the stage, being more frequent in advanced disease (Gsell 1974). Others have failed to establish any correlation between the presence of bacteriuria and the progression of disease (Cove-Smith and Knapp 1978) and, in a recently published study, the frequency of a history of urinary tract infections in patients with AN did not differ significantly from comparable controls (Thiel *et al.* 1989). In patients with renal diseases related to NSAIDs, urinary tract infection seems to be rare (Clive and Stoff 1984; Garella and Matarese 1984).

10.2.3 Hypertension

Hypertension occurs in 15–70 per cent of patients with classical AN; it may increase in severity with declining renal function (Kincaid-Smith and Nanra 1988). In the end stage renal population, hypertension is more frequent with AN than in other diagnoses (Theil *et al.* 1989), but differences in the frequency of hypertension become less obvious when the degree of kidney impairment is considered (Mihatsch *et al.* 1982*b*). Results from one study suggest that hypertension does not increase mortality from all causes in patients with AN (Cove-Smith and Knapp 1978).

Malignant hypertension has been observed in about 7 per cent of patients with underlying classical AN (Prescott 1982*a*; Kincaid-Smith and Nanra

1988), but it may also be found in analgesic-induced vasculitis. In AN it may occur suddenly and disappear spontaneously (Dawborn *et al.* 1966; Kincaid-Smith 1986*b*). Malignant hypertension may precipitate patients into terminal renal failure (Kincaid-Smith and Nanra 1988). Severe hypertension has been seen with acute RPN.

The role of hypertension in patients with NSAID intake is a subject of controversy (Clive and Stoff 1984). NSAIDs exert a number of influences on the regulation of systemic blood pressure, including effects on natriuresis, the renin–aldosterone axis, arterial smooth muscle tone, and interference with pharmacological actions of antihypertensive agents (Garella and Matarese 1984).

10.2.4 Papillary necrosis and calculus formation

RPN is the most frequent lesion in analgesic-associated kidney disease and can be caused by compound analgesics (Spühler and Zollinger 1953; Bengtsson 1962; Arger *et al.* 1976; Burry 1978; Gloor 1978*a*; Kincaid-Smith and Nanra 1988), perhaps single antipyretic–analgesics (Krikler 1967; Prescott 1982*a*; Segasothy *et al.* 1984, 1988) and NSAIDs (Munn *et al.* 1982; Mitchell *et al.* 1982; Clive and Stoff 1984; Garella and Matarese 1984; Caruana and Semble 1984; Carmichael and Shankel 1985). RPN related to analgesic drugs cannot be differentiated with certainty by contrast urography from that due to other causes (Kincaid-Smith and Nanra 1988; Chapter 8). Drugs other than analgesics have been implicated occasionally (Lai *et al.* 1987) and RPN has been documented in children treated with NSAIDs for chronic arthritis (Allen *et al.* 1986).

The appearance of calculi, and changes in the renal cortex, as seen in AN, depends on the fate of the necrotic renal papillae (Goldberger and Talner 1975; Burry 1978; Gloor 1978; Mihatsch 1989). If there is rapid demarcation, which is rare, necrotic papillae can remain in the pelvis or be passed causing renal colic and gross haematuria. Under these conditions, cortical changes may be absent. If the papillae remain *in situ* calcification, or even ossification, may develop. Fragments of necrotic papillae which are retained provide a nidus for precipitation which may lead to obstruction, stasis, and infection which may be recurrent or followed by pyonephrosis (Kincaid-Smith and Nanra 1988; Mihatsch 1989). Either protracted shedding or retention *in situ* of necrotic papillae is followed by progressive cortical atrophy which causes the pattern of shrinking and irregularity of the renal surface detectable by imaging techniques.

10.2.5 Urinary obstruction

Urinary obstruction due to RPN, uroepithelial tumour, calculus, or rarely inflammatory stricture or retroperitoneal fibrosis, is a serious complication seen mostly in patients with long-term intake of compound analgesics

(Bengtsson 1962; Lewis *et al.* 1975; Arger *et al.* 1976; Mihatsch *et al.* 1980*a*; Nanra 1980; Mihatsch and Knüsli 1982; Kincaid-Smith and Nanra 1988). Clinically, recurrent colic with the passage of papillary fragments or calculi is common in this group. However, obstructive uropathy may develop silently, resulting in unexplained decrease of renal function. Coincidental urinary tract infections may lead to pyonephrosis and septicaemia. If associated with painless haematuria, obstruction is suggestive of carcinoma of the renal pelvis or ureter.

10.3 The value of renal biopsy

Percutanous renal biopsy is a basic tool in the assessment of analgesic and NSAID-associated nephrotoxicity (Prescott 1982*b*; Mustonen *et al.* 1984; Reeves *et al.* 1984; Kleinknecht *et al.* 1986; Cotran *et al.* 1986). The type of renal lesion due to analgesic exposure is unpredictable and the various analgesic substances may induce different clinical and histological patterns (Table 10.3).

Acute renal failure after exposure to NSAIDs, salicylates, pyrazolons, and anilide substances may be due to acute interstitial nephritis, or tubular or cortical necrosis (Rupp *et al.* 1983; Clive and Stoff 1984; Mignon *et al.* 1984; Reeves *et al.* 1985; Kleinknecht *et al.* 1986; Björck *et al.* 1988; Chapters 14 and 15). In allergic interstitial nephritis, the lymphocyte transformation test can identify the causative drug (Brattig *et al.* 1988). Nephrotic and, less frequently, nephritic syndromes with interstitial and glomerular changes can be caused by NSAIDs and pyrazolones (Esparza *et al.* 1981; Clive and Stoff 1984; Abt and Gordon 1985; Artinano *et al.* 1986). Systemic vasculitis with renal involvement has been observed after exposure to pyrazolones (Leung *et al.* 1984) and NSAIDs (Garella and Matarese 1984; Hurault de Ligny *et al.* 1984; Carmichael and Shankel 1985). Chronic renal insufficiency with interstitial fibrosis and secondary glomerulopathy are typical of classical AN but may be seen after recurrent exposure to NSAIDs (Abraham and Keane 1984; Clive and Stoff 1984; Cotran *et al.* 1986). Renal biopsy is not indicated in classical AN if clinical evaluation and morphological assessment by imaging techniques is diagnostic.

10.4 Renal transplant failure

The effect of analgesic and NSAID intake in patients with kidney grafts has been rarely investigated. Graft function may be altered by three different mechanisms: long-term intake of analgesic compounds may result in AN of the renal graft; intake of NSAIDs and non-narcotic analgesics may harm transplant function by functional changes involving renal blood flow and glomerular regulatory mechanisms; or the nephrotoxicity of immunosuppressive agents may be enhanced.

Table 10.3 *Spectrum of renal lesions related to analgesic and non-steroidal anti-inflammatory drugs*

Clinical syndrome	Drugs responsible	Pathology
Acute renal failure	Salicylates	TN; AIN; PN
	Anilides[1]	TN; PN
	Pyrazolones	AIN; PN
	NSAIDs	TN; AIN; PN
Nephritic syndrome	Salicylates	AIN
	Pyrazolones	AIN; GN
	NSAIDs	AIN; GN
Nephrotic syndrome	Pyrazolones	GP; GN
	NSAIDs	GP; GN; CIN; AIN
Vasculitis (with renal impairment)	Pyrazolones	MV
	NSAIDs	MV
Chronic renal failure	Anilides[2]	CIN; PN; GS
	NSAIDs	CIN; PN; GS
Renal graft failure	Anilides[2]	CIN; PN
	NSAIDs	TN; CIN; AIN
Tumours	Anilides[2]	TCC; RAC

[1] In combination or single drugs; [2] in combination drugs only. Abbreviations: AIN = acute interstitial nephritis; CIN = chronic interstitial nephritis; GN = glomerulonephritis; GP = glomerulopathy; GS = glomerulosclerosis; MV = microscopic vasculitis; PN = papillary necrosis; RAC = renal adenocarcinoma; TCC = transitional cell carcinoma; TN = tubular necrosis.

Continuing analgesic intake has been proven by detection of salicylates and acetaminophen in repeated urine samples from about 30 per cent of the West Berlin transplant population (Pommer *et al.* unpublished). More than 40 per cent of patients who formerly suffered from AN nephropathy have been found to continue analgesic intake (Furman *et al.* 1976), but no evidence was given in these patients for resulting renal damage. One case of irreversible renal transplant failure after ketoprofen intake has been reported (Windeck and Bock 1983), and in another, enhancement of cyclosporin nephrotoxicity due to diclofenac was observed (Deray *et al.* 1987). Recurrent or *de novo* AN in renal grafts seems to be rare because of the long induction time of the disease (Brunner and Thiel 1986).

10.5 Analgesic intake in patients with intrinsic renal disease

In addition to the potential effect of analgesic substances in causing a specific drug-related renal failure, the harmful role of analgesic exposure in patients

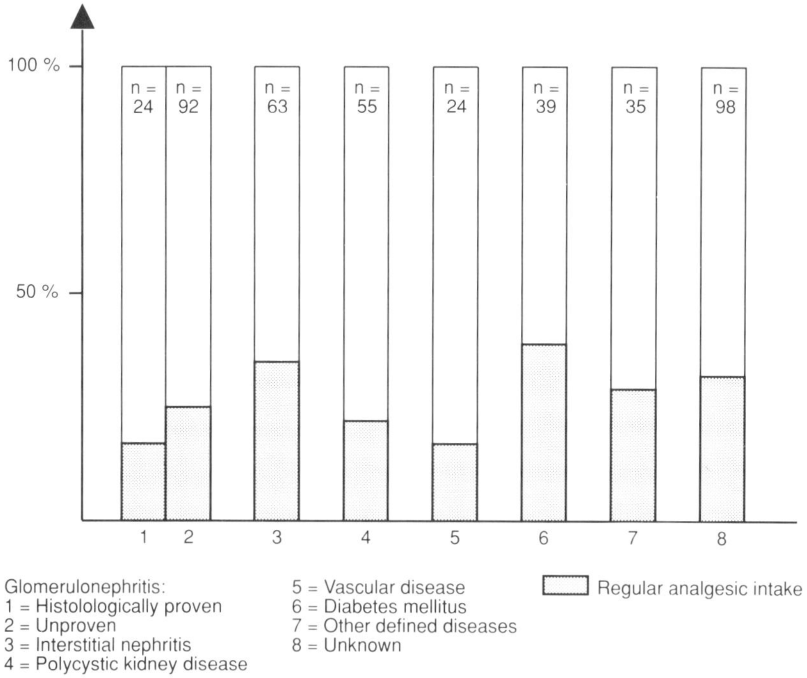

Fig. 10.2 History of regular analgesic consumption in patients with end stage renal failure due to different causes. From Pommer *et al.* (1989).

with other renal diseases, which may progress with analgesic intake, should be considered. In patients with glomerular diseases, renal function deteriorated promptly after NSAID intake and improved after cessation of exposure (Abt and Gordon 1985; Ciabattoni *et al.* 1984*a*, Brater 1986; Colin-Jones and Maskell 1986; Whelton *et al.* 1990), and it has been suggested that progression of minimal change glomerulopathy to focal glomerulosclerosis can occur with fenoprofen (Artinano *et al.* 1986).

Regular intake of analgesic compounds was found to various degrees in patients with defined renal diseases in the West Berlin study (Pommer *et al.* 1989) (Fig. 10.2). In a recently published case-control study, the intake of phenacetin-containing mixtures was said to be associated with increased risks of renal impairment in patients with diabetic nephropathy and glomerulonephritis (Sandler *et al.* 1989).

10.6 Summary

Analgesic-associated kidney diseases remain responsible for significant proportions of acute and chronic renal failure. Up to now, compound analgesic preparations are the most widespread cause of the analgesic syndrome which covers a spectrum of disorders including renal failure due to AN, and uroepethelial and renal tumours, the most serious complications caused by regular intake of analgesics.

On the other hand, syndromes due to single analgesics or NSAIDs are more varied and less defined, although probably just as common as classical AN. While the drug history and the clinical response to withdrawal of the drug may clarify the diagnosis, many cases remain uncertain or undetected. More widespread use of renal biopsy in cases of renal failure of uncertain aetiology, and perhaps specific tests for drug sensitivity, will increase the recognition of atypical analgesic-associated renal disease.

11

Treatment of renal failure due to analgesics

Anke Schwarz

As renal parenchymal damage caused by analgesics is itself not reversible, there can be no specific therapy for established analgesic nephropathy. The first reported treatment was a surgical one: decapsulation and denervation of the affected kidney (Brunner and Spühler 1951). This treatment was directed against the early stage of the disease with swelling, was mainly used in Switzerland in the pioneer period, and was not successful (Spühler and Zollinger 1950; Zollinger and Spühler 1950; Spühler and Zollinger 1953). Nowadays, as treatment is directed against progression of renal damage, and the disorders which result, early diagnosis is of first importance.

11.1 Prevention of further abuse

Since the discovery of the correlation between analgesic intake and nephropathy (Spühler 1953; Zollinger 1955), an obvious step has been to stop further analgesic ingestion. For this purpose, the physician in charge must be aware of the abuse which is not always evident and may be denied even on direct questioning (Fig. 11.1).

Analgesic consumption has been understated by 37–60 per cent in epidemiological studies (Horisberger *et al.* 1958; Purnell and Burry 1967; Murray 1978), and recent analgesic intake is denied by 25–80 per cent of consumers, as proved by measuring analgesic metabolites in the urine (Finnigan *et al.* 1974; Landmann-Suter and Dubach 1975; Furman *et al.* 1976; Schwarz *et al.* 1984). Denial of analgesic intake is a major problem in treating nephropathy: the patient wants relief of the symptoms of the disease but not of its cause. Not only should the abuse itself be addressed, but also pain and other circumstances which may have pre-determined or perpetuated the abuse. The patient may require alternative pain relief, social help, peer support, or psychological or psychiatric care; withdrawal of analgesics in a psychiatric clinic may be necessary (Diener 1988*a*,*b*). However, no causal help of this kind is possible in cases of denial.

As many as 24–54 per cent of analgesic abusers are addicted (Gsell *et al.* 1961; Maruta *et al.* 1979). In our experience, 21 per cent of analgesic patients

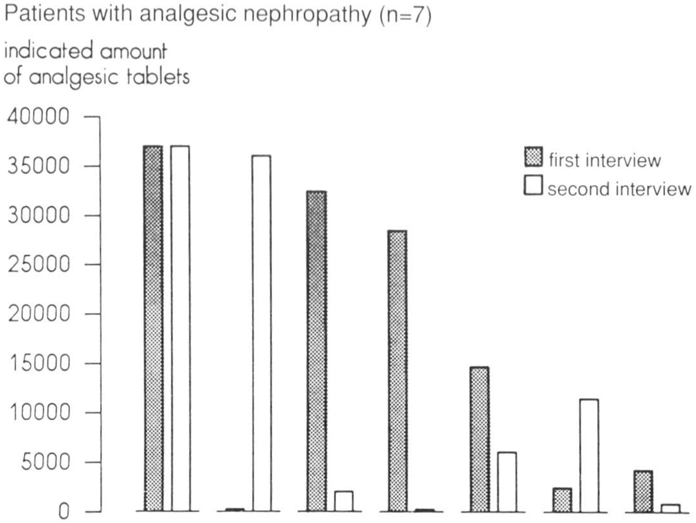

Fig. 11.1 Cumulative analgesic intake in 7 patients as recorded in 2 questionnaires completed with an interval of 6 months. From Drukker *et al.* (1986), with permission from Wichtig Editore.

with renal insufficiency and 25 per cent of those on haemodialysis continued their abuse, as proved by measuring analgesic metabolites in urine or blood (Schwarz *et al.* 1988*a*, 1989). Secret abuse must be kept in mind, as must the frequent concomitant abuse of laxatives, tranquillizers, or hypnotics (Fellner and Tuttle 1969; Murray 1978; Nanra *et al.* 1978*a*; Schreiner *et al.* 1981; Dubach *et al.* 1983; Keller and Schwarz 1983).

Haemodialysis patients with analgesic nephropathy often legitimize their abuse by obtaining prescriptions for at least some of their medicaments (Keller and Schwarz 1983). In a retrospective study in our haemodialysis centre, analgesic patients obtained a significantly higher number of prescriptions for analgesics (63 per cent vs 40 per cent, $p = 0.04$), hypnotics (42 per cent vs 20 per cent, $p = 0.03$), laxatives (42 per cent vs 18 per cent, $p = 0.01$), and all drugs combined (18.2 ± 10.6 vs 14.3 ± 10.1, $p = 0.03$) than age-matched patients with other renal diseases (Schwarz *et al.* 1985*a*). There is no simple solution to this dilemma, but prescribing analgesics and tranquillizers should be limited to acute situations.

However, one should keep in mind that, knowing that they have kidney disease caused by analgesic abuse, some 20–30 per cent of patients manage simply to give up taking analgesics. Subsequently they often become free of headaches, which may have been caused by analgesic metabolites or by caffeine- or drug-withdrawal (Dreisbach and Pfeiffer 1943; Diener 1988*a*,*b*).

11.2 Progression of analgesic nephropathy

11.2.1 Discontinuation of analgesic intake

That progression of renal insufficiency can be prevented by giving up analgesic consumption has been suggested by studies based on the information about abuse given by patients (Bell *et al.* 1969; Nitzsche and Bock 1970; Murray *et al.* 1971*a*; Murray 1972; Steele and Edwards 1971; Porpáczy and Schmidt 1973; Gault 1975) and confirmed in a study using the presence of acetaminophen in urine (NAPAP, Welch and Conney 1965) as the indicator of continuing consumption. Patients with analgesic nephropathy and continued abuse were found to have a more rapid decline of creatinine clearance than all other renal patients and kidney function improved in 9 of 44 analgesic patients who stopped the abuse, but in none of the 13 patients who continued it (Fig. 11.2).

However, renal failure may progress in analgesic nephropathy even without further intake, and in the absence of uncontrolled hypertension or urinary tract infection or obstruction (Schwarz *et al.* 1989). For the most part, the causes will be the same as those which result in progression of other forms of renal failure, but there are likely to be differences due to the characteristic nature of analgesic nephropathy.

11.2.2 Glomerulosclerosis

It is not clear whether glomerulosclerosis is caused by hyperfiltration of the remnant nephrons alone (Brenner *et al.* 1982), or if other mechanisms play a role, for example premature arterial ageing which is characteristic of analgesic nephropathy (Krishnaswamy *et al.* 1974; Kaladelfos and Edwards 1976; Nanra *et al.* 1978*a*, 1980; Mihatsch 1982*b*, 1983*b*; Schwarz *et al.* 1985*a*; Dubach *et al.* 1991). Intrarenal vascular disease and age independently correlate with the occurence of glomerulosclerosis (Kasiske 1987). In animal studies, hyperlipidaemia alone has been found to cause progression of glomerulosclerosis (Schmitz *et al.* 1989; Harris *et al.* 1990). Although there are no objective data confirming the hypothesis, it is conceivable that atheroma or hypercholesterolaemia are risk factors for the development, or progression, of glomerulosclerosis in analgesic nephropathy.

No studies have been done in analgesic nephropathy to test whether a low protein diet or angiotensin-converting enzyme inhibitors have a favourable influence on the progression of renal failure, as has been presumed for other kidney diseases. This may be difficult to prove since patients with analgesic nephropathy may retain an impaired, but unchanged, kidney function for many years.

11.2.3 Renal artery stenosis

Atherosclerotic renal artery stenosis may lead to worsening of renal function directly, or through hypertension. Complete occlusion of a stenotic renal

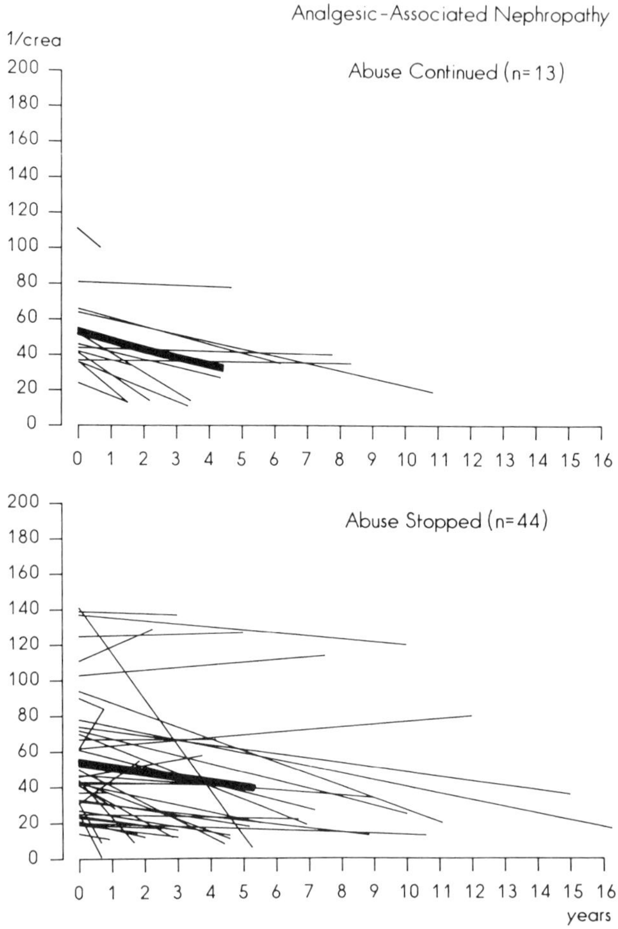

Fig. 11.2 Progression of renal insufficiency in 57 patients with analgesic nephropathy. Clearance loss 6.9 ± 5.5 ml/min/yr in 13 patients who continued analgesic intake (urinary NAPAP positive), and 4.1 ± 11.0 ml/min/yr in 44 patients who discontinued analgesic intake (urinary NAPAP negative). From Schwarz *et al.* (1989), with permission of Karger.

artery leads to a sudden decline of renal function; successful revascularization has been reported up to 47 days after occlusion (Ramsay *et al.* 1983; O'Donohoe *et al.* 1990).

11.2.4 Acute renal failure

Patients with analgesic nephropathy are prone to develop superimposed acute renal failure which may not be reversible. This acute event may overshadow the analgesic background and lead to incorrect diagnosis. Of 48 haemodialysis patients with analgesic nephropathy, 4 had started dialysis because of rapid deterioration of renal function associated with a separate acute disease. Some such patients recover their renal function soon, some after a period of dialysis, and some never.

11.3 Management of complications

11.3.1 Urinary tract infections

Urinary infection is so frequent that it has been mistaken for the underlying disease—chronic pyelonephritis (Reubi 1954; Schweingruber 1955; Cottier *et al.* 1958; Jasinski and Wuhrmann 1958) which may also be suggested by the pyelographic appearances (Lindvall 1978). In our experience, 40 per cent of analgesic patients with end stage renal disease had relapsing or complicated urinary infections. It is recognized that the damaged papillary region may be a nidus for bacterial infection, possibly leading to septicaemia especially in cases of obstruction. For this life-threatening situation, antibiotics may be used in high dosage and, in the case of aminoglycosides, may cause ototoxicity unless care is taken with blood level measurements and adjustment of dosage according to renal function. Treatment continuously with a prophylactic evening dose of antibiotics as determined by *in vitro* sensitivity tests, may be tried. With persistent ureteric obstruction, causing hydro- or pyo-nephrosis, percutaneous nephrostomy or surgery may be required for relief. This condition may necessitate transient dialysis treatment.

11.3.2 Salt-losing nephropathy

A salt-losing tubular syndrome with tubular acidosis may occur early in analgesic nephropathy. In some cases hypokalaemia, often worsened by the use of laxatives, is a permanent and serious concomitant of renal insufficiency requiring massive oral supplements of potassium. Potassium-wasting diuretics should be avoided. Later, in the stage of advanced renal failure or haemodialysis, such potassium loss may become an advantage, allowing a freer diet and thereby improving the quality of life. The loss of sodium chloride is less frequent and less important, except in cases of infection or diarrhoea, when acute dialysis may be necessary due to pre-renal uraemia, electrolyte derangement or acidosis.

11.3.3 Renal osteodystrophy

Patients with analgesic nephropathy often exhibit symptoms and signs of renal osteodystrophy (bone pain and proximal myopathy) relatively early in the course of renal failure. Vitamin D_3 deficiency may be the cause. In a group of patients with renal insufficiency, those with analgesic nephropathy

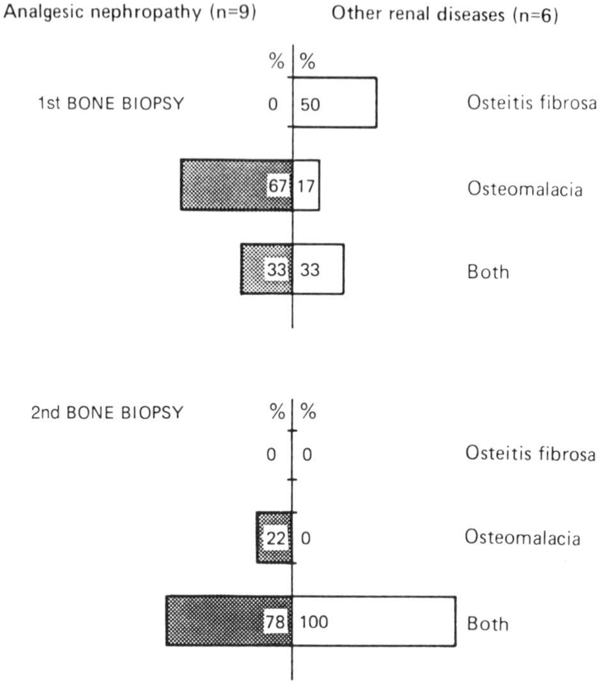

Fig. 11.3 Development of osteodystrophy in 15 patients with renal insufficiency. The predominant early bone lesion was osteomalacia in 9 patients with analgesic nephropathy, and osteitis fibrosa in 6 with other renal disease; the interval between the first and second bone biopsies was 34.4 ± 26.0 months.

had significantly lower 25(OH) vitamin D_3 blood levels than patients with other renal diseases (27 ± 98 vs 54 ± 57 ng/ml, $p = 0.04$). Sixty per cent of the analgesic patients exhibited deficiency compared to only 15 per cent of the other patients ($p = 0.002$). This would explain their lower serum calcium levels (2.0 ± 0.32 vs 2.2 ± 0.2 mmol/l, $p = 0.03$) and, at least at an early stage of osteodystrophy, predominance of osteomalacia in the biopsy (Fig. 11.3).

The low vitamin D_3 status in analgesic patients with renal insufficiency may be due to tubulointerstitial damage causing systemic acidosis (Nanra *et al.* 1978*a*) which, in turn, may enhance the hepatic clearance of vitamin D_3 (Baran *et al.* 1982). This may be intensified by direct liver enzyme induction caused by phenacetin and acetaminophen themselves (Flower *et al.* 1985). In addition, absorption may be disturbed in patients having undergone partial gastrectomy. The condition responds well to orally administered vitamin D_3 or its analogues, with amelioration of myopathy after 6–20 weeks (Offermann 1979).

At the stage of haemodialysis, it should be kept in mind that analgesic patients tend to have high serum aluminium levels from phosphate-binding agents and antacids, and should be given aluminium-free preparations, preferably calcium carbonate (Schwarz *et al.* 1987).

11.3.4 Arterial hypertension

High blood pressure does not occur more often in analgesic nephropathy than in other renal diseases (renal insufficiency 77 per cent vs 76 per cent; haemodialysis 33 per cent vs 37 per cent; Schwarz *et al.* 1985*a*, 1989). Analgesic patients with renal insufficiency took the same number of antihypertensive drugs as patients with other renal diseases (2.7 ± 1.3 vs 2.5 ± 1.3); however, severe hypertension requiring more than one antihypertensive drug occurred more frequently in analgesic nephropathy (60 per cent vs 41 per cent, $p = 0.04$; Schwarz *et al.* 1989). One should keep in mind that secondary arteriosclerotic renal artery stenosis may develop, aggravating hypertension. This condition is found more frequently in analgesic, than in other, renal patients (Horvath *et al.* 1982). The stenosis often develops in the course of years and cannot be excluded by a previous normal arteriogram. A possible treatment, the dilation of the renal artery by angioplastic measures (Vaughan 1985; Jacobson 1988), may lead to worsening of renal function by thrombosis of the renal artery or cholesterol embolism. If hypertension appears to be sustained by a non-functioning kidney, renal arterial embolization may be preferred to nephrectomy (Kunzendorf *et al.* 1990).

11.3.5 Accelerated atherogenesis

Analgesic patients exhibit premature vascular ageing, the cause of which has not been identified (Krishnaswamy *et al.* 1974; Kaladelfos and Edwards 1976; Nanra *et al.* 1978*a*; Nanra 1980; Mihatsch *et al.* 1982*b*, 1983*b*; Schwarz *et al.* 1985*a*; Dubach *et al.* 1991). Risk factors are hyperlipidaemia (Kaladelfos and Edwards 1976; Helber *et al.* 1980; Schwarz *et al.* 1985*a*), nicotine abuse which is frequent (Fellner and Tuttle 1969; Nanra *et al.* 1978*a*, Murray 1978; Dubach *et al.* 1983; Schwarz *et al.* 1985*a*), and hypertension (see above).

The ability to influence these risk factors is limited. It goes without saying than analgesic patients should cease their smoking, but it is not easy to persuade them to do so. Haemodialysis patients especially will answer that they want to keep this remaining pleasure in a life with so many other restrictions.

With regard to the correction of dyslipoproteinaemia, analgesic patients with renal insufficiency usually are not overweight; indeed they tend to have a lower body mass index than other patients with renal insufficiency (Schwarz *et al.* 1989). A cholesterol-restricted diet may be tried, but avoiding further weight loss. Drug therapy with cholestyramine is often associated with gastrointestinal complaints and poor compliance; in transplanted patients, it may alter the bioavailability of immunosuppressive drugs. The usefulness of nicotinic acid is limited by side-effects. Bezafibrate may cause rhabdomyolysis in patients with decreased renal function (Rumpf *et al.* 1976; Pierides *et al.* 1975; Keller *et al.* 1987). Treatment by the hydroxymethylglutaryl coenzyme A reductase inhibitors, lovastatin or simvastatin, seems to be possible in patients with renal insufficiency, but no long-term controlled studies have been performed (Wanner *et al.* 1989; Kasiske *et al.* 1990). Cyclosporin-treated patients given lovastatin have developed rhabdomyolysis (Corpier *et al.* 1988; East *et al.* 1988; Norman *et al.* 1988).

Thus there seems to be as yet no certain way of preventing further arteriosclerosis in analgesic patients at any stage of renal impairment, and thereby to influence this consequential cause of morbidity and mortality.

11.3.6 Anaemia

Anaemia due to haemolysis was the first reported toxic effect of analgesic abuse (Jasinski and Müller 1950; Schaub *et al.* 1953; Lorenzen and Schwartz 1960). Gastrointestinal blood loss, which may be occult, from gastric erosions or ulceration is the most frequent cause of anaemia (Gsell *et al.* 1957; Gault *et al.* 1968*b*; Nanra *et al.* 1978*a*). Some patients, having undergone gastric resection, may develop lack of iron, vitamin B_{12}, and folic acid. Gastric complaints and anaemia are usually signs of continued abuse of aspirin-containing compounds or non-steroidal anti-inflammatory drugs (Alvarez and Summerskill 1958; Roth *et al.* 1963; Gsell 1974).

11.3.7 Carcinoma

In the population of our haemodialysis centre, with a high proportion (30 per cent) of analgesic patients, tumours of the urothelium and the kidney had the highest incidence (2.2 and 1.5 per cent, respectively; Pecqueux *et al.* 1990). Urothelial tumours were significantly more frequent in 97 haemodialysis patients with analgesic nephropathy than in 188 patients with other renal diseases (6.2 per cent vs 0.5 per cent, $p = 0.01$). Phenacetin abuse may lead to the development of urothelial carcinoma, which has been reported to occur in up to 10 per cent of abusers at any stage of renal impairment (Hultengren *et al.* 1965; Angervall *et al.* 1969; Taylor 1972; Johansson *et al.* 1974; Bengtsson *et al.* 1978; McCredie *et al.* 1982*b*, 1986; Gonwa *et al.* 1980; Blohmé and Johansson 1981; Porpáczy and Schramek 1981; Mihatsch and Knüsli 1982; Piper *et al.* 1985).

The urine of former analgesic abusers should be examined regularly for malignant cells, but this is impossible in dialysis patients with no or little residual kidney function. A special problem is the extent to which routine screening for urothelial tumours should be done before renal transplantation. In our clinic, these patients undergo cytoscopy and, when possible, retrograde pyelography and/or ureteroscopy, as well as ultrasound of the kidney, at the time of joining the transplantation waiting list. But the mean waiting time at our centre is one year, ranging up to four years (Schwarz and Offermann 1989), and since these routine tumour investigations are not repeated, the possibility of transplanting and immunosuppressing a patient with cancer cannot be excluded (Vogt *et al.* 1990). Patients with urothelial carcinoma must be free of tumour for at least 3 years after resection before entering the transplant waiting list (Mahony *et al.* 1977). We discovered bladder cancer by routine cystoscopy before transplantation in three women, aged 49–63 years, in a total of 114 analgesic patients. Two of them were transplanted, 2 and 4 years after surgical removal of the tumour. One patient died of myocardial infarction shortly after transplantation; the other developed a new urothelial tumour at a different site of the bladder, in one ureter, and in one kidney 18–41 months after transplantation and 42–65 months after transurethral resection.

Adenocarcinoma of the kidney has been reported as another risk in patients with analgesic nephropathy (McCredie *et al.* 1988; Lornoy *et al.* 1986). Acquired cystic degeneration of shrunken kidneys, which is present in 63 per cent of patients with end stage renal failure, always has to be regarded as a risk factor for adenocarcinoma of the kidney (Gehrig *et al.* 1985; Thomson *et al.* 1986). In our experience, the incidence of adenocarcinoma of the kidney was (perhaps due to small numbers) not significantly different between 97 analgesic and 188 other dialysis patients (2.1 per cent vs 0.5 per cent). The condition was always diagnosed late, usually after frank haematuria or systemic symptoms.

11.4 Haemodialysis

Prior to the introduction of long-term dialysis, patients with chronic pyelonephritis, who were in part representing those with analgesic nephropathy, were preferentially treated with dialysis, for they survived after a temporary period of dialysis longer than comparable patients with chronic glomerulonephritis (Cottier *et al.* 1958; Edel 1966; Losse *et al.* 1966). This is in keeping with the belief that analgesic patients develop severe, but transient, decline of renal function or acidotic electrolyte derangement more easily than patients with other kidney disease.

11.4.1 Acceptance for maintenance dialysis

Due to their high age and co-morbidity, and the fact that analgesic patients are often addicts and unwilling to discontinue the abuse, their suitability for chronic dialysis was at one time doubted (Cove-Smith and Knapp 1978). Since about 1972, the indication for maintenance dialysis has been almost unlimited in Berlin. Analgesic patients are the largest group among the dialysis population (Fig. 11.4). Because of age and reservations regarding transplantation, they are more frequently found in the dialysis than in the

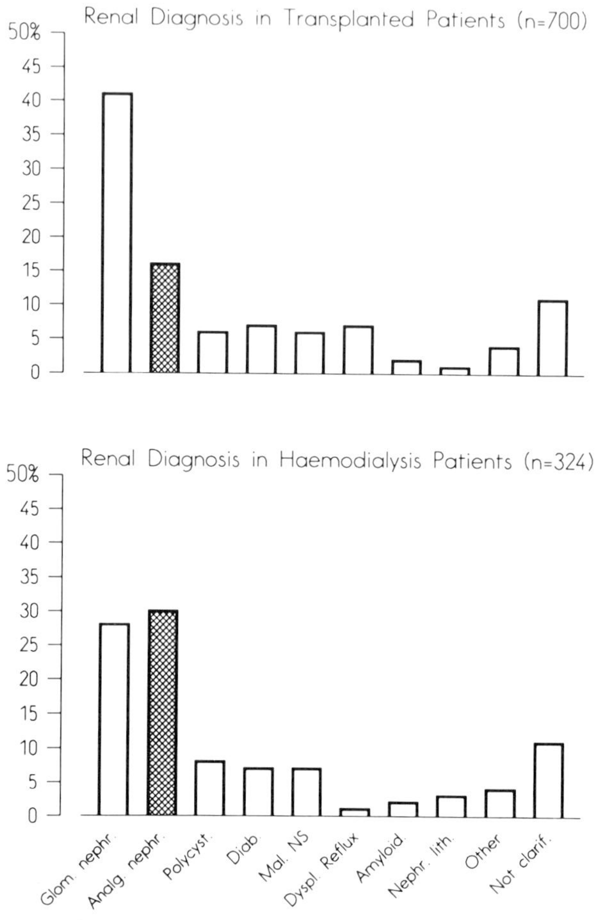

Fig. 11.4 Causes of renal failure in transplant recipients and patients on maintenance haemodialysis. Abbreviations: Glom. nephr. = glomerulonephritis; Analg. nephr. = analgesic nephropathy; Polycyst. = polycystic kidney disease; Diab. = diabetic nephropathy; Mal.NS = arteriopathy due to malignant hypertension; Dyspl. Reflux = renal dysplasia or reflux nephropathy; Amyloid. = renal amyloidosis; Nephr. lith. = nephrolithiasis; Not clarif. = diagnosis uncertain.

transplant population (30 per cent of 324 haemodialysis patients, 16 per cent of 700 transplant recipients).

Besides the increasingly broad indication for dialysis, a number of factors have encouraged us to accept analgesic patients with end stage renal failure. They adapt well, seeming to enjoy the social respect accorded to dialysis patients. Social over-adaptation is one reason for analgesic abuse (Kielholz 1954); it also appears to be the reason for good compliance with the haemodialysis regimen by patients with analgesic nephropathy. The fact that

Table 11.1 *Morbidity in haemodialysis patients according to cause of renal failure*

Morbidity	Analgesic nephropathy[1]	Other kidney disease[1]	Significance (p)[2]
Myocardial infarction	25%	8%	0.028
Angina pectoris	63%	38%	0.014
Atrial fibrillation	21%	4%	0.014
Peptic ulcer	58%	29%	0.011
Diverticulosis	15%	2%	0.027
Haemorrhoids	67%	42%	0.014
Haemoglobin (g/l)	84 ± 19	93 ± 20	< 0.02
Renal osteodystrophy			
radiological signs	67%	38%	0.004
symptoms	28%	8%	0.016
Serum cholseterol (mmol/l)	6.95 ± 1.21	5.70 ± 1.73	0.001
Serum triglyceride (mmol/l)	3.69 ± 3.07	1.60 ± 0.98	0.013
Carpal tunnel compression	23%	8%	0.049
Urinary tract infections	40%	13%	0.0025

[1] Each group comprises 48 age-matched patients; [2] statistical probability by χ^2 or 2-tailed *t*-test; From Schwarz *et al.* (1985*a*), with permission from Schwabe.

analgesic patients are significantly older than other dialysis patients (60 ± 10 vs 52 ± 15 years, $p < 0.001$) and are predominantly women (65 per cent vs 37 per cent, $p = 0.003$) explains why they are less likely to suffer financial disadvantages through their condition than other, younger patients who may lose their jobs (Schwarz *et al.* 1988*a*). Moreover, diet may not need to be as restricted because of tubular potassium loss and the frequent use of laxatives. Reflecting the basically co-operative and contented attitude of the analgesic patients, their compliance in important dialysis parameters, like weight gain between dialyses and diastolic blood pressure, was better than that of other haemodialysis patients (Schwarz *et al.* 1988*a*).

Dialysis patients with analgesic nephropathy have a higher morbidity than others (Table 11.1). Despite their higher age and morbidity, their long-term survival is the same as that of other patients on haemodialysis (Fig. 11.5), perhaps indicating that contentment and compliance are as important for survival as physical condition (Gabriel 1984; Hellerstedt *et al.* 1984).

11.5 Renal transplantation

Age-matched analgesic dialysis patients wanted to be transplanted significantly less often than patients with other renal diseases (6 per cent vs 23 per

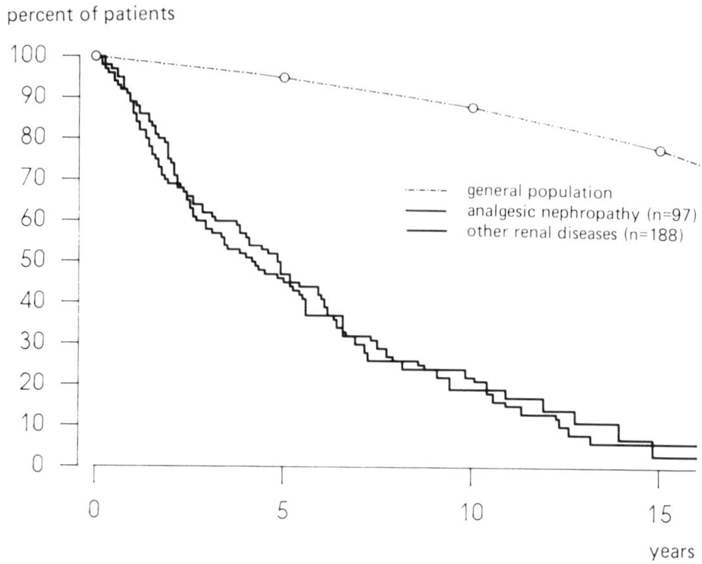

Fig. 11.5 Actuarial survival in patients on maintenance haemodialysis. From Schwarz *et al.* (1988*a*), with permission from Dustri-Verlag.

cent, $p = 0.02$; Schwarz *et al.* 1985*a*). This corresponds to the observation that some analgesic patients after successful renal transplantation seem to miss the constant medical and personal attention of the dialysis centre as well as the social contacts and their status as dialysis patients.

Besides urothelial carcinoma (see above), arteriosclerosis is the main contraindication to transplantation: coronary heart disease is a life-threatening risk at surgery and during the post-transplantation period, and sclerosis of the iliac arteries causing difficulty for the arterial anastomosis. Despite selection before transplantation, the mean age of transplanted analgesic patients is higher than that of other recipients (49.2 ± 7.0 vs 38.7 ± 12.0 years; $n = 700$; $p = 10^{-6}$).

In our experience, analgesic patients less often continue to abuse analgesics after renal transplantation than before or during the time of dialysis (urine test positive for acetaminophen in 2 of 30 transplanted analgesic patients; and in 1 of 54 other transplanted patients). A possible explanation is that those prepared to face the uncertainties of transplantation are the more active and flexible patients who have less difficulty in changing their analgesic habits. Others have reported a higher rate of continued analgesic abuse (Furman *et al.* 1976). Even in patients continuing the analgesic abuse after renal transplantation, recurrence or *de novo* development of analgesic nephropathy is rarely observed, as renal grafts seldom function long enough (Kaude *et al.* 1976; Eknoyan *et al.* 1982; Cameron 1983).

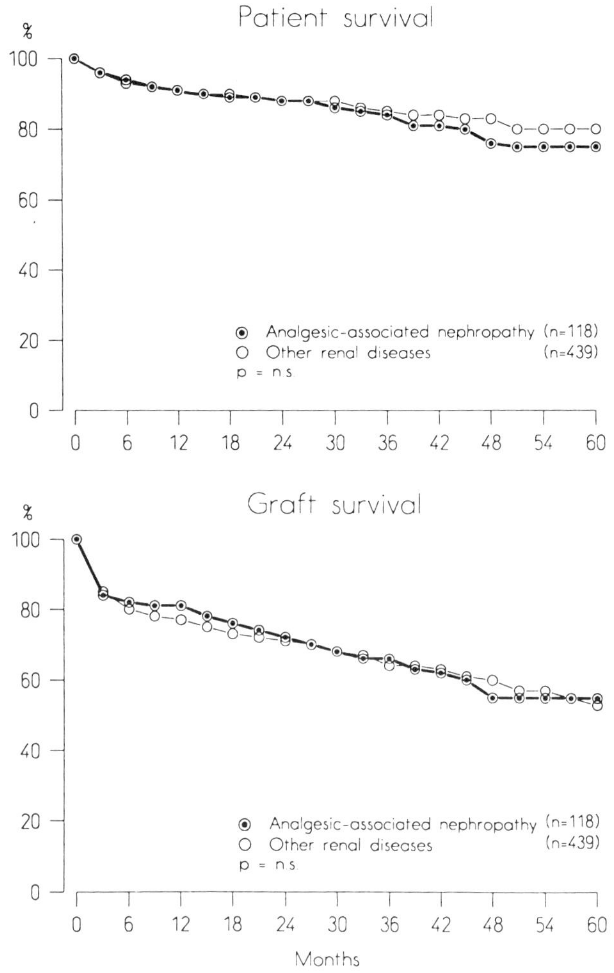

Fig. 11.6 Actuarial survival of patients and grafts after renal transplantation (using cyclosporin in the immunosupressive regimen).

In summary, there is no general reason for excluding analgesic patients from transplantation. Despite the higher age, survival of patient and graft are not different in patients with analgesic nephropathy than with other kidney diseases (Fig. 11.6).

11.6 Summary

Renal tissue, once damaged by analgesics, cannot be restored, hence the prime importance of prevention and of early recognition, for if analgesic consumption can be stopped, remaining renal function can be preserved, often indefinitely. Specific threats to renal function are posed by papillary separation causing obstruction (with or without infection), salt-wasting and acidosis, uncontrolled hypertension, atheromatous renal artery stenosis, and renal pelvic cancer; in the absence of these, renal failure may worsen from non-specific causes, such as hyperfiltration-induced glomerulosclerosis. Urinary infection, tubular acidosis, and premature appearance of renal bone disease relatively frequently complicate management of renal insufficiency in analgesic nephropathy.

Despite a number of theoretical contraindications, there are no grounds to discriminate against patients because of analgesic nephropathy in acceptance for maintenance dialysis; and only the possibility of significant atheroma or of urothelial cancer should influence consideration of this group of patients for transplantation.

12

Biochemistry and pharmacology of non-steroidal anti-inflammatory drugs and renal prostaglandins

Francesco Pugliese and Giulio A. Cinotti

Currently available non-steroidal anti-inflammatory drugs (NSAIDs) comprise a large number of compounds that have been subdivided into different classes according to chemical structure (Table 12.1). Despite their different structures, NSAIDs share a similar: (1) spectrum of pharmacological activities (antipyretic, anti-inflammatory, analgesic, anti-platelet); (2) spectrum of adverse side-effects (gastric mucosal damage, nephrotoxicity, disorders of haemostasis); and (3) mechanism of action. The last is likely to be inhibition of cyclooxygenase (Vane 1978), the enzyme which generates cyclic endoperoxides (prostaglandin (PG)H_2, PGG_2) from arachidonic acid, ultimately leading to the production of PGs, thromboxane A_2 (TxA_2) and prostacyclin (PGI_2). This belief is supported by: (1) PGs and Tx play a prominent role as humoral mediators of the inflammatory response (Stork *et al.* 1986); (2) at therapeutic concentrations, all NSAIDs inhibit PG and Tx production both *in vivo* and *in vitro* (Pugliese and Ciabattoni 1984; Pugliese and Ciabattoni 1987); (3) all share the property of inhibiting cyclooxygenase; (4) other classes of drugs generally do not influence this enzyme; and (5) the degree of inhibition of cyclooxygenase agrees with the efficacy of NSAIDs as anti-inflammatory agents (Ferreira and Vane 1974).

Due to their analgesic and antipyretic effects, NSAIDs are extensively used for the treatment of inflammation, pain, and discomfort. Consequently, they have become the most frequently prescribed drugs in western countries, even if aspirin (the most used and abused drug of our society) is not counted. Their toxicity to the stomach and to the first portion of the small intestine has long been known, but their effects on renal function have only been recognized in the last 10–15 years. The low prevalence of renal complications, the multiplicity of mechanisms by which they can occur (prerenal azotaemia, acute intrinsic renal failure, allergic acute interstitial nephritis, papillary necrosis), and the relatively recent understanding of their pharmacokinetic and pharmacodynamic characteristics, are major factors that have contributed to scant awareness of them by prescribing physicians.

Table 12.1 *Currently used non-steroidal anti-inflammatory drugs*

Salicylates—acetylated	acetylsalicylic acid (aspirin)
—non-acetylated	sodium salicylate
	magnesium salicylate
	salicylamide
	salsalate
	diflunisal
Pyrazolon derivatives	phenylbutazone
	oxyphenbutazone
	phenazone (antipyrine)
	aminopyrine
	apazone
p-Aminophenol derivatives	paracetamol (acetaminophen)
	phenacetin
Indolacetic acid derivatives	indomethacin
	sulindac
	tolmetin
	zomepirac
Anthranilic acid derivatives	mefenamic acid
	flufenamic acid
	meclofenamic acid
	diclofenac
Propionic acid derivatives	ibuprofen
	naproxen
	fenoprofen
	ketoprofen
	indoprofen
	flurbiprofen
	phenbufen
Oxicam derivatives	piroxicam
	sudoxicam
	isoxicam

The aim of this chapter is to review the available information on the mechanism of inhibition of renal PG synthesis by currently used NSAIDs, and its pathophysiologic importance. The major steps of renal PG and TxA_2 biosynthesis will be described, emphasizing the anatomical and functional compartmentalization in distinct segments of the nephron. Finally, likely mechanisms underlying differential inhibition of cyclooxygenase by NSAIDs in various tissues, including the kidney, and the proper use of selective inhibitors of PG synthesis to achieve less nephrotoxicity, will be addressed.

12.1 Biochemistry and distribution of renal eicosanoids

The kidney is a rich source of the cyclooxygenase and lipoxygenase enzymes which catalyse the conversion of arachidonic acid to eicosanoids (which embrace all oxygenated products of eicosatetraenoic (arachidonic) acid). PGs and other eicosanoids are autacoids which do not have a circulating endocrine function, but rather act in a paracrine or autocrine manner affecting cells close to or at the site of their synthesis (Pugliese and Ciabattoni 1984).

12.1.1 Release of arachidonic acid

Arachidonic acid (AA) exists only bound to cell membrane phospholipids; its release occurs as a consequence of specific hormone–receptor interaction with subsequent activation of phospholipases C and A_2. At least three mechanisms of hormone-evoked arachidonate release from membrane phospholipids can be considered:

1. Sequential activation of phospholipases C and A_2. Upon binding of an agonist, its receptor activates specific guanine nucleotide-binding membrane proteins (G proteins) to stimulate phospholipase C. This effector enzyme leads to hydrolysis of membrane inositol phospholipids, and the generation of two potential second messengers, inositol triphosphate and diacylglycerol. Inositol triphosphate can cause a rapid elevation in intracellular free calcium ion levels ($[Ca^{2+}]_i$) resulting from the release of stored intracellular Ca^{2+} as well as enhanced Ca^{2+} entry through plasma membrane channels. Increased $[Ca^{2+}]_i$ in turn activates phospholipase A_2, a Ca^{2+}-dependent enzyme that releases AA from membrane phosphatidylcholine and phosphatidylethanolamine (Van den Bosch 1980; Lapetina 1982).

2. Direct receptor-mediated activation of phospholipase A_2, as suggested by recent evidence showing that release of AA and increased PG production in response to some agonists may occur prior to any increment of diacylglycerol and inositol triphosphate (Bonventre *et al.* 1988), or without change in $[Ca^{2+}]_i$ (Mené *et al.* 1989*b*).

3. Diacylglycerol lipase action. AA-containing diacylglycerol, formed by the phospholipase C-mediated hydrolysis of inositol phospholipids, can also be freed by the action of a specific lipase (Bell *et al.* 1979).

12.1.2 Oxidation of arachidonic acid

Once released, AA becomes substrate for cyclooxygenase and lipoxygenase enzymes. The oxidative metabolism of AA through the cyclooxygenase pathway leads to the synthesis of PGs and Tx; lipoxygenase produces mono- and di-hydroxylated eicosatetraenoic acid and leukotrienes.

AA cyclooxygenation yields two intermediate compounds, the endoperoxides PGG_2 and PGH_2. These in turn undergo further biotrans-

Table 12.2 *Renal distribution of prostaglandins and thromboxane*

Eicosanoid	Sites of synthesis	Sites of action
PGI_2	Glomerulus, arterioles	Mesangium, vascular smooth muscle, juxtaglomerular cells
TxA_2	Glomerulus	Mesangium, vascular smooth muscle
PGE_2	Glomerulus, tubules, medullary interstitium	Mesangium, collecting tubule, loop of Henle, vascular smooth muscle
$PGF_{2\alpha}$	Glomerulus, tubules, medullary interstitium	Mesangium, collecting tubule, vascular smooth muscle(?)

formation by specific isomerases catalysing the conversion of PGH_2 into PGE_2 (endoperoxide isomerase), $PGF_{2\alpha}$ (endoperoxide reductase), PGI_2 (prostacyclin synthetase), and TxA_2 (thromboxane synthetase). That NSAIDs inhibit, in roughly equal measure, the formation of all derivatives of PG-endoperoxides, indicates that they are inhibitors of the first enzymatic stage of the biotransformation of AA, namely cyclooxygenase.

Lipoxygenase converts AA into hydroperoxide acids from which many compounds are derived, including leukotrienes B_4, C_4, D_4, and E_4. However, this pathway has not been unequivocally demonstrated in, at least the human, kidney.

12.1.3 Degradation and elimination of eicosanoids

PGs synthesized within the kidney are degraded locally by enzymes acting on the δ-13,14 double bond (13,14-PG reductase) and hydroxyl group C-15 (15-OH-PG dehydrogenase). The resulting 13,14-dehydro-15-keto-metabolites are biologically inactive, and are removed from the kidney in the lymphatic and venous drainage or by excretion into the urine. Further biodegradation is achieved by β-oxidation and Ω-oxidation with the production of dicarboxylic derivatives which are exclusively excreted in the urine.

The metabolism and inactivation of leukotrienes are largely unknown but seem to involve bioconversion by peptide cleavage from one active compound to another with less biological activity (Dunn 1983).

12.1.4 Renal distribution of eicosanoids

Because the various specific isomerases are variously represented according to cellular type, there are qualitative and quantitative differences in PG distribution in the kidney (Table 12.2). Human isolated glomeruli and papillary homogenates synthesize PGI_2, PGE_2, $PGF_{2\alpha}$, and TxA_2 (Sraer *et al.*

Table 12.3 *Main renal actions of prostaglandins and thromboxane*

Target structure	Eicosanoid	Action
Vasculature	PGI_2	Vasodilation
	TxA_2	Vasoconstriction
	$PGF_{2\alpha}$	Vasoconstriction (?)
Glomerulus	PGI_2, PGE_2	GFR preservation
	TxA_2	GFR reduction
	$PGF_{2\alpha}$	GFR reduction (?)
Collecting tubule	PGE_2	Increased excretion of sodium and water; decreased urea permeability

1982). PGI_2 and TxA_2 are the most abundant metabolites of AA in human glomeruli, and PGE_2 and $PGF_{2\alpha}$ in the papilla (Schlondorff 1986).

Functionally, it is convenient to consider PGs and TxA_2 as originating from two renal compartments: (1) the cortex whose structures (glomeruli, arterioles, and cortical collecting tubules) synthesize compounds which regulate cortical functions, that is renal blood flow (RBF), glomerular filtration rate (GFR) and renin release; and (2) the medulla whose structures (interstitial cells, collecting tubules) elaborate PGs capable of modulating medullary events, such as medullary blood flow, and salt and water excretion. Thus, the functional consequences of changes in PG and Tx synthesis will be different in the various segments of the nephron (Table 12.3).

12.2 Synthesis and physiology of glomerular eicosanoids

12.2.1 Synthesis

Detailed information regarding glomerular eicosanoid biosynthesis has been provided by *in vitro* techniques involving isolation of glomeruli and glomerular cell cultures. Human glomeruli generate the vasodilator PGI_2, usually measured as the stable hydrolysis product 6-keto-$PGF_{1\alpha}$, and the vasoconstrictor TxA_2, measured as the hydrolysis product TxB_2. These are the most abundant products of cyclooxygenase in human glomeruli, whereas PGE_2 and $PGF_{2\alpha}$ are the major AA metabolites in rat glomeruli (Ciabattoni and Pugliese 1989).

Since the glomerulus is a complex microvascular structure composed of at least three major cell types—endothelial, epithelial, mesangial—and since PGs are autacoids, identifying their sites of synthesis (by cell culture) indicates their potential physiological role.

PGE_2 is the major PG of rat glomerular epithelial cells, while $PGF_{2\alpha}$, PGI_2, and TxA_2 are produced in smaller amounts (Petrulis *et al.* 1981; Sraer *et al.* 1979). However, when these cells are cloned, the principal PG synthesized is PGI_2 (Kreisberg *et al.* 1982). Whether this difference reflects distinct cell populations, or changes in the PG biosynthetic capacity depending on the number of passages the cells undergo, remains to be seen. Negligible amounts of PGs and Tx are produced by human glomerular epithelial cells (Ardaillou *et al.* 1983).

Primary cultures and cloned populations of rat mesangial cells synthesize large amounts of PGE_2, but less $PGF_{2\alpha}$ and PGI_2 (Sraer *et al.* 1979; Kreisberg *et al.* 1982). Human mesangial cells yield predominantly PGI_2, and no TxA_2 (Ardaillou *et al.* 1985).

Data are lacking on PG synthesis by glomerular endothelial cells, but endothelial cell cultures from extra-glomerular vasculature produce predominantly PGI_2 and PGE_2 (Terragno *et al.* 1978; Kirschenbaum *et al.* 1985).

12.2.2 Vasomotor action of glomerular eicosanoids

The glomerulus serves as target organ for, and site of synthesis of, a variety of vasoactive hormones which participate in the regulation of renal haemodynamics (Dunn 1983) (Table 12.3). There is good evidence that a balance between vasoconstrictor and vasodilator agents modulates the vascular tone of renal arterioles and thereby controls RBF and GFR (Brenner *et al.* 1981; Schor *et al.* 1981; Edwards 1983). Moreover, due to their capacity to promote mesangial cell contraction (Kreisberg 1983; Kreisberg *et al.* 1985), vasoactive agents may influence the total glomerular capillary area available for filtration, and hence the glomerular ultrafiltration coefficient (Dworkin *et al.* 1983). *In vivo* and *in vitro* evidence suggests that vasodilatory PGs modulate the systemic and intrarenal vascular action of vasoconstrictor substances (Scharschmidt *et al.* 1983). Agents that induce renal vasoconstriction as well as mesangial cell contraction, stimulate the glomerular synthesis of vasodilator PGI_2 and PGE_2 (Scharschmidt and Dunn 1983; Ardaillou *et al.* 1985), probably through phospholipase C-stimulated hydrolysis of inositol phospholipids. Furthermore, inhibition of renal PG synthesis by NSAIDs potentiates both renal vasoconstriction (Scharschmidt *et al.* 1983) and mesangial cell contraction (Foidart and Mahieu 1986; Scharschmidt *et al.* 1986) induced by numerous vasoconstrictor substances. Thus, it would seem that glomerular PGs play a critical role in the dynamic balance between vasodilator and vasoconstrictor forces controlling renal haemodynamics. Decreased glomerular synthesis of vasodilator PGs, or exaggerated vasoconstrictor stimuli to the kidney, may alter this balance, thereby inducing renal functional alterations.

12.2.3 Modification of inflammatory responses by glomerular eicosanoids

In addition to the control of renal haemodynamics, eicosanoids appear to play an active role in both acute and chronic inflammatory states, including glomerulonephritis (Stork *et al.* 1986). Renal PG and Tx synthesis is altered in many forms of clinical and experimental glomerular disease (Ciabattoni *et al.* 1984*a*; Patrono *et al.* 1985*b*; Rahman *et al.* 1987). Vasoconstrictor TxA_2 is also considered to be an important mediator of inflammation (Kitchen *et al.* 1978), and its selective inhibition has been shown to ameliorate renal function and glomerular histology in some models of progressive glomerulosclerosis (Salvati *et al.* 1990). Vasodilator PGE_2 and PGI_2 may influence glomerular filtration of macromolecules and thereby contribute to the vascular-exudative component of glomerular inflammation (Vriesendorp *et al.* 1986*c*). Moreover, PGs of the E series have direct anti-inflammatory, immunoregulatory effects on both cellular and humoral immune responses (Goodwin and Webb 1980; Goodwin and Ceuppens 1983). Finally, it should be pointed out that recent studies have attributed to eicosanoids a regulatory action on mesangial cell proliferation (Mené and Cinotti 1989), suggesting a potential involvement in at least some forms of proliferative glomerulonephritis.

12.3 Synthesis and physiology of tubular eicosanoids

12.3.1 Synthesis

Proximal tubules and the thick ascending loop of Henle have little capacity to synthesize PGs. Along the other segments of the nephron, the important sites of synthesis are the cortical and medullary collecting tubules, both of which generate predominantly PGE_2, less $PGE_{2\alpha}$ and PGI_2, and negligible TxA_2 (Schlondorff 1986).

12.3.2 Functions

If the concept of anatomical and functional compartmentalization of renal eicosanoid synthesis is valid, then tubular PGs will be local regulators of tubular physiology (Table 12.3). Numerous studies *in vivo* and *in vitro* have shown that cyclooxygenase products may influence several aspects of the renal concentrating mechanism (Stokes 1981) to promote free water excretion, the chief influence appearing to be interference with the cellular action of arginine vasopressin (AVP). Studies in microperfused nephron segments (Torikai and Kurokawa 1983; Edwards *et al.* 1981), toad urinary bladder (Omachi *et al.* 1974; Schlondorff *et al.* 1981) and *in vivo* (Lum *et al.* 1977; Licht *et al.* 1981), have shown that AVP stimulates the synthesis and excretion of PGE_2, which in turn acts in the medulla of the kidney to decrease water reabsorption in response to AVP. This effect seems to be achieved through the capacity of PGE_2 to interfere with the production of AVP-stimulated cyclic adenosine monophosphate (AMP) (Anderson *et al.* 1985). On the other hand, PGE_2 itself is a stimulus for cyclic AMP production by renal tubular cells (Torikai and Kurokawa 1983; Edwards *et al.* 1981), and cyclic AMP is capable of inhibiting both phospholipase and cyclooxygenase activity, at least in dog renal tubular cells (Hassid 1983). These data point to a modulatory effect of cyclic AMP on PG synthesis, acting as a negative feedback pathway.

Other studies on primary cultures of rat and rabbit renal collecting tubule cells have reported that AVP does stimulate cyclic AMP production while it does not affect PGE_2 synthesis (Grenier *et al.* 1981). Furthermore, in renal papillary collecting tubule cultures, inhibition of cyclooxygenase by NSAIDs does not potentiate AVP-stimulated cyclic AMP, and exogenous addition of PGE_2 or AA does not reduce the production of intracellular cyclic AMP in response to AVP (Grenier *et al.* 1981; Pugliese *et al.* 1983). Additionally, studies in microperfused rabbit collecting ducts have reported that water permeability is not affected by either inhibition or stimulation of PG synthesis (Stokes 1985).

These conflicting data may be related in part to differences in the experimental conditions involving *in vitro* incubation of renal tissue. In preparations of cortical and medullary collecting tubules (the major target sites for AVP action) uncontaminated by cells from other nephron segments, the existence of an interaction between AVP, PGs, and cyclic AMP seems likely (Schlondorff *et al.* 1985).

In addition to interfering directly with vasopressin action at the cellular level, PGs may influence urinary concentration indirectly through their vasodilator action. As intrarenal vasodilators, PGE_2 and PGI_2 tend to enhance RBF and GFR, increasing delivery of solute and water to distal nephron segments and overwhelming maximal urinary concentrating capacity. Also, by reducing efferent arteriolar resistance, vasodilator PGs may decrease peritubular osmotic pressure and increase peritubular hydraulic pressure, thus impairing proximal tubular reabsorption of salt and water. Lastly, by increasing renal medullary blood flow, PGs tend to wash out solutes, thereby diminishing the papillary hypertonicity required for water reabsorption.

Without denying the importance of the haemodynamic influence of PGs on tubular salt and water handling, some data suggest that they may exert a direct inhibition of sodium reabsorption in several distal nephron sites, especially collecting tubules (Raymond and Lifschitz 1986). Also it has been reported that PGE_2 and $PGF_{2\alpha}$ inhibit urea transport into the interstitium, thus enhancing water excretion (Roman and Lechene 1981).

It is apparent from these data that the contribution of PGs to the regu-

Table 12.4 *Renal side-effects of non-steroidal anti-inflammatory drugs*

Sodium retention and reduced effect of diuretics
Impaired water excretion
Hyperkalaemia
Renal failure due to:
(a) papillary necrosis
(b) chronic interstitial nephritis
(c) acute interstitial nephritis with glomerular lesions
(d) haemodynamic factors

lation of sodium and water balance should be kept in mind when approaching patients with oedema-forming states in which inhibition of PG synthesis could promote sodium retention and reduce diuretic efficacy. The ultimate effect could be an exacerbation of the sodium retention underlying clinical conditions such as heart failure, nephrotic syndrome, and ascites.

12.4 Effects of local inhibition of cyclooxygenase

It is well known that NSAIDs may cause series of undesirable side-effects within the kidney (Clive and Stoff 1984) (Table 12.4).

In normal subjects or experimental animals under physiological conditions, NSAIDs only minimally reduce GFR and RBF (Pugliese and Ciabattoni 1987). This does not rule out a role for basal eicosanoids in regulation of renal function, but rather suggests that under normal conditions, inhibition of renal PGs and Tx synthesis by NSAIDs may not alter the balance between vasodilator and vasconstrictor forces while other regulatory systems (adrenergic tone, renin release, vasopressin, dopamine, bradykinin, histamine, serotonin) are unstressed and can compensate for reduced PG production. However, RBF and GFR may become critically dependent on renal PG synthesis when the administration of NSAIDs takes place after a haemodynamic insult. For instance, anaesthetized experimental animals, especially after laparotomy, respond to the administration of PG synthesis inhibitors with a dramatic reduction in renal haemodynamic parameters (Terragno *et al.* 1977). Similarly, if healthy subjects become sodium depleted, or if a diuretic is administered, NSAIDs may reduce RBF and GFR to the point of acute renal failure (Dunn 1983).

The most impressive effect of NSAIDs on renal function has been observed in patients with hepatic cirrhosis in the ascitic phase, congestive heart failure, or chronic glomerulonephritis (including lupus nephritis) with or without nephrotic syndrome. Such clinical settings share either exaggerated vasoconstricting stimuli to the kidney (Dunn and Zambraski 1980), or a local reduction in the synthesis of PGI_2 (Pugliese and Ciabattoni 1984; Pugliese and Ciabattoni 1987). These patients respond to inhibitors of PG synthesis with an acute, but generally reversible, reduction in RBF, GFR, and sodium excretion.

NSAID administration may also be associated with sodium retention. The pathophysiologic mechanisms underlying this event appear to be multifactorial (see 12.3.2). However, water reabsorption disproportionate to sodium retention may lead to the development of hyponatraemia, especially in patients concomitantly given drugs limiting free water excretion, such as thiazides (Clive and Stoff 1984) or chlorpropamide (Walshe and Venuto 1979).

Due to its incidence and severity, hyperkalaemia is probably the most important adverse clinical effect of NSAIDs which reduce renin and aldosterone secretion (Tan *et al.* 1979). Potassium retention rarely occurs in patients with normal renal function, but it has been well documented in, for example, elderly patients with pre-existing renal disease given indomethacin (Zimran *et al.* 1985).

The mechanisms whereby NSAIDs may cause renal damage, including chronic interstitial nephritis, and acute interstitial nephritis associated with glomerular lesions and proteinuria, are not clear; they may be in some way related to the suppression of anti-inflammatory, immunoregulatory actions of PGs of the E series on cellular and humoral immune responses. Medullary ischaemia due to PG inhibition may contribute to the genesis of renal papillary necrosis (Clive and Stoff 1984).

12.5 Inactivation of renal cyclooxygenase

NSAIDs inhibit cyclooxygenase by competing with AA for non-covalent binding to the enzyme. This process is critically dependent upon systemic plasma drug concentration, and is reversible with drug elimination. Another mechanism, unique to aspirin, is the selective acetylation of the hydroxyl group of a single serine residue within the polypeptide chain of cyclooxygenase (Roth *et al.* 1975), resulting in the irreversible inactivation of the enzyme. The onset, extent, and duration of inhibition of cyclooxygenase depend upon such variables as absorption, distribution and metabolism, and binding to plasma proteins. Removal of drug from the active site of cyclooxygenase (in case of reversible inhibitors), or *de novo* synthesis of the enzyme (in case of irreversible inhibitors), represent the mechanisms by which PG and TxA_2 synthesis may be restored. In platelets and other cell types lacking the biosynthetic machinery necessary to form the enzyme, aspirin causes an irreversible defect for the life of the exposed cells (8–10 days for platelets) (Patrono *et al.* 1985*a*).

Table 12.5 *Inhibition of cyclooxygenase in different tissues*

Drug	Synovia	Gastric mucosa	Kidney	Platelets
Piroxicam	60%	66%	70%	73%
Naproxen	..	68%	60%	88%
Sulindac	69%	33%	0%	77%
Diclofenac	..	72%	62%	79%
Ibuprofen	..	75%	73%	80%

Tested in patients with rheumatoid arthritis. From Pugliesi and Ciabattoni (1987).

Most, if not all, widely used NSAIDs have been shown to inhibit renal PG and TxA_2 synthesis in healthy subjects (Ciabattoni *et al.* 1980; Pugliese and Ciabattoni 1982; Ciabattoni *et al.* 1984*b*) as well as in patients with renal (Ciabattoni *et al.* 1984*a*; Kimberly *et al.* 1978*a,b*; Berg and Talseth 1985), hepatic (Zipser *et al.* 1979; Laffi *et al.* 1986), rheumatic (Pugliese and Ciabattoni 1987; Svendsen *et al.* 1984), and cardiovascular (Svendsen *et al.* 1984; Salvetti *et al.* 1982) disease. With the possible exception of sulindac (see 12.6.2) nearly all these agents have been reported to reduce renal cyclooxygenase activity by up to 60–70 per cent (Pulgiese and Ciabattoni 1987; Pugliese and Ciabattoni 1982), although no detailed dose–response studies have been carried out to determine relative potencies. In general, maximal suppression of renal PG synthesis occurs within 24–48 h of treatment with therapeutic doses, and is fully reversible within 48–72 h of discontinuation, depending upon the pharmacokinetics of the individual agent. Reduced kidney and liver function do not substantially modify the degree of inhibition of renal cyclooxygenase, although they certainly influence plasma survival of NSAIDs. Thus, delayed plasma clearance may jeopardize the reversibility of acute changes in renal function, and should be taken into account by physicians prescribing NSAIDs.

12.6 Differential inhibition of human cyclooxygenase

In addition to inhibiting renal PG and Tx synthesis, NSAIDs given in therapeutic doses reduce cyclooxygenase activity in the various other tissues in which such activity can be measured. Conventional doses of structurally different anti-inflammatory agents (except sulindac) share the capacity to inhibit cyclooxygenase in equal measure at renal, platelet, gastric, and synovial sites in patients with rheumatoid arthritis (Table 12.5). In healthy subjects, there is a similar degree of cyclooxygenase inactivation by different NSAIDs in gastric mucosa (Caruso and Porro 1980; Ciabattoni *et al.* 1984*b*), platelets (Patrono *et al.* 1980; Patrono *et al.* 1985*a*; Ciabattoni and Pugliese 1989), and the kidney (Pugliese and Ciabattoni 1982; Ciabattoni and Pugliese 1989). Thus, it seems that the majority of anti-inflammatory agents act as non-selective inhibitors of cyclooxygenase in all tissues endowed with the enzyme. Nevertheless, exceptions have been recorded, deserving mention because of their pharmocological and pathophysiological implications.

12.6.1 Low-dose aspirin

Low-dose aspirin (0.45 mg/kg/day) has been shown to be capable of selectively inhibiting the synthesis of platelet TxA_2 without modifying the urinary excretion of PGs (Patrono *et al.* 1985*a*), suggesting that renal PG synthesis is not inhibited. The mechanism is likely to be related to the different rate of recovery of cyclooxygenase in kidney and platelets following irreversible acetylation of the enzyme, and possibly to a lesser sensitivity to aspirin of renal cyclooxygenase. Thus, low-dose aspirin represents an ideal antithrombotic tool, even for those patients with underlying renal disease, without the risk of jeopardizing PG-dependent renal function with higher, conventional, doses of the drug.

12.6.2 Sulindac

Sulindac does not seem to inhibit the synthesis of PGs and Tx in the kidney in healthy subjects (Ciabattoni *et al.* 1980; Sedor *et al.* 1986), in patients with Bartter's syndrome (Ciabattoni *et al.* 1980), or in chronic glomerulonephritis, both primary and secondary (Patrono and Pierucci 1986), while it exhibits the same efficacy as other NSAIDs in reducing extrarenal cyclooxygenase activity (Pugliese and Ciabattoni 1987). In contrast with the marked reduction in urinary excretion of PGs and Tx, RBF and GFR caused by ibuprofen, sulindac treatment of patients with renal disease is not associated with any significant modification of renal function (Ciabattoni *et al.* 1984*a*). This suggests a correlation between cyclooxygenase activity and renal function, a view further supported by studies comparing sulindac to a variety of other NSAIDs in physiological, as well as in different clinical, conditions. In healthy subjects, indomethacin has been found to reduce the renal production of PGs and Tx and to diminish the excretion of sodium and water, while sulindac has no effects upon these parameters (Sedor *et al.* 1986). Analogous results have been reported in patients affected by nephrotic syndrome (Vriesendorp *et al.* 1986*a*,*b*,*c*): unlike indomethacin, diclofenac, and flurbiprofen, sulindac does not modify proteinuria, GFR or renal PG synthesis. A similar lack of effect of sulindac on renal function has been noted in chronic liver disease (Daskalopoulos *et al.* 1985; Laffi *et al.* 1986).

However, conflicting data regarding the biochemical selectivity of sulindac have been reported in both health (Brater *et al.* 1985; Roberts *et al.* 1985)

Table 12.6 *Proposed mechanisms of differential inhibition of cyclooxygenase in human tissues*

1. Different sensitivity of cyclooxygenase(s) in the various cell types
2. Different rate of restoration of enzymic activity after irreversible inactivation
3. Different affinities of the drug for the binding, and the catalytic, site of the enzyme
4. Different distribution of the drug and its active metabolites in the various tissues
5. Selective inhibition of the active metabolites of the drug at the tissue level

and disease (Daskalopoulos *et al.* 1985), possibly explained by differing conditions of radioimmunoassay, the technique most widely used for measuring urinary PG excretion (Patrono and Dunn 1987).

12.6.3 Tissue specific activities of non-steroidal anti-inflammatory drugs

Numerous mechanisms have been proposed to explain the diverse activities of certain NSAIDs in different tissues (Table 12.6). In respect of sulindac, the inactive pro-drug, sulindac sulphoxide, can be reversibly reduced to its active metabolite, the sulphide, or irreversibly oxidized to the biologically inactive sulphone (Miller *et al.* 1984), depending upon the local tissue redox potential. The active metabolite is produced predominantly in those tissues where oxygen tension is low, as occurs classically in inflammatory foci and in poorly oxygenated tissue. In the kidney, where the redox potential is sharply shifted towards the oxidizing form, it is likely that the sulphide is rapidly reconverted to sulphoxide (sulindac itself), and in turn further oxidized irreversibly to sulphone which will be eliminated in the urine.

Metabolic irregularities of sulindac excretion have been described in patients with hepatic cirrhosis (Juhl *et al.* 1983) or with chronic nephropathy and seriously impaired renal function (Swainson and Griffiths 1985), in whom prolonged plasma survival of sulindac sulphide appears to reduce renal PG synthesis to approximately 50 per cent, without causing significant alteration of renal function.

Sulphinpyrazone, like sulindac, is reduced to a sulphide metabolite more powerful than the drug itself, and lacks the capacity to inhibit renal cyclooxygenase when given to healthy subjects at doses which significantly reduce platelet Tx and extrarenal PG synthesis (Catella *et al.* 1984). These findings accord with the absence of its short-term effects on GFR, both in healthy subjects (Pedersen and FitzGerald 1985), and in patients with myocardial infarction (Choudhury *et al.* 1983).

12.7 Conclusions

PGs synthesized in the kidney modulate many facets of renal function. They contribute to the regulation of RBF, GFR, sodium, water, and potassium excretion. Additionally, as mediators of inflammation, eicosanoids may play a role both in glomerulonephritis and interstitial inflammatory processes. Research in the past 10 years has established that integrity of renal PG synthesis is necessary to maintain renal cortical and medullary function in patients with diverse disease. This is of importance in that the most widely used anti-inflammatory drugs exert their therapeutic and adverse effects by inhibiting cyclooxygenase in all tissues endowed with the enzyme including the kidney, thereby, in some cases, causing severe impairment of renal function. However, due to the particular pharmocodynamic or pharmocokinetic properties of some drugs, it is possible to inhibit selectively the production of PGs in some tissues but not others. Low-dose aspirin has been shown to spare extra-platelet cyclooxygenase, while some, but not all, studies have indicated that at conventional dosage sulindac does not inhibit renal PG synthesis or alter renal function.

13
Effects of non-steroidal anti-inflammatory drugs on renal function

Edward J. Zambraski and Michael J. Dunn

The focus of this chapter will be on the clinical implications of non-steroidal anti-inflammatory drug (NSAID) administration, with emphasis on their effects on renal function. We will briefly define the role of prostaglandins (PGs) in the maintenance of normal renal function, but PG biochemistry and NSAID pharmacology, discussed in Chapter 12, will be excluded. Our intention is to describe situations where kidney function is 'PG dependent', and thus may be adversely affected by NSAID treatment. We will also present information suggesting that in certain diseases NSAIDs may ameliorate renal dysfunction. Differences among various NSAIDs with respect to renal function, and the issue of 'renal PG sparing' drugs, will also be discussed. Lastly, important unresolved issues concerning the use of these drugs, and their potential influence on renal function, will be presented.

13.1 Prostaglandins in the kidney

PGs play an important role in all important facets of renal function (haemodynamic, tubular, endocrine) (Dunn 1984, 1987; Patrono *et al.* 1985*c*; Schlondorff 1986; Patrono 1989; Lote and Haylor 1989).

13.1.1 Modulatory role

The concept that PGs modulate the renal effects of various endocrine and neural stimuli has been widely accepted (Dunn and Zambraski 1980; Schlondorff 1986). This role of PG is most evident, and perhaps clinically relevant, for renal haemodynamics (i.e. renal blood flow, glomerular filtration rate) where vasodilatory PGs (PGE_2, PGI_2) may attenuate the renal vasoconstrictor effects of angiotensin II, arginine vasopressin, circulating norepinephrine and/or renal sympathetic nerve activity. In addition, PGs also appear to modulate non-haemodynamic events influenced by these factors, such as renal hormone release, endocrine effects on the glomerulus, and tubular transport. Consequently, the effects of a decrease in renal PG due to NSAID administration are dependent upon the levels of these other stimuli. Situations where these stimuli may be elevated have been described as 'PG dependent' states. In contrast, a renal PG independent state would exist when these other factors or stimuli are minimal, and/or when basal renal PG synthesis is not elevated. Predictably, in these settings NSAID administration would have minimal or no impact on kidney function.

13.1.2 Processes regulated by basal levels of prostaglandins

However, there are several renal processes that are regulated by PG in basal or control situations. Examples would include some specific pathways for renal renin release (namely the macula densa mechanism) (Henrich 1981), the synthesis and release of erythropoietin (Lote and Haylor 1989), and some aspects of glomerular and mesangial cell function (Mené *et al.* 1989*a*). Consequently, regardless of the presence or absence of other factors or stimuli, NSAIDs could potentially interfere with these aspects of renal function.

13.1.3 States associated with increased renal prostaglandin synthesis

Predicting the renal response to NSAIDs is also confounded by several factors listed in Table 13.1. As will be discussed, certain disease states are associated with elevated renal PG synthesis, conditions which amplify the effects of a NSAID. A point which must be stressed is that, although there are inherent limitations in our ability to assess renal PG synthesis *in vivo* (Patrono and Dunn 1987), the best estimates of the decrements in renal PG synthesis with the most efficacious NSAIDs are in the range of 50–60 per cent, with the highest values approaching only 80 per cent (Patrono and Pierucci 1986; Patrono and Dunn 1987; Patrono 1989). This decrement in renal PG may be less with certain NSAIDs. Consequently, regardless of the drug used, all NSAID therapy leaves a significant amount of renal PG synthesis intact, an amount which may delay or minimize an adverse effect on renal function even in a PG dependent state. The fact that all NSAIDs are to an extent renal PG sparing suggests that new, yet to be developed NSAIDs, which could be more effective renal cyclooxygenase inhibitors, may cause more prevalent and serious renal complications than are seen with existing drugs.

Despite the complexity of the renal PG system, there are two major points that we will illustrate: (1) renal PGs are extremely important in determining renal function, and (2) there are well-defined physiological and pathological states in which NSAID therapy will adversely affect the kidneys.

13.2 The effect of prostaglandins on renal function

13.2.1 Renal haemodynamics

PGs, either through direct vasodilation (PGE_2, PGI_2), or the attenuation of non-PG vasoconstrictors, can alter the diameters of the afferent and efferent

Table 13.1 *Factors which complicate the prediction of the effects of non-steroidal anti-inflammatory drugs upon kidney function*

I	PG 'independent' and 'dependent' conditions in various normal and pathophysiological states
II	Differing basal synthetic rates of renal PG biosynthesis
III	Incomplete suppression of renal PG synthesis with current NSAIDs
IV	'Renal PG sparing' effects of selective NSAIDs
V	Removal of PG directly responsible for renal processes (as distinct from those acting through haemodynamic effects)
VI	Predominant removal of vasodilatory (PGE_2, PGI_2) or vasoconstrictor (TxA_2) actions
VII	Differences between acute and chronic renal PG inhibition
VIII	NSAID shunting of arachidonic acid towards lipoxygenase and epoxygenase metabolic pathways
IX	Direct influence (independent of PG) of NSAIDs on kidney structures or function

arterioles. This capacity appears to be greater at the afferent arteriole. Consequently, PG-mediated vasodilation of pre-glomerular resistance vessels will elevate glomerular capillary hydrostatic pressure, promoting filtration. By influencing contractility of either the afferent or efferent arterioles, renal blood flow will also be affected. As the concentrations of PG are highest in the medullary region of the kidney, they are believed to be critical in maintaining medullary and papillary blood flow (Roman and Lianos 1990).

13.2.2 Glomerular function

Because of recently devised techniques enabling the study of isolated glomeruli and of the various cell types derived from glomerular structures, a large amount of information has been obtained on PG control of glomerular function (Schnermann and Briggs 1981). As indicated earlier, PGs may determine glomerular capillary hydrostatic pressure. They may also increase the glomerular permeability coefficient (*Kf*) through attenuation of angiotensin II or arginine vasopressin-induced mesangial contraction (Scharschmidt *et al.* 1986). In certain diseases, PGs may also modulate the constrictor effects of thromboxane A_2 (TxA_2) and possibly other factors, such as platelet activating factor and the leukotrienes C_4 and D_4 (Patrono and Pierucci 1986). Whereas regulation of mesangial contraction affects the surface area component of the *Kf*, PGs may also directly influence the hydraulic conductivity of the glomerular membrane. A recent report suggests that PGs may be involved in the control of mesangial growth and proliferation (Mené and Dunn 1990).

Lastly, PGs are important determinants of glomerular membrane barrier function (Dunn 1990*a*). This effect on the movement of macromolecules, such as albumin, across the glomerular capillary membrane appears to involve a complex interaction between angiotensin II and PG. Over 15 years ago patients with nephrotic syndrome were treated with NSAIDs to reduce proteinuria (Arisz *et al.* 1976; Donker *et al.* 1976). Since exogenous angiotensin II may cause proteinuria, while angiotensin converting enzyme inhibition may decrease proteinuria, an involvement of angiotensin II has been implicated. It has been hypothesized that in conditions where angiotensin II is elevated. NSAIDs may augment its constrictor effects by removing PG, and thereby alter glomerular capillary pressure or other factors so as to ameliorate the proteinuria (Dunn 1990*a*,*b*). Although the exact mechanism is unknown, it is clear that PGs can mediate proteinuria and that NSAID therapy may decrease this condition in a variety of disease states.

13.2.3 Tubular processes

PGs are well known for their natriuretic properties, when infused intrarenally an increase in sodium excretion is seen. However, a direct effect of PG inhibiting tubular sodium transport has been controversial (Bonvalet *et al.* 1987). More direct and conclusive evidence exists for PG-attenuating active chloride transport in the thick ascending limb of the loop of Henle (Stokes 1981).

PGs may regulate the excretion of water via several different mechanisms. By reducing sodium reabsorption in the proximal tubule, isosmotic reabsorption of water may be altered. It has been well documented that PGs attenuate the hydro-osmotic effects or arginine vasopressin in the collecting tubule (Stokes 1981). Lastly, the tonicity of the medullary interstitium, the driving force for the abstraction of water from the collecting duct, will be influenced by sodium chloride reabsorption, vasa recta blood flow, and urea reabsorption (Bonvalet *et al.* 1987). In the medullary zone, the high basal rates of PG synthesis will alter all of these factors in a direction that will decrease urine osmolality and increase free water clearance.

13.2.4 Endocrine effects

PGs are known to modulate the effects of various hormones acting within the kidney including angiotensin II, arginine vasopressin, the kallikrein–kinin system, and catecholamines. They do not appear to be involved with the renal actions of atrial natriuretic peptide (Salazar *et al.* 1988). In addition, PGs appear to be directly responsible for the renal synthesis or release of several hormones.

There are numerous pathways that may stimulate renal renin release. Although the baroreceptor and neural mechanisms seem not to involve PG, the macula densa sensing mechanism appears to require PG (Henrich 1981). Consequently, a reduction of renal PG synthesis could decrease renin release driven by this tubular feedback mechanism.

Erythropoietin release by mesangial cells, and possibly peritubular vascular endothelium, may also be mediated by PGs (Mené *et al.* 1989*a*). It is believed that hypoxia, which is a known stimulus for renal PG synthesis, may stimulate synthesis of erythropoietin via the activation of adenylate cyclase (Lote and Haylor 1989).

Recent studies have dealt with the renal effects of endothelin (Banks 1990; Corner *et al.* 1990; Stacey *et al.* 1990). Because it is a potent renal vasoconstrictor reducing renal blood flow and glomerular filtration rate, Cornet, *et al.* (1990) have shown that endothelin induces proteinuria. PGs attenuate the renal vascular and glomerular effects of endothelin, and NSAIDs accentuate endothelin-induced vasoconstriction. Zoja *et al.* (1990) and Simonson and Dunn (1990) demonstrated that endothelin is a potent stimulus for the synthesis of PGE_2 and PGI_2 in cultured mesangial cells.

13.3 Renal effects of non-steroidal anti-inflammatory drugs

13.3.1 Normal individuals

In healthy individuals, the reduction of renal PG synthesis after the acute administration of a NSAID may have little measurable effect on renal function. Renal blood flow (RBF), glomerular filtration rate (GFR), sodium excretion, and urine volume are usually unaltered.

This response can change if various pressor system are activated. For example, if a patient is stressed with hypovolaemia, such as due to blood loss or dehydration, activation of the blood pressure homeostatic systems (renin–angiotensin, sympathetic nervous system) will occur. Under these conditions, NSAIDs will significantly reduce renal function. The most marked effect will be a decrease in GFR; RBF is usually less affected. Changes in water and sodium excretion are variable, but with increased duration of treatment, and depending upon the decrease in GFR, an antinatriuresis and antidiuresis will occur. This role of PGs as modulators of angiotensin II-mediated vasoconstriction was established using sodium deprived dogs by Blasingham *et al.* (1980) and Blasingham and Nasjletti (1980), who demonstrated that the decrease in GFR with NSAID treatment was correlated with plasma renin activity. Recently, it has been shown in man that with sodium deprivation there is a selective increase in renal sympathetic nerve activity, as estimated by renal norepinephrine overflow (Friberg *et al.* 1990). Consequently, the renal response to NSAIDs in sodium deprivation may also involve the removal of PG attenuation of the vasoconstrictor effects of renal sympathetic nerve activity. An exaggerated renal response to NSAIDs is also seen in animals with experimentally induced volume depletion or low cardiac output, conditions known to activate both renin and the sympathetic nervous system (Izumi *et al.* 1985; Oliver *et al.* 1981; Riegger *et al.* 1989). Thus, a detrimental renal response to NSAIDs is predictable in states where renal sympathetic tone, or circulating norepinephrine or renin–angiotensin-II activity, is elevated.

13.3.2 Disease states

In certain disease states, consistent and markedly deleterious changes in renal function have been documented following suppression of renal PG synthesis with NSAID treatment. Since the initial reviews describing a protective or supportive role of PG on renal function (Dunn and Zambraski 1980; Patrono *et al.* 1985*a*), the number of conditions in which NSAIDs are known to have a deleterious effect on the kidneys has increased (Table 13.2). For most, NSAID-induced renal vasoconstriction, with concomitant retention of sodium and water, has been demonstrated in man. Many of these studies on humans were preceded or confirmed by animal studies using experimentally induced cirrhosis (Zambraski and Dunn 1984), heart failure (Oliver *et al.* 1981; Riegger *et al.* 1989), diabetes mellitus (Moel *et al.* 1987), and other states in which deleterious renal effects of NSAIDs had been observed.

13.3.2.1 Nephrotic syndrome

Arisz *et al.* (1976) reported a 35 per cent decline in GFR with indomethacin in nephrotic syndrome, and Donker *et al.* (1976) observed a 20 per cent decrease in patients with miscellaneous forms of renal disease. GFR declined approximately 30 per cent with NSAID therapy in patients with chronic glomerular diseases (Patrono *et al.* 1986). More recently, Whelton *et al.* (1990) evaluated the effects of ibuprofen (800 mg three times per day) in 12 women with various types of renal disease and mild, but stable, chronic renal failure. The majority showed significant renal deterioration by day 12.

13.3.2.2 Hepatic cirrhosis

Numerous studies in experimental animals and man have established that the renal synthesis of PGE_2 and PGI_2 is elevated in hepatic cirrhosis (Zambraski and Dunn 1984; Zipser *et al.* 1979; Uemura *et al.* 1986; Laffi *et al.* 1986), in which condition PGs acting as vasodilators are essential in maintaining GFR and sodium and water excretion. The administration of NSAIDs consistently adversely affects the kidneys in patients with hepatic cirrhosis and ascites, in whom decreases in GFR of approximately 50 per cent after 24 h of indomethacin or ibuprofen treatment are observed (Boyer *et al.* 1979; Zipser

Table 13.2 *Renal prostaglandin-dependent states: conditions of increased risk for the adverse effects of non-steroidal anti-inflammatory drug therapy*

Sodium deprivation/dehydration
Low renal perfusion pressure
Diuretic induced hypovolaemia
Congestive heart failure
Nephrotic syndrome
Diabetes mellitus
Miscellaneous renal disease with hypertension
Mild stable chronic renal failure
Cirrhosis (decompensated with ascites)
Chronic glomerular disease
Systemic lupus erthymatosus
Arteriosclerotic cardiovascular disease
Reduction of renal mass/nephron number
Old age (?)

et al. 1979; Uemura *et al.* 1986). The reduction in filtration was correlated with decrements in renal PGE_2 synthesis and the fall in GFR was accompanied by a 42 per cent decrease in sodium excretion; in contrast, indomethacin did not significantly change GFR in cirrhotics without ascites (Uemura *et al.* 1986). More recently, Antillon *et al.* (1990) reported similar decreases in GFR in patients with cirrhosis and ascites after indomethacin treatment, as well as a 65 per cent decline in sodium excretion. The fact that these responses were observed within 4 h emphasizes the rapidity with which these dramatic changes can occur.

13.3.2.3 Other diseases

There are disease states such as arteriosclerotic cardiovascular disease, systemic lupus erythematosus, and chronic glomerular nephritis, where there may be a decline in basal renal PG synthesis (Dunn 1987). Individuals with these conditions are also susceptible to adverse renal effects of NSAID therapy. In systemic lupus erythematosus, aspirin or ibuprofen treatment decreases GFR by 60 per cent (Patrono *et al.* 1986). Significant reductions in GFR have been reported in systemic lupus erythematosus after indomethacin (ter Borg *et al.* 1989), and in chronic glomerulonephritis after ibuprofen (Patrono *et al.* 1986).

In otherwise healthy subjects, decreased functional renal mass also results in a PG dependent state. In animal models with ligation of branches of the renal arteries (Kirschenbaum and Serros 1981), and in human renal transplant donors (Donker 1983), NSAID treatment will significantly reduce RBF and GFR.

13.3.3 Special populations

13.3.3.1 The elderly

The elderly comprise a large percentage of those persons taking NSAIDs, as well as a large fraction of those with the various conditions associated with increased renal susceptibility to NSAIDs (Cameron 1988; Clive and Stoff 1984; Patrono and Dunn 1987; Whelton *et al.* 1990). There are several reasons why one would predict an increased likelihood of renal complications with NSAIDs in the elderly.

First, peripheral and renal sympathetic activity rises with age (Izzo 1989). This would escalate the potential role of PG in attenuating age-related increases in renal constrictor tone. With ageing, there is also a decline in functional nephron numbers, perhaps analogous to the experimental reductions in renal mass which amplify the renal vasoconstriction observed with NSAIDs. The elderly are more likely to develop hyperkalaemia, possibly because of concomitant hyporeninaemic hypoaldosteronism. Although one should adopt a conservative approach, the conclusions being drawn about NSAIDs, renal function and the elderly, are not yet proven, having been based more on association than direct experimental evidence.

13.3.3.2 Neo-natal infants

Approximately fifteen years ago, the first reports of renal complications in infants who were being treated with indomethacin for patent ductus arteriosus appeared (Friedman *et al.* 1976; Heymann *et al.* 1976); symptoms included transient oliguria and azotaemia. Recently Lindsley and Warady (1990) reviewed the renal toxicity of NSAIDs in children. Cases of NSAID-induced acute renal insufficiency, interstitial nephritis, and papillary necrosis have been reported, and although the incidence of these complications is low, physicians should be aware of the factors in children that lead to increased renal vulnerability to NSAIDs. One factor of particular concern is dehydration because of its occurrence even in healthy children.

13.4 Clinical syndromes resulting from non-steroidal anti-inflammatory drugs

The possible consequences of NSAID administration in individuals who are at risk are illustrated in Fig. 13.1. The major problems are the possibility of acute renal failure, sodium and water retention, and plasma electrolyte alterations. In addition, it should be emphasized that certain NSAIDs may cause glomerular and/or tubular damage which may be independent of changes in renal PG synthesis.

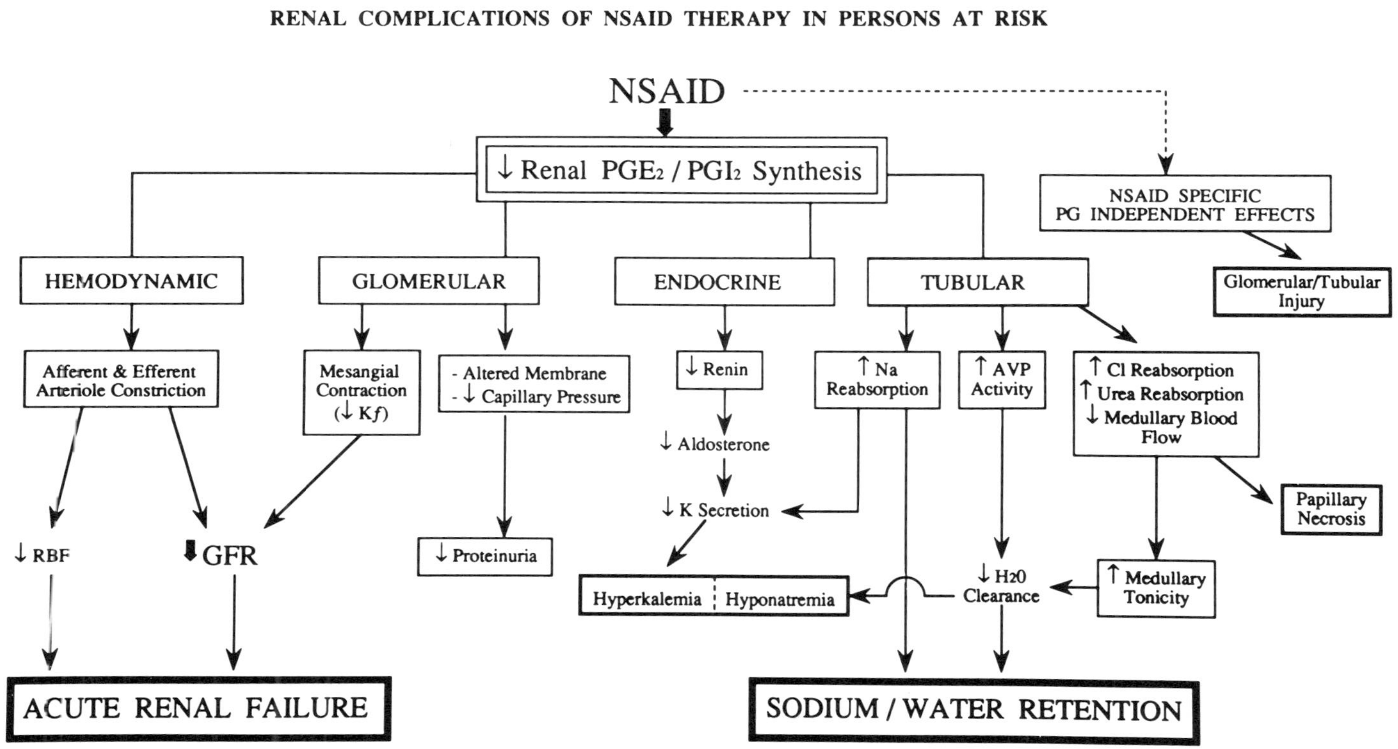

Fig. 13.1 The possible complications, and their mechanisms, associated with non-steroidal anti-inflammatory drug therapy in persons at risk (see Table 13.2).

13.4.1 Potassium, sodium, and water retention

NSAIDs can induce hyperkalaemia as a result of decreased renal excretion of potassium (Carmichael and Shankel 1985; Whelton *et al.* 1990). The mechanism responsible for this effect is complex, but includes suppression of renin and aldosterone, and direct inhibition of distal tubular potassium secretion.

One of the major renal effects of NSAIDs, especially when considering longer treatment (i.e. days, weeks), is sodium retention. The mechanisms responsible for this effect undoubtedly involve haemodynamic factors (decreased GFR and filtered sodium load) and enhanced tubular reabsorption of sodium chloride. The magnitude and importance of this effect has been emphasized by Clive and Stoff (1984) who note that oedema may occur in as many as 25 per cent of patients with arthritis receiving aspirin or fenoprofen chronically, and 10 per cent of those receiving ibuprofen.

The possibility of hyponatraemia exists (Clive and Stoff 1984), due to the disproportionately greater decrease in free water clearance than in sodium excretion. This condition may be exacerbated by diuretic therapy.

13.4.2 Intrinsic kidney disease

Besides these purely functional renal effects, NSAIDs may cause nephrotoxicity (Chapter 14). Carmichael and Shankel (1985) reviewed the worldwide literature and cited 274 cases of renal complications due to NSAIDs. Unspecified renal failure was described for 37 per cent of those cases, followed by papillary necrosis (20 per cent), acute interstitial nephritis (19 per cent), nephrotic syndrome (12 per cent), acute tubular necrosis (11 per cent), and acute glomerulitis (5 per cent).

Recently, Warren *et al.* (1989) evaluated the records of 55 patients with minimal change glomerulopathy over a 6-yr period. Nine per cent were using NSAIDs, and all demonstrated complete remission after discontinuing NSAID use. Tubulointerstitial nephritis, with or without minimal change glomerulopathy, may also be induced by NSAID therapy (Cameron 1988).

13.5 Renal sparing non-steroidal anti-inflammatory drugs

Since many patients requiring NSAID therapy fall into one or more of the categories for increased risk of renal complications (Table 13.2), considerable efforts have been made to identify 'safe' NSAIDs. With the increasing number of chemically dissimilar NSAIDs, initiatives are being made to quantitate relative toxicities and the therapeutic effectiveness of the various compounds, as well as to directly evaluate the renal effects of specific NSAIDs in patients at risk (Clive and Stoff 1984; Patrono and Pierucci 1986).

13.5.1 Sulindac

With its unique pharmacology, sulindac has received considerable attention as a possible renal PG sparing NSAID (Patrono and Dunn 1987; Patrono 1989; Chapter 12). While there are reports variously showing that sulindac does, or does not, inhibit renal PG synthesis, there are clearly demonstrable and clinically important renal functional differences with this particular NSAID. Compared to drugs such as indomethacin, the acute administration of sulindac to persons at risk may not cause significant renal vasoconstriction, decrements in GFR, or sodium retention. Despite these encouraging findings, there are concerns about the effects of more prolonged sulindac treatment, and of changes in sulindac metabolism which, in certain patients such as cirrhotics, could potentially increase nephrotoxicity (Patrono and Dunn 1987; Whelton *et al.* 1990).

13.5.2 Salicylates

Another class of compounds, which may be renal PG sparing, are the non-acetylated salicylates which do not significantly decrease renal PG excretion (Reimann *et al.* 1985). Also, in contrast to compounds such as indomethacin or meclofenamate, non-acetylated salicylates do not cause renal vasoconstriction, or sodium retention in animals which are sodium deprived (Zambraski *et al.* 1988*a*) or in a decompensated ascitic state with hepatic cirrhosis (Zambraski *et al.* 1988*b*). A key element appears to be the lack of acetylation, since aspirin (acetylsalicylic acid) may adversely affect the kidneys under these circumstances. This possibility of a therapeutic advantage of salicylates was recently supported by the work of Antillon *et al.* (1989) who compared the non-acetylated salicylate, diflunisal, to indomethacin in 9 patients with alcoholic cirrhosis and ascites. In these renal PG dependent individuals, indomethacin significantly decreased GFR and PGE_2 excretion, and the natriuretic response to frusemide was blunted. None of these deleterious changes were observed with diflunisal.

Compared to compounds such as indomethacin, both aspirin and non-acetylated salicylates are relatively weak renal PG synthesis inhibitors, and would appear to have less nephrotoxicity (Dunn and Zambraski 1980; Clive and Stoff 1984).

Another potentially important feature of salicylates is that when they bind to cyclooxygenase they limit the ability of the newer NSAIDs to inhibit the enzyme. Although the molecular biochemistry of acetylsalicylate binding to cyclooxygenase has been described (DeWitt *et al.* 1990), the exact mechanism responsible for this unique property of salicylate remains to be determined. This biochemical effect of salicylate is also supported by experimental data in intact kidneys. For example, in sodium-depleted or cirrhotic animals, if salicylate is administrated prior to meclofenamate, no adverse renal effects are seen (Zambraski *et al.* 1988*a*,*b*). The possibility of using salicylates in conjunction with some of the never NSAIDs to minimize their nephrotoxic effects remains to be tested.

13.6 Beneficial renal effects of non-steroidal anti-inflammatory drugs

Although the emphasis of this chapter has been on the potential deleterious effects of NSAIDs on the kidney, it should be pointed out that in certain circumstances NSAIDs may be beneficial. Indomethacin may significantly reduced proteinuria in patients with nephrotic syndrome in which, although acute reductions in GFR may occur, longer-term benefits of a reduction in proteinuria exist. If NSAIDs decrease proteinuria by lessening glomerular capillary pressure or by directly influencing glomerular membrane structure or permeability, they could slow the progression of glomerular damage. Vriesendorp *et al.* (1986*c*) observed less end stage renal failure in those nephrotic patients treated with indomethacin over 10 yr. In addition, meclofenamate has been used to prevent renal disease in transplant recipients with a history of focal glomerulosclerosis (McCoy *et al.* 1985). Until we understand the role of PG in either mediating or preventing long-term glomerular disease, it will be difficult to predict possible long-term benefits of NSAID therapy.

13.7 Long term renal effects of non-steroidal anti-inflammatory drugs

Most of the studies we have discussed have examined short-term NSAID administration. Although in persons at risk, the deleterious effects become apparent within hours or days, the effects of long-term NSAID therapy and a 60–80 per cent reduction in renal PG synthesis for an extended period of time, are largely unknown. This also is true for normal persons or those not considered to be at risk. For example in healthy, normally hydrated individuals, NSAIDs given acutely will not cause a significant change in sodium excretion, yet in persons with arthritis, but with presumably normal kidneys, chronic renal PG inhibition with NSAIDs may cause sodium retention in as many as 25 per cent (Clive and Stoff 1984).

With NSAID treatment and the resultant inhibition of cyclooxygenase, free arachidonic acid may be metabolized in the kidney by at least two alternative metabolic pathways. A lipoxygenase pathway will result in the synthesis of leukotrienes, and a less well understood epoxygenase pathway may produce dihydroxy- and trihydoxy-fatty acids (Schlondorff and Ardaillou 1986). The renal effects of increased leukotrienes and/or hydroxy metabolites of arachidonic acid, due to NSAID inhibition of cyclooxygenase, are not yet known.

13.8 Summary

The potential deleterious effects of NSAIDs on various aspects of renal function have been reviewed (Fig. 13.1). Well defined states in which the maintenance of normal kidney function is PG dependent, and therefore susceptible to complications from NSAIDs, have been identified (Table 13.2).

In the general population, it has been stated that the risk of renal problems due to NSAIDs is low; the incidence has been estimated at less than 1 per 1000 patient days of therapy (Corwin and Bonventre 1984). Although this would appear to be a relatively low rate, this estimate has been questioned by Murray and Brater (1990). If the end point utilized to define a renal risk is the diagnosis of renal disease, this would exclude patients demonstrating acute adverse effects such as increased serum creatinine or decreased GFR, since their NSAID therapy would be discontinued. Also, several epidemological studies of NSAIDs that have excluded the elderly, diabetics, and persons with congestive heart failure or renal insufficiency, would clearly be underestimating the relative risk of renal complications, since a significant percentage of the complications would be seen in these groups.

Until the actual relative risks of NSAIDs are known, physicians should be acutely aware of the various conditions that increase the probability for adverse renal effects of their use. With the current availability of over-the-counter NSAIDs, and the likelihood of an increased number of NSAIDs becoming available without prescription, the public must also be educated about their adverse effects on renal function.

Acknowledgements

The authors thank and acknowledge the secretarial assistance of Jan Houtman in the preparation of this chapter.

14

Diseases of the kidney caused by non-steroidal anti-inflammatory drugs

D. Kleinknecht

Non-steroidal anti-inflammatory drugs (NSAIDs) are now in widespread use, sometimes as an over-the-counter preparation. They can produce a wide spectrum of tubular, interstitial, glomerular, and vascular lesions (Table 14.1). The most common disorder is functional, prerenal insufficiency, due to decreased synthesis of renal vasodilatory prostaglandins (Chapter 13). An increasing number of structural renal diseases associated with the use of NSAIDs has been reported in the past ten years and they will now be detailed.

14.1 Incidence

The real incidence of nephrotoxicity due to NSAIDs is unknown because we have no accurate method of detection. The overall incidence could be very low, considering that up to 40 million people in the United States take NSAIDs regularly (Henrich 1988). Brezin *et al.* (1979) found that the reported incidence of renal abnormalities with fenoprofen, a drug usually taken on prescription, was less than one case per 5300 patient-years of treatment. In the 10-yr period 1972–1982, 8 million prescriptions for mefenamic acid were given, and only 23 cases of nephropathy were attributed to this drug (Nicholls *et al.* 1985).

The incidence of nephrotoxicity is higher in selected and prospective studies. Renal impairment occurred in 18 per cent of 1908 patients treated with ibuprofen in general medical practice (Murray *et al.* 1990). Corwin and Bonventre (1984) found that renal insufficiency secondary to NSAIDs accounted for approximately 6 per cent of acute renal failure seen during a 2-yr period. In a prospective collaborative study, NSAIDs represented 15.6 per cent of patients with drug-induced acute renal failure, and 2.8 per cent of all acute renal failure (Kleinknecht *et al.* 1986). In a later study, half of the prescriptions for NSAIDs could be considered as therapeutic errors, that is, excessive or prolonged doses were given to older or high-risk patients (Kleinknecht *et al.* 1989).

14.2 Acute interstitial nephritis

Interstitial nephritis due to NSAIDs was diagnosed in 1 per cent of 460 renal biopsies reviewed by Abraham and Keane (1984), and 2 per cent of 398 (10 per cent of biopsied) patients with drug-induced acute renal failure collected in a collaborative study (Kleinknecht *et al.* 1986).

14.2.1 Drugs involved

About 100 cases of documented acute interstitial nephritis, related to some 20 different NSAIDs, have been reported. Some were observed with phenylbutazone and other pyrazolon derivatives (Pommer *et al.* 1983; Grünfeld *et al.* 1988).

Propionic acid derivatives were responsible for nearly half the reported cases, mainly fenoprofen (Curt *et al.* 1980; Handa 1980,1986; Regester 1980; Wendland *et al.* 1980; Finkelstein *et al.* 1982; Mourad *et al.* 1982; Magil 1983; Stachura *et al.* 1983; Bender *et al.* 1984; Feinfeld *et al.* 1984; Jao 1986; Kleinknecht *et al.* 1986; Warren *et al.* 1989), ibuprofen (Regester 1980; Bender *et al.* 1984; Kleinknecht *et al.* 1986; Moss *et al.* 1986; Marasco *et al.* 1987; Pirani *et al.* 1987; Tolins and Seel 1987), and naproxen (Brezin *et al.* 1979; Wasser *et al.* 1982; Bender *et al.* 1984; Adams *et al.* 1986; Pirani *et al.* 1987; Robinson *et al.* 1990). Fewer were associated with pirprofen (Hurault de Ligny *et al.* 1986; Eugène *et al.* 1987), ketoprofen (Ducret *et al.* 1982), and benoxaprofen (Onwubalili 1983).

Indoleacetic derivatives, accounting for 20 per cent of reported NSAID-associated interstitial nephritis, included indomethacin (Gary *et al.* 1980; Kleinknecht *et al.* 1983; Pommer *et al.* 1983; Green *et al.* 1985; Handa 1986), sulindac (Whelton *et al.* 1983; Lins *et al.* 1986), clometacin (Lavaud *et al.* 1984; Kleinknecht *et al.* 1986; Lang *et al.* 1986), tolmetin (Chatterjee 1981; Katz *et al.* 1981; Bender *et al.* 1984), and zomepirac (McCarthy *et al.* 1982; Mease *et al.* 1982; Ratner 1982; Bender *et al.* 1984; Cummings *et al.* 1984).

There are about 10 instances of interstitial nephritis ascribed to mefenamic acid (Venning *et al.* 1980; Dixon *et al.* 1981; Woods and Michael 1981; Englert *et al.* 1982; Brunner *et al.* 1985*b*; Nicholls *et al.* 1985; Adams *et al.* 1986; Jenkins *et al.* 1988; Boletis *et al.* 1989; Joh *et al.* 1990), and one case each to niflumic acid and mefenamate (Kleinknecht *et al.* 1983).

Some patients developed interstitial nephritis while taking phenylacetic acid derivatives, either diclofenac (Rossi *et al.* 1985; Wolters and van Breda Vriesman 1985; Campistol *et al.* 1989), alclofenac (Vereerstraeten *et al.* 1982), or fenclofenac (Raftery *et al.* 1985). Lastly, a handful of cases have been associated with the use of piroxicam (Mitnick and Klein 1984; Fellner 1985; Sarma 1989), or the salicylic acid derivatives, aspirin or diflunisal (Grünfeld *et al.* 1988). Sometimes two or more different NSAIDs were

Table 14.1 *The various renal lesions associated with non-steroidal anti-inflammatory drugs*

Non-steroidal anti-inflammatory drug	Acute interstitial nephritis	Acute tubular necrosis	Minimal change nephrotic syndrome[1]	Membranous nephropathy	Proliferative glomerulonephritis	Papillary necrosis
Pyrazolon derivatives	+	+	+	+	+	+
Indolacetic derivatives						
indomethacin	+	+	+	..	..	+
sulindac	+	..	+	+	..	..
clometacin	+	+	..	..	..	..
tolmetin	+	..	+	..	..	..
zomepirac	+	+	+	..	..	..
Propionic derivatives						
fenoprofen	+	+	+	+	+	+
ibuprofen	+	+	+	..	..	+
naproxen	+	+	+	..	..	+
ketoprofen	+	+	..	+	..	..

pirprofen	+	+	+	..	..	..
benoxaprofen[2]	+	..	..	..	..	+
fenbufen	..	+	..	..	..	..
Phenylacetic derivatives						
diclofenac	+	+	+	+	..	+
alclofenac	+	..	+	..	..	..
fenclofenac	+	..	..	..	+	..
Piroxicam	+	+	+	..	..	+
Mefenamates						
mefenamic	+	..	..	..	+	+
niflumic acid	+	+	..	..	..	..
Salicylic derivatives						
aspirin	+	+	+	..	..	..
diflunisal	+	..	..	..	..	..
salsalate	..	..	+	..	..	..

Excluding prerenal failure, [1] without interstitial nephritis, [2] withdrawn from the market, .. = not reported.

Table 14.2 *Comparison of acute interstitial nephritis due to non-steroidal anti-inflammatory drugs and β-lactam antibiotics*

	Non-steroidal anti-inflammatory drugs	β-lactam antibiotics
Age	generally > 60 yr	any
Male : female	1 : 2	3 : 1
Latent interval (mean)	5 months	15 (range 2–60) days
Fever, rash, eosinophilia, eosinophiluria	rare	frequent
Non-oliguric renal failure	frequent	frequent
Requiring dialysis	30–40%	15–20%
Nephrotic syndrome	80%	< 1%
Interstitial cellular infiltrates		
lymphocytes	common	common
eosinophils	rare	frequent
epithelioid cell granulomas	rare	sometimes
Circulating anti-tubular basement membrane antibodies	absent	inconstant
Renal recovery	frequent	usual
Efficacy of steroid therapy	uncertain	uncertain

given, and it was not possible to identify the main offending agent (Adams *et al.* 1986; Kleinknecht *et al.* 1986; Lévy *et al.* 1987; Schwarz *et al.* 1988*b*).

14.2.2 Clinical features

A rather characteristic clinical picture of NSAID-associated acute interstitial nephritis is given when the patient presents with heavy proteinuria (Clive and Stoff 1984; Garella and Matarese 1984; Carmichael and Shankel 1985; Pirson and van Ypersele de Strihou 1986; Grünfeld *et al.* 1988). The picture is somewhat different from that observed in β-lactam-related allergic interstitial nephritis (Pirani *et al.* 1987; Grünfeld *et al.* 1988) (Table 14.2).

One-third of patients share some risk factors with those who develop prerenal failure due to inhibition of prostaglandin synthesis (Chapter 13), including older age, hypertension, concomitant use of diuretics or aspirin, pre-existing renal insufficiency, and diabetes (Abraham and Keane 1984; Kleinknecht *et al.* 1986, 1989).

Extrarenal signs may occassionally be present. One patient taking diflunisal had erythroderma (Chan *et al.* 1980). Hepatitis was commonly associated with clometacin nephrotoxicity (Lavaud *et al.* 1984; Lang *et al.*

Table 14.3 *Clinical features of acute renal failure associated with non-steroidal anti-inflammatory drugs*

	Prerenal failure	Tubular necrosis	Interstitial nephritis
Mean age	70 yr	60 yr	60 yr
Proteinuria	no	absent or mild	heavy
Signs of hypersensitivity	0	10%	15%
Mean duration of renal failure	6 days	10 days	15 days
Pre-existing renal lesions	20%	20%	0
Predisposing factors	≥ 90%	70%	35%
Reversibility	≥ 90%	80%	50–70%
Class of NSAID commonly responsible	nearly all	propionic and indole derivatives	nearly all

1986). Vasculitis was reported in a few cases of interstitial nephritis associated with the use of fenoprofen (Finkelstein *et al.* 1982), indomethacin and niflumic acid together (Kleinknecht *et al.* 1983), and diclofenac (Lévy *et al.* 1987). Most of the patients taking mefenamic acid had abdominal pain, diarrhoea and vomiting before renal failure was diagnosed (Nicholls *et al.* 1985; Jenkins *et al.* 1988).

Dialysis was required in one-third of patients. In most cases, interstitial nephritis and the nephrotic syndrome improved within days or weeks after discontinuing the offending drug, but the time course of resolution may extend up to one year (Colvin and Fang 1989). Complete remissions are often observed, sometimes after a period of several years (Warren *et al.* 1989). Stachura *et al.* (1983) demonstrated, in a repeat biopsy, resolution of the inflammatory infiltrate and restoration of normal foot processes.

However, full renal recovery is not the rule. In our experience, a higher percentage of patients had permanent renal damage than in those suffering from other types of NSAID-associated renal lesion (Table 14.3). Persistent renal damage has also been documented by several workers (Adams *et al.* 1986; Kleinknecht *et al.* 1986; Boletis *et al.* 1989; Cameron 1988; Schwarz *et al.* 1988*b*). Chronic dialysis was sometimes required (Wasser *et al.* 1982; Boletis *et al.* 1989) and deaths have been reported (Finkelstein *et al.* 1982; Wasser *et al.* 1982; Adams *et al.* 1986; Sarma 1989).

A beneficial effect of steroids is not clearly established, since renal function frequently improves before steroid administration. However, Finkelstein *et al.* (1982) and Campistol *et al.* (1989) found that prednisone seemed to hasten the resolution of renal failure and proteinuria in some of their patients.

Recurrence of acute renal failure may occur after resuming therapy with the same (Vereerstraeten *et al.* 1982; Abraham and Keane 1984; Lavaud *et al.* 1984; Raftery *et al.* 1985) or a different NSAID (Bender *et al.* 1984). On the other hand, Warren *et al.* (1989) observed no relapse when their patient was rechallenged with the same NSAID.

14.2.3 Pathology

Detailed renal biopsy analyses can be found in several reviews (Pirani *et al.* 1987; Grünfeld *et al.* 1988; Colvin and Fang 1989). By light microscopy, there is a diffuse or patchy infiltration of the interstitium by small lymphocytes, with few plasma cells and eosinophils. Interstitial epithelioid granulomas with giant cells are sometimes found (Dixon *et al.* 1981; Magil 1983; Onwubalili 1983; Kleinknecht *et al.* 1983, 1986; Schwarz *et al.* 1988*b*). Focal tubular atrophy and cell degeneration is common and correlates roughly with the degree of renal insufficiency (Abraham and Keane 1984). Extensive necrosis of the tubular epithelium is sometimes associated. 'Tubulitis', defined as invasion of tubular cells by lymphocytes through breaks of the tubular basement membrance, is rarely seen (Pirani *et al.* 1987). Enlarged nuclei in cells of the collecting duct have been found in three patients with NSAID-induced interstitial nephritis (Bender *et al.* 1984), but it is open to question whether this feature has diagnostic value.

Glomeruli are normal, except in cases with pre-existing chronic nephropathy. In all cases with a nephrotic syndrome, electron microscopy reveals diffuse spreading of epithelial foot processes, which has occasionally been seen in biopsies of non-nephrotic patients. Mild mesangial proliferation or mesangial electron-dense deposits have been observed in a few patients, sometimes associated with membranous and subendothelial deposits (Abraham and Keane 1984; Mitnick and Klein 1984; Marasco *et al.* 1987; Jenkins *et al.* 1988). Immunofluorescence is normal in most studies. Linear C'_3 or IgA staining along the tubular basement membrane has been reported only twice (Chan *et al.* 1980; Bender *et al.* 1984).

14.2.4 Diagnosis

NSAID-associated interstitial nephritis should be suspected when the nephrotic syndrome and renal insufficiency appear together after a few days or weeks of drug exposure. In many cases, renal insufficiency is slowly progressive, and proteinuria is discovered after months of NSAID therapy. Moreover, more than one drug has sometimes been given, and other causes of nephrotic syndrome are then entertained. Features suggestive of an allergic reaction are rarely present; however, they may occur in cases with predominant tubular necrosis (Tables 14.2, 14.3). Patients with NSAID-induced interstitial nephritis often have low fractional excretions of sodium, as is seen in prerenal failure due to the same drugs (Abraham and Keane

1984). This may be misleading when the nephrotic syndrome is absent. Lastly, immunological studies are of little help.

Therefore, when the clinical picture and laboratory tests are not diagnostic, a renal biopsy is indicated. In addition, a search for history of NSAID intake should be made in any patient presenting with unexplained acute renal failure (Adams *et al.* 1986).

14.2.5 Pathogenesis

There is evidence that cases of NSAID-associated interstitial nephritis result from a cell-mediated immune response, as suggested by the prolonged drug exposure, the low incidence of clinical and laboratory signs of hypersensitivity, and the finding that the predominant cells in the interstitial infiltrates are T-lymphocytes with a high proportion of cytotoxic-suppressor (CD8) cells (Finkelstein *et al.* 1982; Stachura *et al.* 1983; Bender *et al.* 1984). Cheng *et al.* (1989) have found that the percentage of CD8 cells and the tubular expression of HLA-DR were greater in the early, than in the late, stages of NSAID-related interstitial nephritis.

It has been postulated that inhibition of prostaglandin synthesis could facilitate lymphokine release by infiltrating lymphocytes and the development of a delayed hypersensitivity reaction, by removing the inhibitory effect of prostaglandins on T-cell function or by shunting arachidonic acid catabolism toward the lipoxygenase pathway (Clive and Stoff 1984). Pro-inflammatory substances, especially leukotriences, are then produced. These substances could, for example, stimulate macrophage adherence to glomerular basement membrane in Bowman's space (Baud *et al.* 1985), explaining the massive proteinuria. The additional necrotizing vasculitis found in a few patients could also occur through a T-cell-dependent mechanism (Finkelstein *et al.* 1982).

Some investigators have made the point that B-lymphocytes can also be seen in the interstitial infiltrates of patients who had taken NSAIDs (Cheng *et al.* 1989), and that their number may be underestimated because recognition with monoclonal antibodies is sometimes unreliable (Pirani *et al.* 1987). Indeed the presence of eosinophils in the blood and in the interstitial infiltrates of a significant number of patients, and the occasional finding of elevated serum IgE levels, suggest that humoral (reaginic) immune factors are also involved in the development of the renal lesions.

In this setting, renal failure could result from the haemodynamic effects of NSAIDs (see Chapter 13) and changes in the glomerular filtration barrier, aggravated by volume contraction due to the nephrotic syndrome, and from the additive effects of interstitial nephritis (Abraham and Keane 1984).

14.2.6 Treatment

Guidelines for management of patients with NSAID-related nephrotoxicity, including interstitial nephritis, are given in Table 14.4. The value of

Table 14.4 *Management of non-steroidal anti-inflammatory drug-associated nephropathy*

1. Withdraw the responsible drug(s)
2. Avoid structurally related drugs and any other NSAIDs
3. Use supportive care and dialysis (if needed)
4. Use corticosteroids if no improvement within 2 weeks
5. Perform renal biopsy if:
   no improvement within 2 weeks of drug withdrawal
   evidence of a glomerular lesion other than minimal change nephrotic syndrome
   unexpected functional deterioration of previously diagnosed renal disease
   active lesions susceptible to treatment likely to be present

According to Pirani *et al.* (1987).

prednisone therapy is unknown. However, there is some evidence that prednisone may hasten recovery in drug-induced acute interstitial nephritis with epithelioid granulomas, when the outcome is more severe and residual renal damage more frequent than in cases without granulomas (Kleinknecht *et al.* 1988).

Although rare and unpredictable, episodes can be prevented or curtailed by monitoring for proteinuria and rising serum creatinine or urea nitrogen in any patient in whom NSAID therapy is initiated.

14.3 Acute tubular necrosis

Tubular necrosis is frequently found in NSAID-induced nephrotoxicity (Table 14.5). Renal tubular toxicity has been mentioned after large doses of NSAIDs in animal studies and suggested in humans taking NSAIDs by the presence in the urine of desquamating epithelial cells and of brush border enzymes of tubular origin (Stygles and Iuliucci 1981). This lesion can be found on biopsy or autopsy following exposure to most NSAIDs available on the market, especially fenoprofen and indomethacin (Carmichael and Shankel 1985; Kleinknecht *et al.* 1986) (Table 14.1). A review of our experience and data from the literature demonstrates that patients with NSAID-induced tubular necrosis and prerenal failure share many features (Table 14.3). Acute tubular necrosis probably represents the most severe expression of the haemodynamic injury due to NSAIDs (Garella and Matarese 1984).

Pathological studies show that there is an overlap between tubular necrosis and other structural renal lesions associated with NSAIDs. Some degree of superimposed interstitial inflammation has been reported (Doyle *et al.* 1983; Thomsen *et al.* 1983; Jao 1986). Minimal change glomerulopathy (Jao 1986), membranous nephropathy (Zech *et al.* 1982), endocapillary proliferation

Table 14.5 *Renal syndromes associated with non-steroidal anti-inflammatory drugs*

	Number	Per cent
Hypoperfusion with acute renal failure	40	14.6
Acute interstitial nephritis	51	18.6
Nephrotic syndrome	34	12.4
Acute tubular necrosis	29	10.6
Papillary necrosis	53	19.3
Acute glomerulonephritis or vasculitis	13	4.7
Uncertain	102	37.2

According to Carmichael and Shankel (1985). Total number of patients = 274; some had more than one syndrome.

(Kleinknecht *et al.* 1989), and mesangial proliferative lupus glomerulopathy (Fong and Cohen 1982; Trèves *et al.* 1983) were associated lesions in other cases. Multi-organ involvement, especially hepatic, was present in the patients described by Monnin *et al.* (1984), Patmas *et al.* (1984), and Marsepoil *et al.* (1987). However, no renal biopsy was perfomed in the two patients reported by Patmas *et al.* (1984). Since a majority of patients with NSAID-associated renal failure do not undergo renal biopsy (Kleinknecht *et al.* 1986, 1989), acute tubular necrosis is often diagnosed clinically.

Rhabdomyolysis has been reported in some patients taking clometacin, pirprofen (Kleinknecht *et al.* 1986), ibuprofen (Ross and Hoppel 1987), and niflumic acid (Desvignes *et al.* 1988). A partial deficiency of muscle carnitine palmitoyl-transferase-A was associated in the case of Ross and Hoppel (1987).

Intravascular haemolysis with acute renal failure has been described after taking naproxen, zomepirac (Patmas *et al.* 1984), and aspirin (Hubert *et al.* 1984). In the last case, an IgM anti-aspirin antibody was present in serum.

14.4 Minimal change nephrotic syndrome

Patients taking NSAIDs may develop nephrotic syndrome without interstitial nephritis. This was the case in 11 per cent of the patients reviewed by Abraham and Keane (1984), and 12 per cent of patients in the series of Carmichael and Shankel (1985). In the experience of Warren *et al.* (1989), 9 per cent of adult patients with minimal change disease had taken NSAIDs.

The drugs involved include phenylbutazone (Greenstone *et al.* 1981), fenoprofen (Stillman *et al.* 1982; Artinano *et al.* 1986; Warren *et al.* 1989), and tolmetin (Chatterjee 1981; Feinfeld *et al.* 1984; Warren *et al.* 1989). Anecdotal reports have implicated ibuprofen (Regester 1980), naproxen

(Schwartzman and D'Agati 1987), pirprofen (Hannedouche *et al.* 1986), zomepirac (Bander 1985), alclofenac (Vereerstraeten *et al.* 1982), diclofenac (Beun *et al.* 1987), piroxicam (Kleinknecht *et al.* 1989), sulindac (Lomvardias *et al.* 1981), salsalate (Vallès and Tovar 1987), aspirin (Kleinknecht *et al.* 1986; Stavanc and Favre 1986), and a combination of aspirin, indomethacin, and diclofenac (Joh *et al.* 1990). In some cases, a combination of four (Kleinknecht *et al.* 1986), or even eight, different NSAIDs had been taken (Robinson *et al.* 1990).

Patients, in general, were female and had received NSAIDs for months before proteinuria was discovered. Acute renal failure may or may not have been present. No patient developed fever, rash, or eosinophilia. A complete remission was usually achieved within 3–4 weeks of simply discontinuing the drug. Some patients had a second episode of proteinuria after resuming the same drug (Vereerstraeten *et al.* 1982; Vallès and Tovar 1987), and a spontaneous relapse of nephrotic syndrome without drug re-exposure has once occurred (Schwartzman and D'Agati 1987). In only two instances was there a progression to focal glomerulosclerosis with severe renal failure (Artinano *et al.* 1986; Pagniez *et al.* 1988).

Renal biopsies examined by light microscopy showed normal glomeruli, sometimes with mild or moderate mesangial cellularity (Warren *et al.* 1989). The only ultrastructural finding was spreading of epithelial cell foot processes. Immunofluorescence studies showed no significant glomerular deposits. This form of NSAID-induced renal damage cannot be distinguished pathological from idiopathic minimal change disease.

14.5 Other glomerulopathies

14.5.1 Membranous nephropathy

A few cases of membranous nephropathy have been attributed to the use of diclofenac (Ducret *et al.* 1980; Hurault de Ligny *et al.* 1984; Clèdes *et al.* 1988; Campistol *et al.* 1989), fenoprofen (Zech *et al.* 1982), ketoprofen (Sennesael *et al.* 1986) and sulindac (Champion de Crespigny *et al.* 1988). Acute interstitial nephritis (Clèdes *et al.* 1988; Campistol *et al.* 1989), and tubular necrosis were sometimes associated in the renal biopsy (Zech *et al.* 1982). All patients had proteinuria which diminished within weeks when the responsible NSAID was stopped, but persistence of mild proteinuria was observed in 3 patients after a period of 12 weeks to 3 yr.

These cases demonstrate that an immune-complex pathogenetic mechanism may operate in some NSAID-related nephropathies, in addition to a reaginic or to a cell-mediated type.

14.5.2 Proliferative glomerulonephritis

Focal or diffuse proliferative glomerulonephritis, with or without crescents, has been found in a few patients taking NSAIDs (Hamilton *et al.* 1979;

Bender *et al.* 1984; Jenkins *et al.* 1988; Kleinknecht *et al.* 1989). Glomerulonephritis was usually associated with other renal lesions, either interstitial infiltrates or tubular necrosis. It is to be recalled that mild or moderate mesangial hypercellularity is not unusual in typical NSAID-induced interstitial nephritis, and that some patients have clinical features that overlap into three different categories of renal damage (see above). The pathophysiology of these findings is unclear.

14.6 Papillary necrosis and chronic renal failure

Prolonged administration to animals of many NSAIDs has caused papillary necrosis (Clive and Stoff 1984; Garella and Matarese 1984; Chapter 3), but there are few reports of histologically or radiographically confirmed human cases. Aspirin, with or without other NSAIDs, phenylbutazone, and indomethacin, accounted for most of the earlier cases (Carmichael and Shankel 1985; Chapters 3 and 4). More recently, chronic interstitial nephritis or acute renal failure associated with papillary necrosis has been documented after fenoprofen (Husserl *et al.* 1979), ibuprofen (Shah *et al.* 1981; Rossi *et al.* 1988), naproxen (Caruana and Semble 1984), mefenamic acid (Robertson *et al.* 1980), and piroxicam (Adams *et al.* 1986).

Papillary necrosis was sometimes diagnosed a few weeks or months after receiving the drug. Renal failure was often irreversible or partially reversible. No other cause for papillary necrosis, such as diabetes or sickle cell anaemia, was present in these patients. Nanra (1989*b*) recently reported 26 patients who had taken (often multiple) NSAIDs continously for periods of 9 months to over 20 yr. He found that papillary necrosis developed in 8, and chronic interstitial nephritis in 16. Four patients whose renal function had deteriorated, had pre-existing analgesic nephropathy. The clinical syndrome was very similar to that described in analgesic nephropathy.

Medullary ischaemia seems an initiating factor in producing papillary necrosis, and drugs that inhibit cyclooxygenase are prone to reduce medullary blood flow. Indeed, given to anaesthetized animals, NSAIDs cause medullary ischaemia (Clive and Stoff 1984), and in other experiments, indomethacin aggravates the hypoxic cellular damage to the thick ascending limb of Henle (Heyman *et al.* 1988). In addition, pre-existing analgesic nephropathy (Nanra 1989*b*), and acute pyelonephritis (Atkinson *et al.* 1986), seem to favour the nephrotoxicity of NSAIDs, further suggesting that in this setting impaired medullary circulation may play a critical role in inducing papillary necrosis and chronic renal injury.

14.7 Other lesions

Two cases of renal cortical necrosis have been reported after the use of zomepirac (Darwish *et al.* 1984) and ibuprofen (Schneider 1986), possibly related to an anaphylactoid reaction.

A generalized vasculitis was attributed to piroxicam in two patients, and to mefenamate in one. The lesion was reversible in the first two cases after discontinuing the drug (Garella and Matarese 1984).

Two patients developed reversible Schönlein-Henoch purpura after taking piroxicam (Goebel and Mueller-Brodmann 1982).

14.7.1 Tubular obstruction

14.7.1.1 Glafenin

This aminochloroquinoline derivative, formerly used as an analgesic in France and a few other European countries, caused 15–20 per cent of drug-induced acute renal failure reported from French nephrology units (Kleinknecht *et al.* 1986, 1989). Only one-third used the drug for therapeutic reasons, the remainder taking high doses for suicide. Acute renal failure was non-oliguric and of short duration, and renal recovery was the rule. Biopsy, when performed, showed mild focal tubular necrosis rather than interstitial nephritis (Kleinknecht *et al.* 1986).

The drug acts through intratubular obstruction, but also through inhibition of prostaglandin formation. Treatment is directed at inducing diuresis with saline and frusemide.

14.7.1.2 Suprofen

Severe flank pain, haematuria, and reversible acute renal failure have been described in previously healthy individuals after only a few doses of suprofen (Hart *et al.* 1987), a new NSAID of the phenylpropionic acid group, now withdrawn from the market. This drug is chemically related to tricrynafen, a uricosuric diuretic, but it is not clearly stated whether or not suprofen can induce intratubular obstruction by uric acid crystals.

14.7.1.3 Myeloma

Three patients with unrecognized myeloma presented with severe acute renal failure after taking naproxen (Wu *et al.* 1987; Shpilberg *et al.* 1990). None was dehydrated. Autopsy on the last patient revealed large hyaline casts around proximal and distal tubular cells. Whatever the mechanism of this lesion, naproxen, and possibly all NSAIDs, should be avoided in myeloma, even in patients with normal renal function.

14.8 Conclusions

The effect of NSAIDs on intrarenal prostglandin synthesis seems to be the chief factor, in the majority of instances, of their nephrotoxicity, whether acute or chronic. However in a proportion of cases, an immunological component which appears to involve T-lymphocyte and/or macrophage dysfunction, dominates the acute renal lesion, resulting in a condition which comprises interstitial nephritis and minimal change nephrotic syndrome to varying degrees. In others, toxicity which resembles classical analgesic nephropathy characterized by papillary necrosis, or the acute nephrotoxic effects of paracetamol with tubular necrosis (Chapter 15), is seen.

15
Paracetamol-induced renal tubular cell necrosis

Staffan Björck

The effects of overdoses of paracetamol (acetaminophen), a widely used anti-pyretic–analgesic are well characterized. Large doses result in liver cell necrosis which is likely to be an effect of a toxic metabolite formed within the liver (Potter *et al.* 1973). A significant proportion of patients with severe intoxication also develops acute renal failure. This is not surprising since hepatic failure, irrespective of cause, may be accompanied by renal failure due to hypotension, infection, or a hepatorenal syndrome. Recently, however, cases have been reported with acute renal failure after paracetamol ingestion in the absence of hepatic failure, indicating that paracetamol can be directly nephrotoxic. The nephrotoxic potential of high dose paracetamol is supported by experimental studies demonstrating that renal lesions can appear independently of liver damage.

15.1 Experimental evidence

It had been reported that paracetamol intoxication did not result in renal toxicity (Calder *et al.* 1971; Peters *et al.* 1972; Mitchell *et al.* 1973*a*), but histological renal damage has since been described (Mitchell *et al.* 1977). McMurtry *et al.* (1978), after initial failures, developed an animal model for paracetamol induced renal failure. In a carefully controlled study, they found varying degrees of renal tubular necrosis in Fischer rats after acute paracetamol intoxication. The lesions appeared as early as 6 h after injection when secondary renal effects are unlikely to have occurred. Besides paracetamol alone, additional groups of animals were either treated with an inhibitor of cytochrome p450 or a hepatic enzyme inducer. Enzyme induction markedly exaggerated the liver damage without affecting the degree of renal injury, but the enzyme inhibitor reduced the severity of both liver and kidney damage. The results indicate that the renal lesions were not secondary to hepatic failure, and might be produced by a different mechanism.

Recently, Bartolone *et al.* (1989) showed in mice that paracetamol binds covalently to proteins in liver, lung, and kidney. These organs expressed toxicity in their experiment. Protein binding did not occur in spleen and heart which did not undergo necrosis. This supports the view that a paracetamol metabolite prone to bind covalently to macromolecules mediates toxicity, and that tissues capable of producing reactive metabolites are subject to necrosis when the detoxifying pathways are saturated. The ability of the kidney to activate paracetamol metabolically has been shown in several studies (Hart *et al.* 1980; Carpenter and Mudge 1981; Moldéus *et al.* 1982; Newton *et al.* 1983*a*). Variability in the extent of renal involvement can be attributed to unexplained differences between strains or species (Newton *et al.* 1983*a*; Tarloff *et al.* 1988). Several metabolic pathways have been proposed to lead to the formation of toxic metabolites (Potter *et al.* 1973; Carpenter and Mudge 1981; Moldéus *et al.* 1982). Even within the kidney, different structures may be damaged by different mechanisms (Henry and Tange 1987).

15.1.1 Histological findings in experimental animals

The first lesions seen appearing within 12 to 24 h are nuclear pyknosis and karyorrhexis, followed by necrosis confined primarily to the distal portions of the proximal tubules, while the glomeruli remain uninvolved (McMurtry *et al.* 1978). The findings thus seem non-specific and resemble those from other toxic substances. The distribution may vary between species or strains, and both medullary and cortical lesions are described. Ultrastructurally, Henry and Tange (1987) found epithelial cell necrosis in the distal third of the proximal convoluted tubule. In the papilla they found epithelial cell necrosis and also involvement of the vascular endothelium with swelling and some cellular degeneration, adhesion of platelets, dilatation of organelles, and fibrin in the capillary lumens. Although beyond the scope of this review, in another study, chronic paracetamol administration resulted in loss of interstitial cells, and necrosis of the walls of the thin limbs of Henle's loop and of blood vessels in the papilla (Molland 1978). Cortical changes were not sought in this study.

15.2 Clinical observations

Patients with liver failure due to paracetamol intoxication often develop renal failure (MacLean *et al.* 1968; Prescott *et al.* 1976; Prescott 1980; Smith *et al.* 1978; Hamlyn *et al.* 1978 Jeffery and Lafferty 1981; Keaton 1988). In a series of 38 patients, 4 developed biopsy-proven acute renal failure (Douglas *et al.* 1976). The details of the findings were not reported. In another study, 6 of 11 patients surviving intoxication developed renal failure, and these showed varying degrees of acute tubular necrosis on histology (Dixon 1976). Only 3 of these 6 patients had hepatic failure. Whether or not the renal failure is due to a direct nephrotoxic effect of paracetamol, or is in some way secondary to the hepatic failure has been debated. In a survey of 160 patients with fulminant liver failure, 53 with paracetamol intoxication, the frequency of renal failure was similar irrespective of the origin of the liver damage

(Wilkinson *et al.* 1977). In patients with less severe liver damage and no encephalopathy, the frequency of renal failure after paracetamol was 6 per cent, and in viral hepatitis 7 per cent. In patients with hepatic failure, 53 per cent in the paracetamol group and 38 per cent in the viral hepatitis group had a serum creatinine above 400 μmol/l. Endotoxinaemia, demonstrated in most cases, was suggested to be a pathogenetic factor. It was concluded that renal failure is not more common in paracetamol intoxication than in liver failure from other causes.

In a retrospective study, Cobden *et al.* (1982) identified 10 patients with acute renal failure in the absence of fulminant liver damage. A poor correlation was found between the severity of the liver damage and the development of renal failure. Since then, more patients are described with acute renal failure despite absence of hepatic failure (Prescott *et al.* 1976; Prescott 1980; Kleinman *et al.* 1980; Curry *et al.* 1982; Dabbagh and Chesney 1985; Pillans and Hall 1985; Denison *et al.* 1987; Björck *et al.* 1988; Davenport and Finn 1988).

15.2.1 Nephrotoxicity with no or little liver damage

There are also a few published cases of acute renal failure without signs of liver damage (Kher and Makker 1987). Gabriel *et al.* (1982) described two patients with normal liver function tests and moderate renal failure. The paracetamol dose was within the therapeutic range and renal biopsies showed only healing tubular necrosis.

We have seen nine cases of renal failure in which the causal effect of paracetamol seems likely (Table 15.1). Seven have been previously described (Björck *et al.* 1988). Only three of the patients had severe liver damage and one of these had cerebral symptoms with somnolence. In most cases the intake was associated with other drugs or alcohol.

15.3 Clinical presentation

The rise in liver enzymes after paracetamol ingestion is seen within 24 h, and peak values after 2–4 days (Proudfoot and Wright 1970). The serum creatinine rises more slowly than the liver enzymes; this does not necessarily reflect later onset of the kidney damage but the rate of accumulation of creatinine in serum. When severe, the peak is seen after 6–12 days (Boyer and Rouff 1971; Curry *et al.* 1982; Dabbagh and Chesney 1985; Björck *et al.* 1988), and earlier when milder. Gastrointestinal discomfort or pain is frequent, and sometimes there is pain, which may be severe, localized over the kidneys, appearing within 24 h after ingestion (Kleinman *et al.* 1980; Gabriel *et al.* 1982; Pillans and Hall 1985; Björck *et al.* 1988). There may be microscopic hematuria (Gabriel *et al.* 1982; Björck *et al.* 1988). Renal function is reported to return to normal, even in severe cases (Kleinman *et al.*

Table 15.1 *Clinical observations in nine patients with paracetamol-induced tubular necrosis*

Age/sex	Paracetamol dose	Exposure time	Maximum serum creatinine	Maximum serum alanine aminotransferase[1]	Day of renal biopsy
(yr)	(g)	(days)	(μmol/l)	(μkat/l)	
28/M	7.5	1	350	0.4	8
40/M	0.8	1	907	0.5	8
54/M	20	7	1264	1	..
18/M	88	47	442	1.2	53
39/M	8	1	1274	1.9	..
44/F	5–10 daily	> 30	533	6.5	..
51/M	45	7	1190	75	..
37/M	23	1	991	88	..
34/M	10	2	1237	230	..

[1] Normal < 0.7 μkat/l.

1980; Dabbagh and Chesney 1985; Björck *et al.* 1988). Repeat biopsies have not been reported. An increased susceptibility to liver and kidney damage has been suspected in alcoholics (Kaysen *et al.* 1985; Leist *et al.* 1985; Seeff *et al.* 1986; Denison *et al.* 1987), but not confirmed when the relation between dose and toxicity has been compared between alcoholics and non-alcoholics in a larger number of patients (Rumack 1983).

15.4 Histological findings in patients

Microscopic examination has been performed on renal tissue, obtained either by percutaneous needle biopsy or at autopsy. The interpretation of the findings may be confounded by the confused clinical settings, commonly with hypotension and septicaemia. Most often the histological appearances are mentioned briefly and are described as tubular necrosis (Proudfoot and Wright 1970; Douglas *et al.* 1976; Gabriel *et al.* 1982; Kaysen *et al.* 1985; Davenport and Finn 1988). Kleinman *et al.* (1980) however reported in more detail of a case with only slight liver damage after paracetamol ingestion. A biopsy revealed severe focal coagulation necrosis of the proximal convoluted tubules. Electron microscopy showed normal glomerular structure and varying degrees of tubular damage. The renal function returned to normal despite severe renal failure.

In our series of nine patients with paracetamol associated renal failure we performed renal biopsies of cortical tissue in three. We also found focal

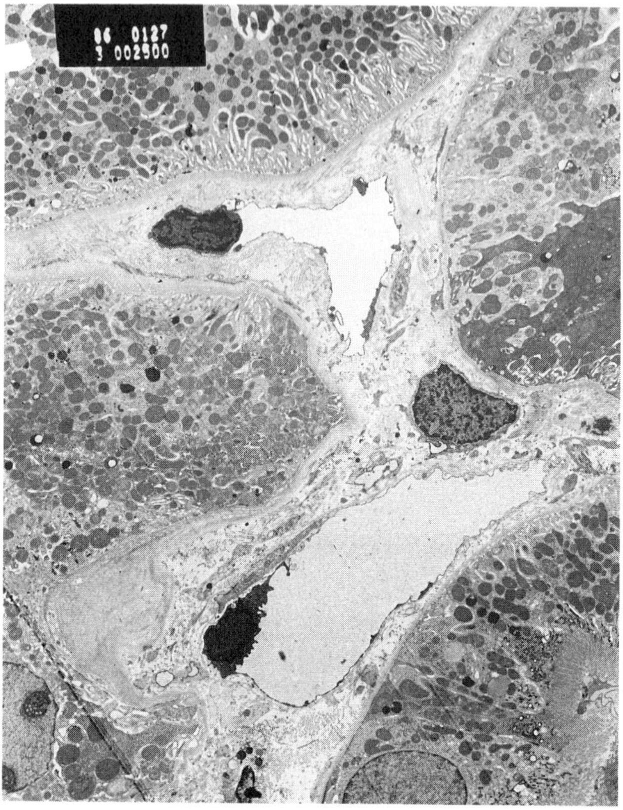

Fig. 15.1 Two peritubular capillaries showing varying degrees of endothelial cell damage and pericapillary oedema. In the lower capillary, note different electron density of adjacent endothelial cell lining of capillary lumen. High density indicates severe damage. Tubular epithelium is also damaged with intracellular oedema and, to the right, partial dissolution of intracellular components. (Electron micrograph; magnification × 3000).

tubular necrosis in both the proximal and the distal tubules. In addition, we unexpectedly found evidence for vascular damage, with arteriolar endothelial necrosis or pyknosis in the peritubular vessels in all three patients, and damage to vascular smooth muscle cells in two. Endothelial lesions were also found in pertubular capillaries (Fig. 15.1). In one patient, necrotic endothelium was found in otherwise normal glomeruli adjacent to normal endothelial cells (Fig. 15.2). Whether these vascular lesions are of pathogenetic importance is not clear, but similar vascular damage has been proposed to lead to secondary renal interstitial fibrosis in cyclosporin-treated patients

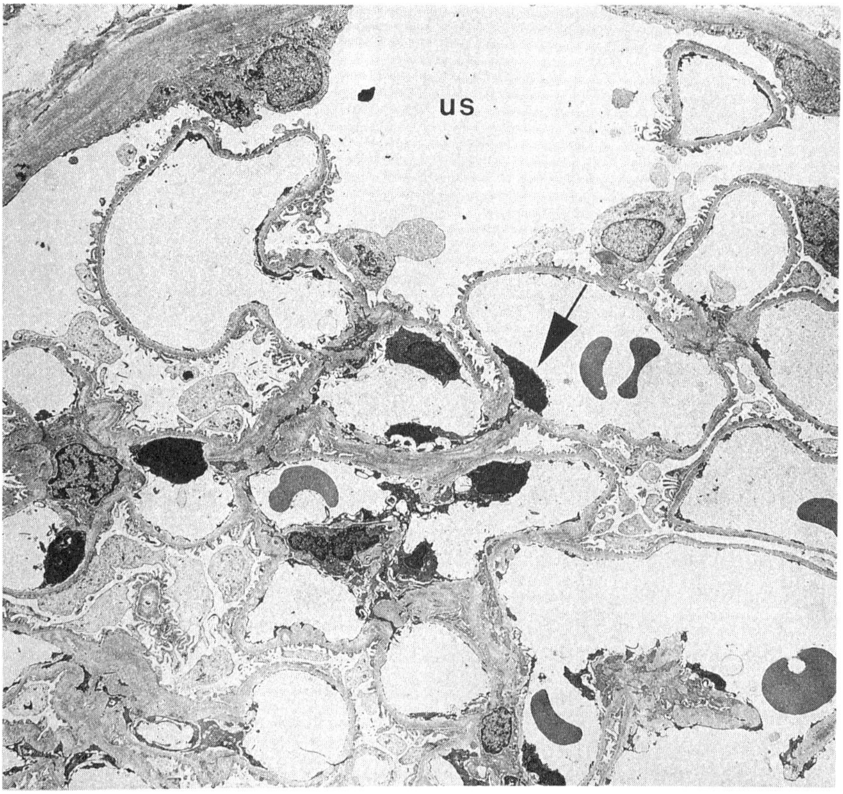

Fig. 15.2 Glomerular capillary lined by damaged endothelial cells, one of which is indicated by arrow. Epithelial and mesangial cells are intact. (Electron micrograph; magnification × 1750). us = Urinary space.

(Mihatsch *et al.* 1985), and as a mechanism leading to chronic analgesic nephropathy (Mihatsch *et al.* 1983*a*).

15.5 Summary

In summary, evidence shows that acute tubular necrosis can be produced by paracetamol intoxication in experimental animals and in humans. Renal toxicity is usually obscured by the greater susceptibility of the liver to toxic damage but in occasional patients, for unknown reasons, renal failure is the dominating lesion. The renal damage is most likely produced by a toxic metabolite, but whether the mechanism is similar to that in the liver is unknown.

16

Experimental evidence and the biochemical basis for the role of analgesics in cancer

Peter H. Bach

Urothelioma represents a small proportion of all human malignancies (Hicks 1980), the background incidence of upper urothelial carcinoma (UUC) being between 1 : 183 000 and 1 : 156 000 (Bengtsson *et al.* 1968, 1978). Renal pelvic, ureteral, and bladder neoplasms occur more commonly in patients who have abused mixed analgesics or who suffer from Balkan endemic nephropathy (Chernozemsky *et al.* 1977). There are, however, marked differences between the clinical features and the gross pathology in these two nephropathies, and it is difficult to find aetiological factors in common. Whereas renal papillary necrosis (RPN) is the earliest and main lesion associated with analgesic abuse (Bach and Bridges 1985), patients with Balkan nephropathy show extensive degenerative changes in the renal cortex, and the medulla does not appear to be primarily affected (Hall and Dammin 1978). Its aetiology is thought to be associated with mycotoxins (Chernozemsky *et al.* 1977; WHO 1979; Berndt *et al.* 1980).

That the tumours are typically multiple, diffuse, poorly differentiated, and rapidly spreading (Lomax-Smith and Seymour 1980*a*,*b*; Mihatsch and Knüsli 1982) makes UUC in analgesic abusers particularly pernicious (Bach and Bridges 1985; Eknoyan *et al.* 1982).

16.1 Urothelial tumours—induction and initiation

Our understanding of the processes of chemically-mediated carinogenesis (Williams and Weisburger 1986) has been derived largely from animal investigations (Lijinsky 1988) which have focused on the multistage model, involving chemical induction by a genotoxic event and promotion by one or more modulating factors (Farber and Sporn 1976; Farber 1976, 1984; Kunze 1979; Hicks 1980, 1983*a*,*b*; Rice and Frith 1981; Cohen 1985). These models are being revised to take into account the role of oncogenes (Willman and Fenoglio-Preiser 1987).

Most research in urothelial malignancy has been on the bladder. The transitional epithelium that lines the bladder, ureter, renal pelvis, calyces, and papillae is derived from one embryological structure (Melicow 1945) and has a similar histological appearance throughout, although there are differences in thickness and surface characteristics (Newman and Hicks 1981). It has been common to grade UUC on the same basis as bladder cancer, and to extrapolate concepts of urinary bladder carcinogenesis to the ureter and renal pelvis.

16.2 The aetiological role of analgesic abuse

The statistical association between long-term analgesic abuse and UUC is strong (Bengtsson *et al.* 1968; Johansson *et al.* 1974; McCredie *et al.* 1982*a*, 1983*a*,*b*), and that with renal papillary necrosis even stronger (McCredie *et al.* 1986). However, that Balkan nephropathy does not have such an aetiology demonstrates that other factors cannot be excluded from the genesis of UUC. For instance, there are rare reports of a genetic susceptibility to transitional cell carcinoma of the renal pelvis (Frischer *et al.* 1985; Orphali *et al.* 1986).

16.2.1 Phenacetin—an aetiological red herring

Despite the fact that it was co-formulated with other analgesics, many of the early investigations were undertaken on the assumption that phenacetin was the primary cause of RPN and (by implication) UUC. It is now generally appreciated that phenacetin is one of a series of papillotoxic agents (Table 16.1). Several hypotheses have been put forward to explain analgesic nephropathy (Rosner 1976; Shelley 1978; Prescott 1982*a*), some of which can be disregarded (Bach and Bridges 1985).

Early speculation on the mechanisms of phenacetin nephrotoxicity favoured the formation of biologically reactive intermediates through cytochrome p450-mediated metabolism (Nery 1971; Mudge *et al.* 1978; Hinson 1983; Fischbach and Lenk 1985*a*,*b*; Veronese *et al.* 1985) (Table 16.2). None is now thought to be implicated in the lesion of RPN or UUC because of the absence of the mixed function oxidase enzymes from the medulla. As the ultimate toxicant(s) or carcinogens must be highly reactive, their half-life(s) must be short, and their toxic effects local.

Attention has shifted towards the key role of paracetamol (acetaminophen) in the development of RPN and UUC (Hiraga and Fujii 1985). Up to 80 per cent of phenacetin is metabolized to paracetamol, which in turn is excreted in the urine as glucuronide (55 per cent) and sulphate (30 per cent) conjugates (Clissold 1986). *O*-glucuronides may react directly with urothelium, whereas *N*-glucuronides can be hydrolysed to free *N*-hydroxy-aromatic amines, which can be metabolically activated (Kadlubar *et al.* 1977; McQueen *et al.* 1987).

Conflicting data are yielded by carcinogenicity bioassays due to such variables as species differences, purity of test chemical, and dietary and environmental factors. Macklin and Szot (1980) have argued that the formulation

Table 16.1 *Drugs and chemicals that have been associated with papillotoxicity in animals*

Antipyretic–analgesics	Non-steroidal anti-inflammatory drugs	Other drugs	Chemicals, etc.
aminopyrine	aclofenac	cyclophosphamide	2-bromoethanamine HBr
5-aminosalicylic acid	bucloxic acid	dapsone	3-bromopropanamine HCl
antipyrine	fenoprofen	phenothiazine	2-chloro-*N*, *N*-dimethylethanamine
aspirin	flufenamic acid	sulphinpyrazone	diphenyl
A P C	ibuprofen	L-tri-iodothyronine	diphenylamine
A P Codeine	indomethacin		diphenylmethyl alcohol
glafenine	ketophenbutazone		etoxuquin
paracetamol	ketoprofen		ethyleneimine
phenacetin	meclofenamic acid		4-isopropylbiphenyl
	mefanamic acid		mono-*N*-methylaniline
	naproxen		1-naphthol
	niflumic acid		phenylalkanoic acid
	oxyphenbutazone		*N*-phenylanthranilic acid
	phenylbutazone		propyleneimine
	piroxicam		tetrahydroxyquinoline
	sudoxicam		
	tolfenamic acid		
	tolmetin		

Updated from Bach and Bridges (1985) and Bach and Gregg (1988).

Table 16.2 *Possible reactive metabolites of phenacetin generated by cytochrome p450 and related mixed functional oxidase enzymes*

N-hydroxyphenacetin
N-hydroxy-4-phenetidine
Phenacetin *N*-hydroxylation
N–O sulphate
N–O glucuronic acid conjugates
O-de-ethylation to paracetamol
Paracetamol quinolimine
N-hydroxylation
O-de-ethylation
3,4-epoxide

of phenacetin into pellets or cubes would result in the generation of *N*-oxide and *N*-nitroso compounds. Thus studies using powdered diet typically give negative carcinogenicity data for phenacetin, whereas those using pelletted or cubed diets cause ear and nasal, liver, mammary, bladder, and renal parenchymal tumours, a pattern characteristic of *N*-nitroso compounds. The relevance of studies using pelleted phenacetin-containing diets to UUC in man appears to be limited.

16.2.2 Analgesics as carcinogens

The potential for single and mixed analgesics to cause cancer has been reviewed by the International Agency for Research on Cancer (IARC 1980, 1982, 1987):

1. The data from humans are not as clear as initially considered (Hultengren *et al.* 1965; Angervall *et al.* 1969; Mahony *et al.* 1977), because many of the early epidemiological conclusions were biased by recording only phenacetin intake, not that of other analgesics.
2. There has been no consistent evidence from short-term tests to suggest that mixed analgesics were carcinogens, and only limited evidence to implicate phenacetin (Table 16.3).
3. In animal studies, numerous investigations have been undertaken on phenacetin, but relatively few on mixed analgesics (Table 16.4). The results are equivocal, the IARC concluding that analgesic mixtures containing phenacetin were probably carcinogenic, although most tumours so induced were elsewhere than in the urinary tract. There was limited evidence to implicate phenacetin alone, only phenazone appearing to be carcinogenic on its own.

Table 16.3 *Potential mutagenic effects of phenacetin in a panel of* in vitro *tests*

Salmonella typhimurium (Strain TA 100)	
presence of hamster liver microsomes	+ ve Ames test
presence of mouse or rat liver mocrosomes	– ve Ames test
urine from phenacetin-treated hamsters	+ ve Ames test
N-hydroxyphenacetin	+ ve Ames test
Chinese hamster fibroblasts	+ ve chromosomal aberrations
rat lymphocyte chromosomal aberrations	marginal increase
sister chromatid exchange	doubling
mouse erythrocytes exposed *in vitro*	no micronuclei
Drosophilia melanogaster	no recessive lethal defects

From IARC (1980, 1982).

4. Long-term rat bioassays have failed to implicate caffeine or aspirin in malignant changes, and there are no adequate epidemiological or bioassay data from which the possible role of other single or mixed analgesics, or any NSAIDs, could be linked to the development of UUC.

16.3 Experimental models of renal papillary necrosis

Part of the problem in understanding the role of analgesics and RPN in the genesis of UUC is due to rodents (the most frequently studied species for carcinogenicity bioassays) being resistant to the papillotoxic effects of many analgesics and NSAIDs, but sensitive to ulcerogenicity (Bach and Hardy 1985). However, papillotoxins such as 2-bromoethanamine (BEA) hydrobromide cause a selective, dose related, RPN within 24 h (Bach *et al.* 1983). The BEA model shows many functional and morphological changes that parallel those seen in animals treated chronically with analgesics and NSAIDs, and in human analgesic nephropathy (Bach and Hardy 1985).

The early morphological changes caused by BEA are useful to understand the progression of RPN in human analgesic abusers. The initial BEA-induced changes in the staining characteristics of the medullary mucopolysaccharide matrix (Bach *et al.* 1983; Gregg *et al.* 1990*a*,*b*) are similar to those reported in the human disease (Burry *et al.* 1977; Burry 1978; Gloor 1978*a*). The absence of matrix staining continues in animals for more than 6 months, suggesting a permanent change in the medullary mucopolysaccharide. The interstitial cells at the tip of the papilla are the first to undergo degenerative change (Fig. 16.1(a)); followed by involvement of the fine elements of the medulla, such as the loops of Henle and the collecting duct. Microvascular changes appear late in the development of the acute lesion (Gregg *et al.* 1990*b*), although they have been given prominence in the genesis of analgesic

Table 16.4 *Experimental studies for the assessment of mixed and single analgesic carcinogenicity*

Evidence in favour of phenacetin carcinogenicity	
Isaka *et al.* 1979	rats had urothelial hyperplasia and UUC; M : F = 3 : 1
Johansson 1981	rats had renal pelvic and bladder tumours
Evidence against phenacetin carcinogenicity	
Johansson and Angervall 1976*a*,*b*	87% of rats had urothelial hyperplasia and microvascular changes[1]
Macklin and Szot 1980	C57BL/6 mice had no UUC
Nakanishi *et al.* 1982	B6C3F1 mice had no RPN or UUC, but bladder hyperplasia[1]
Ham and Calder 1983	rats had no urothelial tumours[1]
Evidence in favour of mixed analgesic or caffeine carcinogenicity	
Johansson 1981	rats given phenacetin and phenazone had renal pelvic and bladder tumours
Evidence against mixed analgesic or caffeine carcinogenicity	
Johansson 1981	rats given phenazone or phenacetin with caffeine had same number of bladder, but fewer renal pelvic, tumours than with analgesic alone[1]
Macklin and Szot 1980	C57BL/6 mice given APC, or any 2 of the 3 ingredients, had no UUC
Evidence in favour of other single analgesic carcinogenicity	
Johansson 1981	rats given paracetamol or phenazone had renal pelvic or bladder tumours
Evidence against other single analgesic carcinogenicity	
Macklin and Szot 1980	C57BL/6 mice given aspirin had no UUC
Ham and Calder 1983	rats given paracetamol had no UUC[1]
Hiraga and Fujii 1985	rats given paracetamol had no cancers

[1] Caused other organotropic tumours: renal parenchymal, mammary, ear duct, oral and nasal, liver, pituitary, forestomach carcinomas, and myeloid leukaemia, desmoplastic fibroma, sarcoma. Duration of studies 72–110 weeks; analgesics given orally at 2.5% of food intake for phenacetin, 900 mg/kg body weight for phenazone, paracetamol, and caffeine, 840 mg/kg for salicylamide, 250 mg/kg for aspirin.

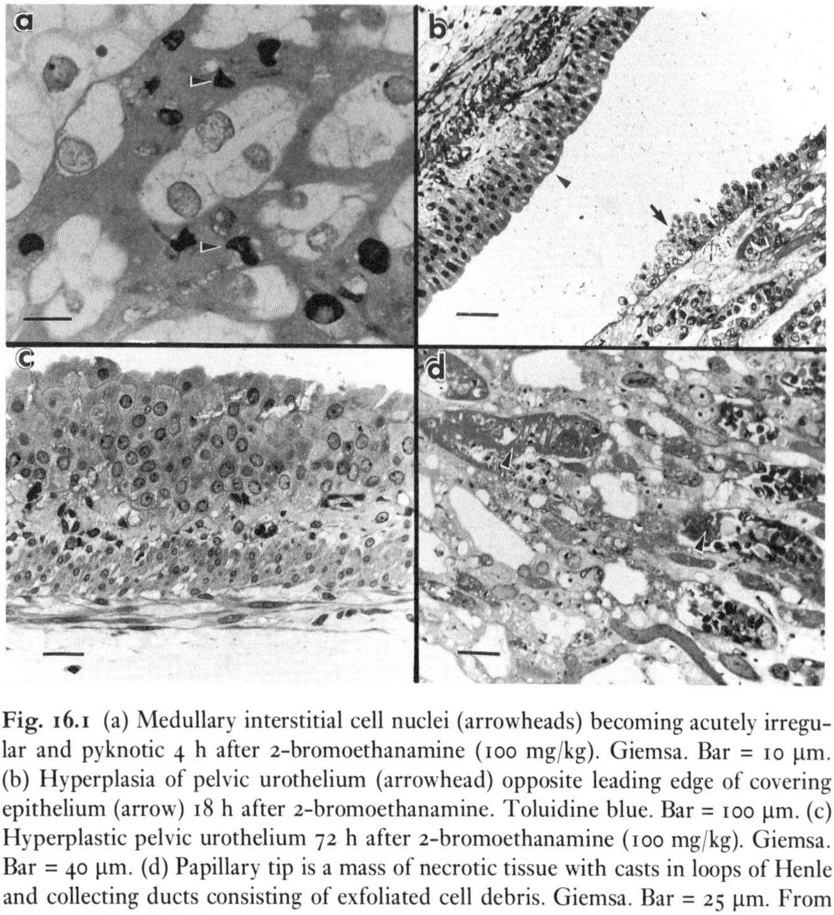

Fig. 16.1 (a) Medullary interstitial cell nuclei (arrowheads) becoming acutely irregular and pyknotic 4 h after 2-bromoethanamine (100 mg/kg). Giemsa. Bar = 10 μm. (b) Hyperplasia of pelvic urothelium (arrowhead) opposite leading edge of covering epithelium (arrow) 18 h after 2-bromoethanamine. Toluidine blue. Bar = 100 μm. (c) Hyperplastic pelvic urothelium 72 h after 2-bromoethanamine (100 mg/kg). Giemsa. Bar = 40 μm. (d) Papillary tip is a mass of necrotic tissue with casts in loops of Henle and collecting ducts consisting of exfoliated cell debris. Giemsa. Bar = 25 μm. From Gregg *et al.* 1989*b* with permission from Plenum.

nephropathy. Active repair occurs between viable tissue and necrotic papillae and there are mitoses in the collecting ducts and loops of Henle; also there is always a marked papillary and pelvic hyperplasia (Fig. 16.1(b,c)).

After a single dose of BEA or *N*-phenylanthranylic acid, the RPN (even if focal) progresses in the long-term, and the kidney undergoes a series of degenerative changes involving the cortex (Sherwood *et al.* 1971; Shimamura *et al.* 1974; Shimamura and Bonk 1976; Bach and Gregg 1988; Bach 1989; Gregg and Bach 1990; Gregg *et al.* 1990*a,b*).

16.3.1 Papillotoxin-induced histochemical changes in renal papillae

A number of histochemical changes may be important because of their diagnostic potential, and because similar staining properties are common in pre-

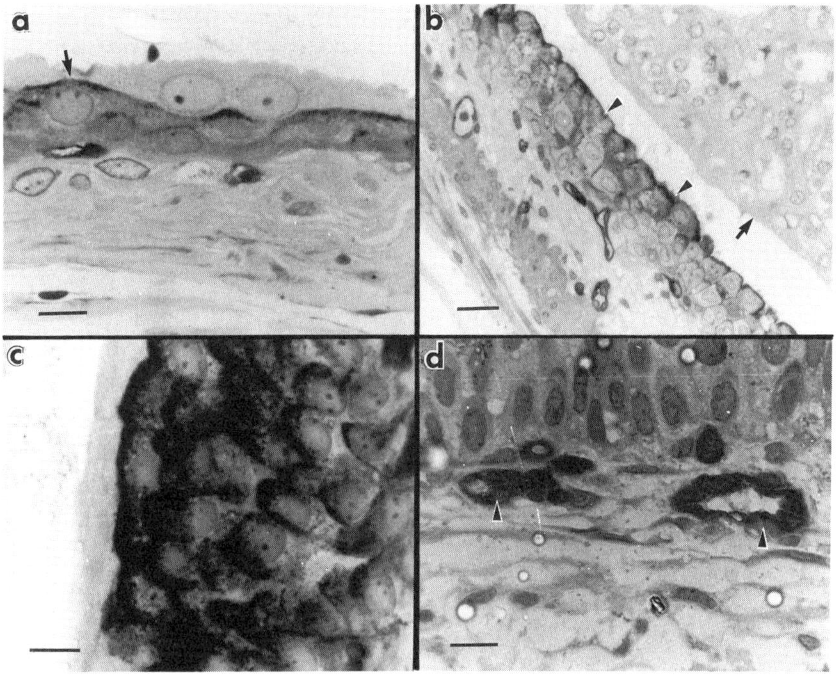

Fig. 16.2 (a) Alkaline phosphatase staining in control bladder urothelium (arrow). The superficial 'umbrella' cell layer is devoid of stain. Bar = 10 μm. (b) Increased alkaline phosphatase staining in pelvic urothelium (arrowheads) opposite denuded covering epithelium (arrow) 8 h after 2-bromoethanamine. Bar = 20 μm. (c) Mosaic pattern of alkaline phosphatase staining in hyperplastic urothelium 18 h after 2-bromoethanamine. Bar = 10 μm. (d) Sub-urothelial capillary endothelium stained with ATPase, with thickness increasing to occlude lumen (arrowheads). Bar = 10 μm. From Gregg *et al.* 1989*b* with permission from Plenum.

malignant and malignant urothelial tissue. BEA causes a change in alkaline phosphatase (Fig. 16.2 (a,b,c)) that is reminiscent of pre-malignancy, but reverts to normal when the burst of urothelial proliferation subsides. By contrast adenosine triphosphatase (ATPase), not normally present in the capillaries, remains in the endothelium of the pelvic microvasculature (Fig. 16.2 (d)) for protracted periods (Gregg *et al.* 1989*b*, 1990*a*,*b*). There is a progressive deposition of neutral lipid material in the capillaries, and then a marked accumulation in the epithelial cells (which normally lack such lipids). These changes extend into the outer medulla which would be assessed as normal by haematoxylin and eosin staining (Bach *et al.* 1991). This pattern of lipid staining appears to be pathognomonic for RPN induced by several methods (Bach *et al.* 1987; Gregg *et al.* 1991*a*). It is also seen in human analgesic abusers (Munck *et al.* 1970), but not as a consequence of other types of renal injury (Bach *et al.* 1991). There is also an intracellular accumulation of PAS-positive inclusion bodies (Gregg *et al.* 1990*a*,*b*), as reported in bladder carcinoma (Hukill and Vidone 1965). These lipid and carbohydrate abnormalities in animals with papillary necrosis are similar to those seen in hyperplastic and dysplastic epithelial cells associated with other malignancies (Kunze and Schauer 1971, 1977; Bannasch 1986*a*,*b*).

16.3.2 The probable mechanism of renal papillary necrosis

The most attractive hypothesis for selective targeting of papilla, pelvis, and upper ureter relates to local medullary metabolic activation of compounds whose effects would be augmented by urine stagnation in the pelvis.

While the absence of cytochrome p450 from the medulla rules out activation by mixed function oxidase systems, many peroxidative enzymes such as the hydroperoxidase activity associated with cyclooxygenase (Marnett *et al.* 1977, 1978; Eling *et al.* 1983; Marnett and Eling 1984) are capable of activation of chemicals (Bach and Bridges 1984, 1985) including the major metabolites of phenacetin, *p*-phenetidine (Andersson *et al.* 1983; Ross *et al.* 1985), and paracetamol (Zenser *et al.* 1979*a*,*b*; Nelson *et al.* 1981*a*; Mohandas *et al.* 1981*a*; Moldéus *et al.* 1982). All of the enzymes involved in prostaglandin synthesis are localized not just to the medullary interstitial cells, but also in the endothelial cells of arteries and arterioles, and in the collecting ducts (Zenser *et al.* 1983*a*; Bach and Bridges 1984). That the medullary interstitial cells contain the high levels of those polyunsaturated fatty acids (Bojesen 1974, 1980) that would predispose to lipid peroxidation if reactive intermediates were generated locally (Bach and Bridges 1984), probably explains why papillotoxins affect predominantly one cell type initially despite the almost ubiquitous distribution of activating enzymes. However, neither paracetamol nor *p*-phenetidine causes RPN in the experimental situation with any degree of reproducibility.

N-phenylanthranylic acid (an analogue of the fenamate NSAIDs) causes a dose-related RPN and almost identical changes in renal function and morphology as do analgesics, NSAIDs, and BEA (Hardy and Bach 1984). Both horseradish peroxidase and prostaglandin synthase from medullary microsomes produce biologically reactive intermediate(s) from *N*-phenylanthranilic acid (Feldman and Bach, unpublished data).

16.3.3 Urothelial hyperplasia following renal papillary necrosis

There is now considerable evidence that urothelial hyperplasia and dysplasia will be found in analgesic abusers (Blohmé and Johansson 1981; Lomax-Smith and Seymour 1980*a*,*b*). It is generally agreed that there is a progression from hyperplasia to dysplasia to malignancy (Williams and

Weisburger 1986); but the earlier stage from proliferative repair to hyperplasia or dysplasia is not clearly established.

Urothelial proliferation is a common, but frequently overlooked, consequence of both chemically induced and spontaneously occurring RPN (Bach and Bridges 1985). Examples include BEA (Axelsen 1978; Bach *et al.* 1983), aspirin (Molland 1976; Henry and Tange 1983), paracetamol (Henry and Tange 1987), *N*-phenylanthranilic acid (Hardy and Bach 1984), ethyleneimine (Ham and Tange 1969, Axelsen 1978), diphenylamine (Hardy 1970*a*,*b*, 1974) and in ageing mice (Gorer 1940), those with amyloid deposits (Dunn 1944), rats fed a fat-free diet long-term (Molland 1982), and the Gunn rat (Axelsen and Burry 1972; Axelsen 1973, 1975; Harper and Axelsen 1982; Henry and Tange 1982; Henry *et al.* 1983).

Papillary urothelial hyperplasia also develops in the absence of RPN, including following phenacetin (Johansson and Angervall 1976*a*,*b*; Isaka *et al.* 1979; Johansson 1981), an indeneacetic acid analogue (Bokelman *et al.* 1971), and feeding with high levels of sodium chloride, monosodium glutamate (Lalich *et al.* 1974), Aroclor 1242 (Bruckner *et al.* 1974), or saccharin (Murasaki *et al.* 1982).

16.3.3.1 Mechanical injury causing urothelial hyperplasia

A role for mechanical and physical injury (glass beads, ulceration by freezing, incisions) has long been established in cell proliferation and hyperplasia in experimental bladder carcinogenesis (Mobley *et al.* 1966). Recently, Cohen and Ellwein (1989, 1990*a*,*b*) and Ellwein and Cohen (1990) have highlighted the importance of mechanical microabrasion from silicate crystals as a contributor to the proliferative bladder changes seen in high dose, long-term, saccharin exposure.

Treatment with BEA causes an intense, but short-lived, magnesium ammonium phosphate crystalluria shortly after dosing (Bach 1990). Birefringent crystals can been seen, but only in neutral red-stained sections of kidney. The most likely explanation is supersaturation of the urine with solute, possibly released from the medullary matrix undergoing degenerative changes (Bach *et al.* 1983). It is not clear if BEA itself affects the urothelium or if the hyperplasia is a consequence of mechanical effects of the crystals.

16.3.3.2 The kinetics of urothelial proliferation following papillary necrosis

The BEA-induced lesion offers an ideal way of assessing urothelial kinetics following papillary injury, and the long-term consequence of RPN in animals with urothelium exposed to a cancer initiator. Renal and urothelial cell proliferation has been assessed in male Wistar rats, with subcutaneously implanted mini-osmotic pumps providing a zero order infusion of ^{3}H-thymidine to amplify cell divisions (Mattingley *et al.* 1991). Autoradiography

Table 16.5 *Comparison of renal cell grain count in kidneys from control and 2-bromoethanamine treated animals after 144 h of ^{3}H-thymidine infusion from subcutaneously implanted mini-osmotic pumps*

Region of kidney	Increase in grain count
Papillary epithelium	> 3 ×
Pelvis adjacent to lesion	> 3 ×
Pelvis adjacent to tip of papilla	> 3 ×
Pelvic fornix	> 15 ×
Collecting duct	> 8 ×
Mouth of ureter	> 3 ×
Proximal tubule	> 3 ×
Distal tubule	> 2 ×
Glomeruli	> 2 ×

of renal sections up to 144 h after dosing showed that proliferation was increased most in the proximal and distal tubules, and in the collecting duct epithelium in the mid-medullary region. The turnover of cells was progress-ively less in pelvic fornix and origin of the ureter, in the pelvis opposite the tip of the papilla and opposite the zone of papillary injury, and least in the area of papillary injury (Table 16.5). The marked pelvic response to an acute RPN, in the absence of major ureteric or bladder change, highlights the focal nature both of the injury and of the urothelial proliferative response.

These data suggest that upper urothelial hyperplasia is an acute response to either RPN, or the release of cellular debris into the pelvis, or a combination of factors. However, the proliferative change is short lived, the hyperplasia returning to normal within 6 months of BEA-induced RPN (Gregg *et al.* unpublished).

There is preliminary evidence that some of the other changes caused in the kidney by papillotoxic substances can exacerbate hyperplasia and contribute to the development of malignancies. This localized proliferative change in the upper urothelium could therefore represent an injury that promoted uncontrolled cell proliferation in any cell population that had already been subjected to genotoxic initiation. In confirmation, Johansson *et al.* (1989) showed an increase in the labelling index of bladder and kidney urothelium associated with urothelial hyperplasia and vacuolated cells after 6 weeks of administration of paracetamol, antipyrine, or phenacetin.

16.4 Experimental models of upper urothelial carcinoma

Based on the current understanding of the mechanism and consequences of acutely induced RPN, the role of two-stage carcinogenesis in upper urothelial carcinoma (UUC) has been reassessed. However, the identification of focal RPN demands painstaking preparation of tissue and careful sectioning to assess the papilla tip (Bach and Hardy 1985). All too often the reported absence of a papillary lesion reflects failure to section the tip, but cortical changes often flag the possibility of such pathology. Changes in the pelvis and ureter of rats are even more subtle, and are rarely systematically addressed.

16.4.1 Spontaneous urothelial carcinoma

Up to 30 per cent of old male Brown Norway rats develop spontaneous bladder tumours (Boorman and Hollander 1974; Boorman *et al.* 1977; Bolhuis *et al.* 1978; Burek 1978), as do up to 50 per cent of male DA/Han rats, with the peak incidence occurring between 25 and 39 months of age; these often are associated with bladder stones (Deerburg *et al.* 1985). There is no information on changes in the ureter or pelvis. Both models have been proposed for studying the human disease, but are unsatisfactory because of variable tumour development, the long latent period, and the low incidence (50 per cent at best).

16.4.2 One-stage models of upper urothelial carcinogenesis

Several complete carcinogens have potential to cause tumours on their own (Williams and Weisburger 1986), possibly due to their ability to initiate, and to promote by causing injury in the same region. All urinary tract carcinogens are thought to be transported to the urothelium via the urine (Cohen *et al.* 1983).

16.4.2.1 FANFT

N-[4-(5-nitro-2-furyl)-2-thiazolyl]formamide (FANFT) has been used as a complete bladder carcinogen (Cohen and Friedell 1979), but more often as the initiating agent for assessing promoters of bladder tumours (Cohen *et al.* 1982). This 5-nitrofuran derivative is nephrotoxic, and the early publications on bladder carcinoma following FANFT treatment reported a few cases of invasive renal pelvic carcinoma and severe hyperplasia of the renal pelvic epithelium (Ertürk *et al.* 1967, 1969). It was suggested that the renal tumours were related to partial urinary obstruction which had caused a significant incidence of hydronephrosis.

Feeding with FANFT causes bladder epithelial hyperplasia in Sprague–Dawley (Ertürk *et al.* 1967, 1969), Fischer (Tiltman and Friedell 1971), and F344 (Jacobs *et al.* 1979) rats at 3 weeks, followed by mitotic activity and squamous metaplasia at 8 weeks, progressing to microscopic papillomata throughout the bladder at 9 weeks and small tumours at 12 weeks, with cellular and nuclear atypia by 25–30 weeks. Tumours enlarge (2 cm at 25 weeks, 3–7 cm by 45 weeks), protrude into the lumen, and invade through to the muscle layer by 45–50 weeks, at which time there is also development of ureteric and renal pelvic tumours with obstruction of ureter and subsequent hydronephrosis in Sprague–Dawley, but not Fischer, rats.

Anderström and Johansson (1983) demonstrated that if male Sprague–Dawley rats were fed 0.2 per cent FANFT for 11 weeks, there was from 30 weeks a 72 per cent incidence of renal pelvic tumours (52 per cent of which were bilateral) as well as a high frequency of tumours in the bladder, the more commonly evaluated target site for FANFT-induced carcinogencity in female rats of this strain.

These data raise several important considerations: upper and lower urothelial carcinoma following FANFT exposure may share a common molecular mechanism; there are major sex- and strain-related differences in the development of tumours; and it seems possible that other bladder carcinogens, which have been overlooked or not reported, could also cause upper urothelial hyperplasia or malignancy.

16.4.3 Two-stage models of upper urothelial carcinogenesis

There is now ample evidence of experimental urothelial carcinoma induction by classical two-stage models, in which various proliferative responses in the upper urothelium represent promotion that will cause cancer following initiation.

16.4.3.1 Bacterial infection as promotion

A high analgesic intake predisposes humans to urinary tract infection (UTI) (Waters *et al.* 1973; Johansson and Wahlqvist 1977; Eknoyan *et al.* 1982) and animals with experimentally induced RPN are prone to UTI (Thiele 1974).

Johansson *et al.* (1987*a*,*b*) showed that a significant number of renal pelvis tumours could be induced in 7 weeks in about one-third of FANFT-exposed female Sprague–Dawley rats given chronic pyelitis or pyelonephritis by means of either a single injection, or sub-chronic doses, of *E. coli* (strain 06K 13H1, known to promote a hyperplastic response in the pelvis and ureter). Possible mechanisms whereby infection promotes UUC include bacterial toxins or their products, mechanical injury, or the metabolic potential of bacterial enzymes. Examples of the latter are nitrosylation of secondary amines (e.g. glucuronidated metabolites of analgesics) to *N*-nitrosamines (Claude *et al.* 1988) which may subsequently hydrolyse to *N*-hydroxylamines (Kadlubar *et al.* 1977), conversion of urinary nitrates into dimethylnitrosamine and other nitrosamines, and deconjugation of glucuronide metabolites (Furman *et al.* 1981) thereby facilitating their local metabolic activation.

Increased cell proliferation, due to chronic inflammation, could play an important part in the localization of the tumours.

16.4.3.2 Pelvic injury as a promoter of upper urothelial cancer

A surgical incision of one renal pelvis stimulates urothelial proliferation, and has been used after subcarcinogenic urothelial initiation (by 6 weeks of 0.2 per cent FANFT feeding) to double the incidence of ipsilateral renal pelvic tumours (Anderström and Johansson 1983).

16.4.3.3 Analgesics as upper urothelial tumour promoters

Phenacetin alone causes a marked urothelial hyperplasia, but UUC has been less frequently reported (Table 16.4) suggesting that phenacetin is not an initiating agent, but a potent promoter. This is supported in experimental animals which, fed on 0.2 per cent FANFT for 6 weeks (an exposure sufficient to cause initiation, but not complete carcinogenesis) followed by 6 weeks of 0.535 per cent dietary phenacetin, developed renal pelvic tumours (both well-differentiated, non-invasive and poorly differentiated, invasive with pulmonary metastases), but not bladder tumours (Anderström *et al.* 1983).

More recently, Johansson and Anderström (1988) have shown that feeding FANFT-initiated animals with antipyrine caused tumours in one-third of the animals, half of which were localized in the pelvis, half in the bladder. One third of the animals had RPN, fewer if antipyrine and caffeine were given together.

16.4.3.4 Cancer promotion by acutely induced renal papillary necrosis

While FANFT has been widely used, its disadvantages are that it is administered in the diet increasing the risk to personnel, the treatment is generally protracted, and because of variable food intake the exact dose of carcinogen is uncertain.

By contrast, *N*-butyl-*N*-(4-hydroxybutyl)-nitrosamine (HO-BBN) is a specific and complete carcinogen (Fukushima *et al.* 1976; Druckrey *et al.* 1964; Herman *et al.* 1985; Fujita *et al.* 1988) acting directly in the bladder (Hashimoto *et al.* 1974) in several species (Ito *et al.* 1969). It can be administered by oral gavage in divided doses over a few weeks and therefore circumvents some of the logistic handicaps of FANFT (Becci *et al.* 1979; McCormick *et al.* 1981*a*,*b*). Wistar rats are more susceptible than mice, hamsters, and guinea-pigs (Hirose *et al.* 1976; Ito 1976), but the malignancy in mice is more likely to be invasive. The number of carcinomas is proportional to the total dose (Ito and Fukushima 1986). Unilateral ureteric ligation in male Wistar rats treated with HO-BBN for 20 weeks caused ipsilateral hyperplasia of the pelvic and ureteric urothelium and induced papillomas and carcinomas (Ito *et al.* 1971). Initiation with HO-BBN, and long-term feeding of phenacetin with or without caffeine (Nakanishi *et al.*

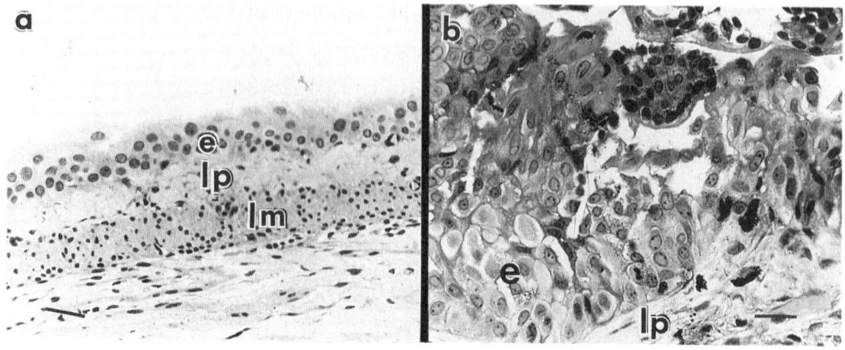

Fig. 16.3 (a) Control urothelium from Wistar rat showing three distinct layers: e = epithelium; lp = lamina propria; lm = lamina muscularis. Giemsa. Bar = 40 μm. (b) Nodular and papillary hyperplasia in ureter from animal 6 weeks after BBN initiation and 2-bromoethanamine promotion. Many areas are dysplastic with extremely basophilic nuclei sloughing into the lumen. Giemsa. Bar = 25 μm. From Gregg *et al.* 1989*b* with permission from Plenum.

1978) enhanced the development of urothelial carcinomas, thus establishing the appropriateness of such a two-stage model.

We have compared rats dosed with a sub-carcinogenic regimen of HO-BBN alone or with BEA to produce an acute PRN, and those dosed only with BEA. Sequential administration causes a sustained hyperplasia leading by 6 weeks to dysplasia that is specifically localized to the upper urothelium (Fig. 16.3(a,b)). The earliest malignancies were present in HO-BBN treated animals at 13 weeks (Fig. 16.4(a,b,c)); by 40 weeks there were macroscopic tumours present in the renal pelvis and the ureter (Fig. 16.4(d)) (Gregg *et al.* 1990*b*, 1991*b*). Upper urothelial changes were not present at 30 weeks in animals treated with similar doses of HO-BBN, although (as expected from published data) bladder carcinomas were seen. BEA alone caused a transient hyperplasia only. Loss of alkaline phosphatase, reminiscent of histochemical features in pre-malignant and malignant bladder urothelium (Kunze and Schauer 1971; Stiller and Rauscher 1971; Kunze 1979, 1987) has been observed in hyperplastic urothelium in the HO-BBN/BEA treated group (Gregg *et al.* 1991*b*).

16.5 The relationship between renal papillary necrosis and upper urothelial cancer in man

The evidence suggests that analgesics predispose to the development of UUC in man through promotion, both directly and by giving rise to RPN (McCredie *et al.* 1986). RPN may accomplish its effects through cellular or

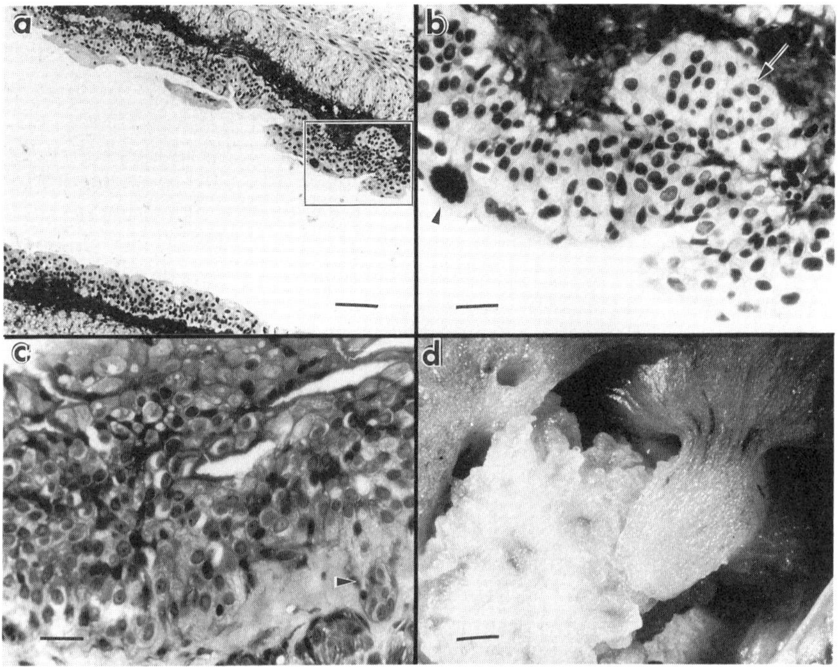

Fig. 16.4 (a) Disorganized hyperplastic ureteric epithelium from animal 13 weeks after BBN/BEA treatment. Giemsa. Bar = 80 μm. (b) Inset from Fig. 16.4(a) showing a nodular 'invasive' area (arrow) and large multinucleated cells (arrowhead). Giemsa. Bar = 20 μm. (c) Papillary and nodular hyperplasia in ureter 13 weeks after BBN/BEA treatment. Toluidine blue. Bar = 20 μm. (d) Macroscopic photograph of tumour found in pelvis 40 weeks after BBN/BEA treatment. Bar = 1 mm. From Gregg *et al.* 1989*b* with permission from Plenum.

crystalline debris, or urinary infection (Ross *et al.* 1989). If so, the question remains as to how carcinogenesis is initiated in the urinary tract of analgesic abusers, as there is little evidence to suggest that analgesics themselves are capable of causing genotoxic injury.

Tobacco is accepted as a cause of bladder cancer (Mommsen and Aagaard 1983) and smoking is highly associated with analgesic abuse in humans with UUC (McCredie *et al.* 1982*b*; 1983*a*,*b*). Polyaromatic hydrocarbons, including 7,8-dihydro-7,8-dihydroxyl-benzo[a]pyrene are excreted via the urine of smokers, and it has recently been established that prostaglandin hydroperoxidase, such as that present in the renal medulla and urothelial cells, activates these compounds to the highly genotoxic 7,8-diolepoxide (Marnett *et al.* 1978).

This hypothesis does not rule out lifestyle factors other than smoking, or occupational exposures, causing cancer initiation within individuals who are taking large amounts of analgesics. Nor does it exclude the possibility that metabolites of individual analgesics, NSAIDs, or caffeine, may contribute to initiation.

The generally higher incidence of chemically-associated carcinomas in the bladder than in the upper urinary tract appears to relate to stagnation of urine allowing an extended contact time with carcinogens and promoters. By contrast, urine does not normally stagnate in the renal pelvis, but this may occur in analgesic abusers, possibly due to decreased prostaglandin and loss of normal pelvic and ureteric peristalsis (Borda *et al.* 1983). However, it is the localization of the promoting influence of RPN in the renal pelvis which is likely to account for the predominance of analgesic-associated tumours at this site.

Acknowledgements

The author's research was supported by The Cancer Research Campaign, The International Agency for Research on Cancer, The Wellcome Trust, The Kidney Research Fund of Great Britain, Johns Hopkins Center for Alternatives to Animals in Testing, The Smith–Kline Foundation, and the Commission of the European Communities. I am indebted to Mimps E. van Ek and Gail Sutherland for preparing the manuscript and to Neill J. Gregg for providing unpublished data or material in press.

17

Analgesics as human carcinogens—clinical and epidemiological evidence

Margaret McCredie

The original observations linking urothelial cancers with abuse of analgesics containing phenacetin were made in a series of patients with renal papillary necrosis (Hultengren *et al.* 1965). Since then many clinical reports have described individual patients, with or without renal papillary necrosis, who had taken excessive amounts of analgesics and subsequently developed cancer of the renal pelvis (e.g. Adams *et al.* 1970; Rathert *et al.* 1975), bladder (e.g. Begley *et al.* 1970), and occasionally, of the renal parenchyma (Anseline and Howarth 1977).

Compound analgesics containing phenacetin were implicated in all but one report, in which renal pelvic cancer was found in two patients who had taken analgesics containing antipyrine (phenazone) but not phenacetin (Schabert *et al.* 1973).

17.1 Case series

The association between renal pelvic cancer and phenacetin-containing analgesics is supported by a substantial number of case series (Table 17.1). These include autopsy studies, patients with urothelial cancer who were questioned about their analgesic intake, and follow-up studies of patients with renal papillary necrosis, chronic pyelonephritis, or analgesic nephropathy. All were consecutive series unless otherwise specified.

Most series were from areas of high prevalence of analgesic abuse where levels of consumption were more extreme than in areas in which this habit was less common (Buckalew and Schey 1986*b*). Without exception, phenacetin was present in the analgesic preparations which had been taken but, as many series reported only the description 'phenacetin-containing analgesics', it is not always possible to identify the other constituents. The mean duration of consumption was 15–28 yr, and the average cumulative dose, 5–25 kg, although in some reports this may have referred to the consumption of phenacetin itself rather than the entire compound. Few of the reports provided information on tobacco consumption by the patients; cigarette smoking is a known risk factor for urothelial cancer and may be unduly

Table 17.1 *Case series of urothelial cancer in patients with excessive analgesic consumption*

Country / Author	Year of study	Criteria for inclusion of cases	Urothelial cancers (no. of analgesic takers)			Analgesic consumption			Smoking history
			CaP*	CaU*	CaB*	Type	Amount (kg)^	Duration (yr)^	
Sweden									
Hultengren 1965	1961	RPN* (*n* = 103)	6(5)	..	2(2)¶	Ph	5.5–> 10	20–30	?
Bengtsson 1968	1958–63	Chronic PN* or RPN				Ph, Pz, C	na	na	?
		anal +ve *n* = 46 *n* = 96	8(8)	..	2(2)				
		anal −ve *n* = 78 *n* = 22	0	..	0				
Bengtsson 1970	1960–7	CaP (surgical; excluding above 8 cases)	20(5)	..	..	Ph	7.5	15	?
Angervall 1969	1960–8	CaP in Jönköping	15(10, ?12)	..	9(2)¶	Ph	..	..	?
Johansson 1974	1960–72	CaP from Göteborg/Jönköping (*n* = 62; 19 reported earlier)	43(43)¶	..	..	Ph, Pz, C	9.1	17	?
Johansson 1977	1962–75	CaB and CaU from Göteborg, with history of analgesic abuse	..	4(4)	42(42)	Ph, Pz, C	7.1	21	?
Walqvist 1980	?	CaP and CaB (urological; *n* = 359)	21(11)	..	148(12)¶	Ph	na	na	10/21 and 94/148 +ve
Australia									
Taylor 1972	1965–9	All CaK, P, U, and B from two Sydney hospitals (*n* = 189)	13(7)	2(0)	144(2)	Ph, A, C	na	na	3/13 +ve
Mahony 1977	1970–6	All CaK, P, U, from a Sydney hospital (*n* = 81)	26(15)	5(2)¶	..	Ph, A, C	24.8	na	17/26 and 5/5 +ve
Orell 1979	1960–76	All CaP from a Newcastle hospital	53(26)¶	..	..	Ph, A, C	na	na	?

Kung 1976	1965–75	Autopsies from Zurich (n = 24 683), including 269 CaK (5 analgesic takers)	15(4)	6(0)	218(11)	Ph	na	na	?
Gloor 1978	1971–6	Autopsies from St Gallen (n = 5350, 60 with RPN)	5(5)	..	..	Ph	na	na	?
Mihatsch 1980*b*	1963–77	Autopsies or biopsies from Basel	46(24)	19(11)	376(38)¶	Ph	na	na	12/46, 6/19 and 80/376 +ve
Denmark									
Høybye 1971	1964–9	Chronic PN (n = 320; 77 with analgesic abuse)	2(2)	..	..	Ph	na	na	?
Palvio 1987	1979–84	Urological CaP or CaU (n = 59)	59(9)¶	..	..	Ph, Pz, C, Co	1–10	10–50	46/59 +ve
Finland									
Juusela 1973	1966–71	CaP	19(5, ?7)¶	..	..	Ph, A, C	na	na	?
Canada									
Handa 1981	1971–9	New Brunswick, AN* (n = 19)	2(2)	..	1(1)¶	Ph, A, C, Co	1.5–6	8–40	?
USA									
Gonwa 1980	1974–9	All CaP, U, B from a North Carolina hospital	5(3)	..	110(3)	Ph	18.3	25.8	?
W Germany									
Steffens 1988	1948–81	CaP or U (surgical, n = 160) Analgesic history available in 118	83(18)	35(4)¶	..	Ph	CaP 5.6 CaU4.9	CaP 24 CaU 26	?
Austria									
Porpáczy 1981	1960–79	Urological cases taking ≥ 0.25 g Ph daily	4(4)	1(1)	26(26)¶	Ph, Pz, C, Co	7.8	27.6	?

* RPN = renal papillary necrosis; PN = pyelonephritis; AN = analgesic nephropathy; Ca = cancer of: P = renal pelvis; U = ureter; B = bladder; K = renal parenchyma; Ph = phenacetin; Pz = phenazone; C = caffeine; Co = codeine; A = aspirin; ˆ average or range; ¶ some patients with multiple urothelial cancers.

common amongst abusers of analgesics. Two-thirds of the series reported cases with tumours at more than one site within the urothelium.

Depending upon the criteria for inclusion in the series, these reports describe either a high prevalence (3–10 per cent) of urothelial tumours amongst patients with analgesic nephropathy, or a high prevalence (20–100 per cent) of analgesic abuse amongst patients with urothelial cancer. While such series are useful in identifying an association, they cannot be used as proof because of publication bias and the absence of a control group.

17.2 Formal epidemiological evidence

17.2.1 Case–control studies

In the last fifteen years, case–control studies have investigated the risk of cancer associated with analgesic abuse (Table 17.2). The majority are population-based and, while some have been carried out in areas of high prevalence of analgesic abuse such as Australia and Denmark, most are from regions where this habit has been less common such as England, Canada, and the United States. The definition of 'regular use' or 'abuse' of analgesics differs between studies as does the extent to which the analyses have been controlled, or adjusted, for the effects of other risk factors such as cigarette smoking or other types of analgesics. However, there appears to be sufficient evidence to assess the risk for various sites within the kidney and urinary tract, and to identify the types of analgesics which are associated with this risk.

The estimate of risk is the 'odds ratio' which compares the risk of cancer in those who have taken analgesics (at a particular defined level) with those who have not (Breslow and Day 1980).

17.2.2 Cohort studies

In 1968, 7311 female volunteers aged 30–49 yr, employed in 88 businesses (watchmaking, pharmaceutical/chemical, metallurgic, textile, food and tobacco, paper, retailing, banking and insurance) in north-west Switzerland were screened for evidence of regular intake of phenacetin-containing analgesics. From this survey a cohort was established comprising a study group of 623 women showing evidence of such consumption (divided into subgroups with high or low intake) and a control group of 621 women showing no such evidence (Dubach *et al.* 1983). These women have been followed for 20 yr (Dubach *et al.* 1991).

A second cohort of almost 14000 elderly residents of a Californian retirement community, who had responded to a mailed questionnaire, were followed for 6½ yr in order to evaluate the associations between use of aspirin and the incidence of cardiovascular disease, cancer, and other chronic diseases (Paganini-Hill *et al.* 1989).

17.2.3 Summary of evidence implicating phenacetin or other analgesic drugs

17.2.3.1 Analgesics—type not specified

In Oxford, although consumption of analgesics (all types considered together) was not associated with renal pelvic cancer, a link was found with cancer of the renal parenchyma (Armstrong *et al.* 1976). This was considered to be non-causal as 6 of the 15 cases had taken analgesics for only 1 yr or less before their diagnosis. Only four had taken analgesics which had previously contained phenacetin, and the effect of smoking had not been taken into account in the analysis.

No association was found between analgesics (all types considered together, and taken for at least 6 weeks in any one year) and renal parenchymal cancer in Los Angeles County, an area where the prevalence of analgesic abuse has been low (Yu *et al.* 1986).

An increased risk of renal pelvic cancer was associated with consumption of analgesics which did not contain phenacetin (considered as a group) in New South Wales (McCredie *et al.* 1982*a*) but no adjustment had been made for the confounding effect of smoking and the control group was not population-based.

17.2.3.2 Phenacetin-containing analgesics

In most countries, phenacetin has never been available as a single agent but has been taken in combination with other drugs, usually aspirin or phenazone, and caffeine and/or codeine.

In 1980, a working group from the International Agency for Research on Cancer evaluating the carcinogenic risk of chemicals to humans reported that: (i) there was 'limited' evidence that phenacetin and *N*-hydroxyphenacetin were carcinogenic in animals; (ii) there was 'limited' evidence that abuse of analgesic mixtures containing phenacetin caused cancer of the renal pelvis in humans; and (iii) it was not possible to specify what component(s) of the analgesic mixtures were responsible for this effect (IARC 1980). All but two of the case–control studies listed in Table 17.2 have been published since that time.

Seven studies made adjustment in their analyses for the effect of smoking which independently increases the risk for urothelial cancer 4- to 8-fold (McLaughlin *et al.* 1983, McCredie *et al.* 1983*a*,*b*; Jensen *et al.* 1988; Ross *et al.* 1989) and may double the risk for renal parenchymal cancer (McLaughlin *et al.* 1984; Yu *et al.* 1986; McCredie *et al.* 1988). These investigations will be considered in more detail than those making no such adjustment.

In New South Wales, a lifetime consumption of at least 0.1 kg phenacetin-containing analgesics increased the risk of cancer of the renal pelvis (4- to

Table 17.2 *Case–control studies investigating the association of analgesics with cancer of the kidney and urinary tract*

Author	Subjects*		Analgesics§ containing	Definition of exposure	Odds ratio	Dose–response	Adjusted for:	
	Cases	Controls					smoking	phenacetin
Renal pelvis								
Armstrong 1976, Oxford	33	33 H matched	Any	Daily, ≥ 6 months	'no association'	–	No	–
McCredie 1982*a*, NSW	67	84 Fr 96 S	Ph Non-Ph	Lifetime total ≥ 0.1 kg ≥ 5 yr before interview	F : 4.1 (1.8–9.2) F : 3.4 (1.4–8.3)	Yes Yes	No No	– Yes
McCredie 1983*a*, NSW	31 F	440 P	Ph Non-Ph	Lifetime total ≥ 0.1 kg	F : 5.4 (2.5–11.7) F : 1.4 (0.5–3.8)	Yes Yes	Yes No	– Yes
McCredie 1983*b*, NSW	29 M	307 P	Ph Non-Ph	Lifetime total ≥ 0.1 kg	M : 8.2 (3.8–17.6) M : 1.6 (0.6–4.3)	Yes No	Yes No	– Yes
McLaughlin 1983, Minnesota	74	697 P	Ph or Pa	≥ every second day for 36 months	M : 3.9 (0.7–20.4) F : 3.7 (0.5–24.7)	No Yes	Yes Yes	– –
McCredie, Stewart 1988, NSW	73#	688 P	Ph Pa	Lifetime total ≥ 1 kg Ph or Pa	7.9 (4.6–13.8) 0.8 (0.4–1.7)	na –	Yes Yes	– Yes
Renal pelvis and ureter								
Jensen 1989, Denmark	96	294 H	Ph A	Ever used, ≥ 5 yr before interview	M : 2.4 (0.9–6.8) F : 4.2 (1.5–12.3) M : 1.8 (0.8–2.2) F : 7.3 (2.1–26)	Yes na na na	Yes Yes Yes Yes	– – Yes Yes
Ross 1989, Los Angeles	187	187 P matched	Ph or Pa A C	> 30 consecutive days at any time	4.0 (0.8–2.1) 2.3 (1.2–4.3) 5.5 (1.2–25)	na na na	No No No	– Yes Yes
Ureter								
McCredie, Stewart 1983*b*, 1988, NSW	36 M	307 P	Ph Non-Ph Pa	Lifetime total ≥ 0.1 kg	M : 1.0 (0.3–3.1) M : 0.8 (0.3–2.0) M : 2.5 (1.1–5.9)	– – No	Yes No Yes	– Yes Yes

Bladder								
Fokkens 1979, Netherlands	1084	1094 H	Ph	> 2 kg Ph in lifetime	4.1; $p = 0.02$	na	No	–
Howe 1980, Canada	632	632 P matched	A	'regularly' for ≥ 6 months	M: 1.5 (1.0–2.3)	–	No	No
					F: 1.1 (0.5–2.4)	–	No	No
			Ph		'no association'	–	No	–
McCredie 1983*a*, NSW	154 F	440 P	Ph	Lifetime total ≥ 0.1 kg	F: 2.3 (1.4–3.9)	Yes	Yes	–
			Non-Ph		F: 0.5 (0.3–0.9)	–	No	Yes
Piper 1985, 1986 New York State	173 F < 50 yr	173 P matched	Ph	≥ 30 days per year for ≥ 1 yr	F: 5.5 (0.9–36)	na	Yes	–
			Pa		F: 1.5 (0.4–7.2)	–	No	No
McCredie, Stewart 1988, NSW	162# F	381 P	Ph	Lifetime total ≥ 0.1 kg Ph or Pa	F: 2.0 (1.1–3.5)	na	Yes	–
			Pa		F: 0.7 (0.4–1.3)	–	Yes	Yes
Renal parenchyma								
Armstrong 1976, Oxford	106	106 H matched	Any	Daily, ≥ 6 months	15 cases, 2 controls¶	na	No	–
McLaughlin 1984, Minnesota	495	697 P	Ph	≥ every second day for 36 months	M: 2.2 (0.6–9.0)	Yes	Yes	–
					F: 2.5 (0.8–7.0)	Yes	Yes	–
Maclure 1985, New York	548	624 P	Ph	≥ 2 per week, no minimum duration given	3.5 (1.0–12.0)	na	?	?
			Pa		'no association'	–	?	?
Yu 1986, San Francisco	160 < 55 yr	160 P	Any	≥ 6 weeks in any year	'no association'	–	No	–
McCredie *et al.* 1988, NSW	360	985 P	Ph	Lifetime total ≥ 0.1 kg	2.2 (1.5–3.1)	Yes	Yes	–
			A (never Ph)			–	Yes	Yes
Asal 1988, Oklahoma	315	336 P	Ph^	≥ 10 times during adult life excluding 3 yr before interview	1.5 (1.0–2.3)	–	No	–
			Ph^^		3.5 (1.7–7.2)	na	No	–
			A		1.7 (1.1–2.7)	na	No	No

* M male F female; P population H hospital Fr friends S screening clinic controls; controls; § Ph phenacetin, Pa paracetamol, A aspirin, C caffeine; # includes previously analysed cases; na not available. ¶ had only taken analgesics for 1 yr or less before diagnosis; only 4 took preparations which previously contained phenacetin. ^ Anacin; ^^ Darvon; phenacetin removed from formulation by 1967 and 1983 respectively but it is not clear when the consumption occurred.

6-fold), bladder (2-fold), and renal parenchyma (2-fold) (McCredie *et al.* 1983*a*,*b*, 1988). A dose–response effect was demonstrated with increasing consumption leading to higher risks. However, no increased risk was found for ureteric cancer (McCredie *et al.* 1983*a*).

In Denmark, phenacetin-containing analgesics taken for at least 30 consecutive days at any time increased the risk of cancers of the renal pelvis and ureter (considered together) by a factor of four in women; the doubled risk in men was not statistically significant (Jensen *et al.* 1989).

For bladder cancer, consumption of phenacetin-containing analgesics on at least 30 days per year more than one year before diagnosis by women aged less than 55 years in New York State, was associated with a 5-fold increase in risk which, however, was not significant (Piper *et al.* 1986).

In Minnesota, phenacetin-containing analgesics taken at least every second day for 3 yr or more doubled the risk of renal parenchymal cancer but the 95 per cent confidence intervals included unity (McLaughlin *et al.* 1984).

Amongst the studies which did not adjust for cigarette smoking, those from areas where excessive analgesic consumption had not been common did not find significantly increased risks for urothelial (Ross *et al.* 1989; Howe *et al.* 1980) or renal parenchymal cancer (Maclure and McMahon 1985). In the data from The Netherlands (Fokkens 1979), division of analgesic intake at the more conventional level of 1 kg (rather than the 2 kg level published in the results) gave an odds ratio of 1.7 which was not statistically significant.

Actuarial analyses of the Swiss cohort after 20 yr, with adjustment for year of birth, cigarette smoking, and length of follow-up, found increased mortality due to cancer (all sites considered together; relative risk 1.9, 95 per cent confidence limits 1.1–3.3) and to urological and renal disease (relative risk 16.1, 95 per cent confidence limits 3.9–66.1) in women who in 1968 had evidence of a regular intake of phenacetin, when compared with those who had no such evidence (Dubach *et al.* 1991). Information is not currently available as to the numbers and sites of the cancers, but one would not expect to detect an increased risk of renal parenchymal or urothelial cancer, given the small size of the cohort (Breslow and Day 1987).

17.2.3.3 Analgesics containing phenacetin or paracetamol

In two studies, the consumption of analgesics containing phenacetin was not separated from those containing paracetamol (acetaminophen). Both in Minnesota (McLaughlin *et al.* 1983) and Los Angeles (Ross *et al.* 1989) there was a 4-fold increased risk of renal pelvic cancer but the 95 per cent confidence interval did not exclude unity. Only the Minnesota study made adjustment for smoking.

17.2.3.4 Paracetamol-containing analgesics

Paracetamol is available as a single drug, or as an ingredient of compound analgesic preparations. It is likely that the molecular effect of paracetamol is altered by the presence of the other constituents of compound analgesics (Chapters 2 and 16), but no epidemiological study has investigated the 'form' of intake as a factor. Moreover, in assessing the risk associated with paracetamol, adjustment must be made for prior or concomitant use of phenacetin-containing analgesics.

No increased risk was found for cancer of the renal pelvis, bladder, or renal parenchyma (Maclure and MacMahon 1985; Piper *et al.* 1986; McCredie and Stewart 1988; McCredie *et al.* 1988). The one positive association, with ureteric cancer, must be viewed with some doubt as there was no dose–response, and when the cut-off was made at a different level of consumption, the result was no longer significant (McCredie and Stewart 1988).

17.2.3.5 Aspirin

Aspirin also can be taken either as a single drug or in compound analgesic preparations, quite possibly with differing carcinogenic potential.

One study of renal pelvic and ureteric cancers (considered together) found an increased risk associated with aspirin which was attributed by the authors to the concomitant intake of phenacetin (Jensen *et al.* 1989). In persons who had never taken phenacetin, there was no increased risk for renal parenchymal cancer from consumption of a lifetime total of at least 0.1 kg of aspirin (McCredie *et al.* 1988).

Three further studies which found an elevated risk associated with aspirin had made no adjustment for the confounding effect of smoking (renal pelvis and ureter: Ross *et al.* 1989; bladder: Howe *et al.* 1980; renal parenchyma: Asal *et al.* 1988).

In the Californian cohort study, daily use of aspirin (of unspecified dose, duration, or timing) was associated with a six-fold increased risk of cancer of the renal parenchyma, but no adjustment had been made for either smoking or phenacetin intake (Paganini-Hill *et al.* 1989). No increase in mortality due to cancer, or urological or renal disease, was found amongst women in the Swiss cohort who in 1968 had evidence of regular salicylate consumption (Dubach *et al.* 1991).

17.2.3.6 Caffeine

In few studies has it been possible to investigate the independent effect of caffeine, as it is commonly taken together with phenacetin and aspirin or an antipyrine derivative in compound preparations.

A 5-fold increased risk of cancer of the renal pelvis or ureter found in Los Angeles was based on a small number of exposed persons and the analysis was not adjusted for smoking (Ross *et al.* 1989).

17.2.4 Evidence implicating renal papillary necrosis

Although renal papillary necrosis (RPN) has been found in a high proportion of subjects with analgesic-associated cancer of the renal pelvis, there is no agreement as to whether RPN is an essential step in the genesis of this cancer. Those who believe that phenacetin itself is a chemical carcinogen, generally have postulated that those tissue changes which precede transitional-cell carcinoma occur separately from, and parallel to, phenacetin's nephrotoxic effect which results in RPN (Bengtsson *et al.* 1978). Thus can be explained the production of urothelial tumours, apparently without coexisting RPN, by feeding phenacetin to rats (Isaka *et al.* 1979), a species which is resistant to the nephrotoxic effects of this drug (Nanra and Kincaid-Smith 1972).

On the other hand, by analogy with transitional-cell tumours which arise in association with chronic urological disease, it has been proposed that RPN, which frequently is associated with urinary obstruction and infection, is an intermediate stage in the development of renal pelvic cancer. In support of this is the observation that in patients who have taken analgesics, renal pelvic cancer has been reported infrequently in the absence of RPN. Indeed, RPN has been found in 75 per cent of the 124 well-documented case reports of the analgesic-associated renal pelvic cancer published up to, and including, 1973 (Rathert *et al.* 1975) and in 92, 87, and 57 per cent, respectively, of one Swedish and two Australian series of such cases published between 1974 and 1979 (Johansson *et al.* 1974; Mahony *et al.* 1977; Orell *et al.* 1979).

To elucidate whether the presence of RPN is a necessary intermediate stage in the development of analgesic-associated cancer of the renal pelvis, a case-control study was undertaken to determine the relative risk associated with the presence of RPN alone, the consumption of phenacetin-containing analgesics alone, or the occurrence of both risk factors together (McCredie *et al.* 1986). Information was obtained from 66 patients with renal pelvic cancer concerning their past consumption of analgesics, and the kidneys from these patients were examined for evidence of RPN. A comparison was made with 86 patients with adenocarcinoma of the kidney. For 751 population-based controls, the prevalence of RPN was taken as that found in autopsy surveys (Burry *et al.* 1974; Burry and Hopkins 1977) and the relative risk for RPN associated with phenacetin-containing analgesics previously found in New South Wales (McCredie *et al.* 1982*b*).

Given that this estimate of the prevalence of RPN in the population was accurate, the results indicated that both RPN and regular consumption of phenacetin-containing analgesics were independent risk factors for renal pelvic cancer, increasing the risk about 7 and 3½ times respectively (Table 17.3). When both were present, the risk was increased 20 times that for persons exposed to neither risk factor.

If the nephrotoxic and carcinogenic effects of phenacetin-containing analgesics occurred separately, the risk for cancer of the renal pelvis associated with consumption of phenacetin-containing analgesics would be unaltered by the presence or absence of RPN. Clearly these date deny this

Table 17.3 *Relative risks (and 95% confidence intervals) for cancers of the renal pelvis and renal parenchyma associated with phenacetin-containing analgesics (PhA) and renal papillary necrosis (RPN)*

		Cancer of the renal pelvis	Cancer of the renal parenchyma
PhA −	RPN −	1.0	1.0
PhA −	RPN +	6.9 (2.1–22)	1.1 (0.1–9.6)
PhA +	RPN −	3.6 (1.6–8.1)	2.5 (1.3–4.9)
PhA +	RPN +	20 (12–34)	0.4 (0.1–2.7)

possibility, for the risk among patients exposed to phenacetin-containing analgesics was more than five times greater in the presence of RPN than in its absence. Each factor had a non-chance association with renal pelvic cancer in the absence of the other; and when both were present, the risk increased in a multiplicative fashion. This suggests that phenacetin-containing analgesics and RPN have independent, and when they coexist sequential, effects. However, the relationship between consumption of phenacetin-containing analgesics and adenocarcinoma of the kidney appears to be entirely a direct one without any intervening effect of RPN (Table 17.3).

17.2.5 Population attributable risks

Case-control studies provide direct estimates of the relative increase in incidence associated with an exposure and, if the control group has been drawn from the population at risk according to a well-defined sampling scheme, they also may give unbiased estimates of the amount of exposure to the risk factor in the general population. The population attributable risk is defined as the proportion of cases occurring in the total population which can be explained by a risk factor (Breslow and Day 1980). Population attributable risks associated with the regular consumption of phenacetin-containing analgesics have been calculated for cancers of the kidney and urinary tract (Table 17.4).

In NSW more than one-third of cases of renal pelvic cancer can be attributed to the regular consumption of phenacetin-containing analgesics (McCredie *et al.* 1983*a*,*b*, 1988). In Denmark the estimate for women is similar in magnitude (Jensen *et al.* 1989) although it was calculated using hospital controls which generally contain a higher proportion of analgesic takers.

17.3 Incidence of renal pelvic cancer

Within Australia (McCredie *et al.* 1990), and internationally (Buckalew and Schey 1986*b*), the incidence of renal pelvic cancer varies considerably and is

Table 17.4 *Population attributable risks associated with phenacetin-containing analgesics*

Author	Population	Relative risk adjusted for tobacco	Percentage of users in control group	Population attributable risk (PAR)
Renal pelvis				
McLaughlin 1983	Minnesota	M: 3.9	1.4	3.9%*
		F: 3.7	6.7	15.3%*
McCredie 1983*a,b*	New South Wales	M: 8.2	9.0	39.3%
		F: 5.4	13.0	36.4%
Renal pelvis and ureter				
Jensen 1989	East Denmark	M: 2.4	6.7	8.6%
		F: 4.2	13.9	30.8%
Bladder				
McCredie 1983*a*	New South Wales	F: 2.3	13.0	14.5%
Piper 1986	New York State	F: 5.5	1.2	5.0%
Renal parenchyma				
McLaughlin 1984	Minnesota	M: 2.2	0.9	1.1%
		F: 2.5	3.7	5.3%
McCredie *et al.* 1988	New South Wales	2.2	11.0	11.7%

* PAR for consumption of phenacetin or paracetamol; # hospital controls used in calculation of relative risk.

Table 17.5 *Withdrawal of phenacetin or compound analgesics and incidence of renal pelvic cancer*

Population	Withdrawal from over-the-counter sales		Incidence (per 100 000 person-years)					
	Phenacetin	Compound preparations	1973–7		1978–82		Most recent[1]	
			M	F	M	F	M	F
Australia New South Wales	1975	1979	0.9	0.9	1.1	1.5	0.7[2]	1.2[2]
Denmark	1961		1.1[3] 1.6[4]	0.6[3] 0.8[4]	1.5	1.0	1.4[5]	1.2[5]
Switzerland Basel	1981		na	na	1.5	1.1	1.2[6]	1.1[6]
Canada Ontario	1973–4		0.7	0.3	0.6	0.3	0.6[7]	0.3[7]
USA Connecticut	1982		1.3	0.6	1.0	0.4	0.5 M and F combined[7]	
England South Thames	1980		0.4	0.2	0.3	0.1	0.3[7]	0.1[7]

[1] Unpublished data obtained through personal communication with population-based cancer registry in each area. [2] 1989; [3] 1968–72; [4] 1973–6; [5] 1983–6; [6] 1985–9; [7] 1983–7; na = not available.

correlated with the prevalence of analgesic abuse. Incidence data for renal pelvic cancer have been obtained from published sources covering the periods centred around 1975 (Waterhouse *et al.* 1982) and 1980 (Muir *et al.* 1987) and from personal communication with population-based cancer registries for more recent periods. Incidence rates, age-adjusted to the 'world' population, are given for populations in areas of high and low prevalence of regular analgesic consumption in Table 17.5.

In women from NSW, Denmark, and Switzerland the incidence of renal pelvic cancer remains high. Although the withdrawal of phenacetin and compound preparations from over-the-counter sales affects the incidence of end stage renal failure due to analgesic nephropathy within 5 to 10 yr (Bengtsson 1979; McCredie *et al.* 1989), one would not expect to see as prompt a reduction in rates of renal pelvic cancer because of its long induction period; moreover, a change in the rate of appearance of cancers caused by analgesics may be masked by unrelated changes in the incidence of the majority of cancers which are due to other exposures, principally tobacco.

In areas of low analgesic abuse, rates of renal pelvic cancer are either low (Ontario, South Thames), or decreasing (Connecticut).

17.4 Summary

The clearly positive results implicating regular consumption of phenacetin-containing analgesics with renal or urothelial cancer have come from areas of high prevalence of analgesic abuse. In these studies, the increased risk associated with phenacetin-containing analgesics is either higher than (renal pelvis), or of the same order as (bladder, renal parenchyma), those of the other major identified risk factor, tobacco. The relationship of analgesics with ureteric cancer is probable but not certain. The association has been more difficult to demonstrate in communities where phenacetin consumption has been neither common nor heavy, although the pattern of these studies also tends to implicate phenacetin-containing analgesics. As phenacetin has almost invariably been taken, at the same or a different time, with other antipyretic-analgesics, a contributory role for, say, aspirin or phenazone remains a possibility.

However, in respect of analgesics other than phenacetin, there is no certain evidence that any is associated with cancer, although some studies have been suggestive—paracetamol in ureteric cancer (McCredie and Stewart 1988) and aspirin in renal parenchymal cancer (Asal *et al.* 1988). While the carcinogenicity of analgesics other than phenacetin cannot be ruled out, clearly their effect must be substantially weaker than that of phenacetin-containing analgesics.

18

Carcinoma of the renal pelvis

J.S. Taylor

Carcinoma of the renal pelvis occurring in association with analgesic nephropathy was first reported from Sweden (Hultengren *et al.* 1965). Subsequently some 12 series and a number of single case reports have appeared in the literature, the total number of reported cases being over 200. Cases have been reported most commonly from Sweden (Bengtsson *et al.* 1968; Johansson and Wahlqvist 1979) and Australia (Taylor 1972; Mahony *et al.* 1977; Orell *et al.* 1979; Lomax-Smith and Seymour 1980*a*,*b*), but also from Switzerland (Leistenschneider and Ehmann 1973) and Germany (Steffens and Nagel 1988). It is now accepted that there is a cause and effect relationship (Chapters 16 and 17).

18.1 Pathology

The tumour may be pedunculated or sessile. The former is fronded, the latter less so. They may arise from anywhere in the renal pelvis or the infundibulum of the calyces, but rarely from the calyceal fornix or the papilla. They may however invade into and obstruct or obliterate calyces. Multiple tumours occur in up to 38 per cent of cases (Johansson *et al.* 1976) (Fig. 18.2).

Microscopically they are transitional cell carcinomas, with some 6–23 per cent showing squamous change (Bengtsson *et al.* 1968). In some, but not all, series, they are less well differentiated than pelvic cancers not associated with analgesic abuse (Mahony *et al.* 1977; Orell *et al.* 1979).

18.2 Incidence

Carcinoma of the renal pelvis generally accounts for some 4–9 per cent of all kidney cancer (Williams 1991), but it may form up to 30 per cent in regions where analgesic nephropathy is common (Taylor 1972; Lomax-Smith and Seymour 1980*a*, Steffens and Nagel 1988). In Newcastle (NSW) there have been 55 cases of renal pelvic cancer amongst some 800 patients with analgesic nephropathy. With the passage of time there is a slow increase in the number of patients with analgesic nephropathy who develop carcinoma of the renal pelvis, with a latency of up to 26 years having been reported (Steffens and Nagel 1988).

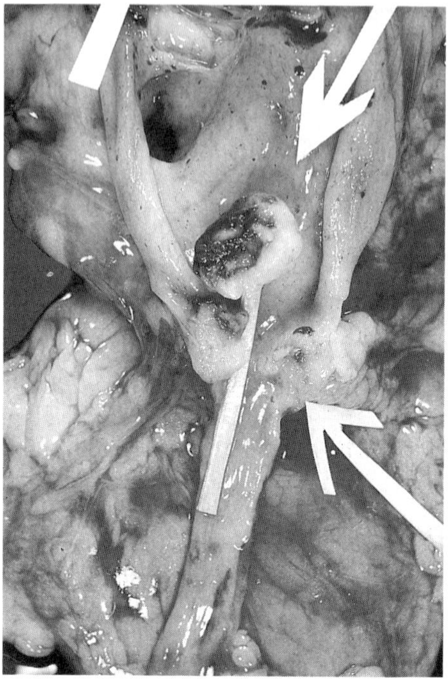

Fig. 18.1 Nephroureterectomy specimen. Note: (1) urothelial tumour at pelvi-ureteric junction (lower arrow); (2) sloughed renal papilla coated with fibrin.

The sex incidence parallels that of analgesic nephropathy, and the tumour develops at a slightly younger age than those occurring in the absence of exposure to analgesics (Mahony *et al.* 1977).

As analgesic abuse has become less common in Australia over the past 10 yr, so too have new cases of analgesic nephropathy, and there appears also to have been a decline in the incidence of analgesic-related carcinoma of the renal pelvis (but see Table 17.5 and Fig. 19.1). A similar situation seems to be the case in Sweden. This indicates that cessation of ingestion of analgesics, even in patients with established analgesic nephropathy, does reduce (but does not abolish) the chance of developing transitional cell carcinoma.

18.3 Clinical aspects

The commonest symptom is macroscopic haematuria, and this occurrence in a patient with known analgesic nephropathy must initiate a search for carcinoma somewhere in the urinary tract. In one series of 110 patients with analgesic nephropathy, 12 developed macroscopic haematuria, and of those 8

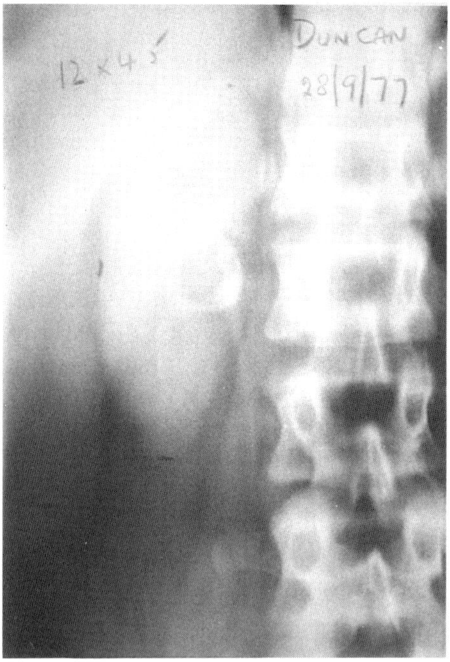

Fig. 18.2 Intravenous urogram showing two tumours of the renal pelvis. Note in this case there is apparent lack of contiguity with the wall of the pelvis, and slight irregularity of the renal outline and calyces indicate analgesic-induced damage.

were shown to have carcinoma of the renal pelvis (Taylor 1972). Persistent microscopic haematuria also should be investigated.

Tumours may present without symptoms and be discovered incidentally, usually by intravenous pyelography. Hence the case for regular screening.

18.3.1 Diagnosis

Contrast radiology is the main diagnostic modality; poor renal function, common in these patients, may necessitate retrograde pyelography. The typical radiological appearance is of an irregular filling defect, constant in position, contiguous to the wall of the renal pelvis or calyceal infundibulum. Irregularity of the surface may allow wisps of contrast to penetrate, resulting in a flare or 'soap-suds' effect which is virtually diagnostic in a patient with analgesic nephropathy (Fig. 18.2).

The other causes of radiolucent filling defects in the renal pelvis are sloughed papillae, radiolucent calculi, blood clot, extrinsic pressure from a blood vessel and, rarely, various hamartomas, cholesteatomas, and fungus balls.

Accuracy of diagnosis is improved if exfoliative cytology on voided urine is positive or, better still, if brush biopsy of the filling defect (taken under image intensification) shows malignant cells (Brown *et al.* 1973).

If doubt exists on the X-ray appearances, the most reliable method of obtaining a definitive diagnosis is by direct visualization and biopsy of the suspicious lesion using a flexible and steerable ureterorenoscope (Papadopoulos *et al.* 1987; Blute *et al.* 1989). This is more definitive than brush biopsy, and more reliable than exfoliative cytology where false positive rates of up to 10 per cent, and false negative rates of up to 60 per cent, have been reported (Sarnacki *et al.* 1971; Dalquen *et al.* 1980).

Sonography is not sufficiently sensitive or specific to be used as a diagnostic tool, but its widespread use necessitates that the clinician must be alert to the appearance that suggests the presence of a tumour, namely a zone that is less echogenic than normal in the renal sinus (Grant *et al.* 1986; Chapter 8).

Computerized tomography and magnetic resonance imaging have no place in the diagnosis except in staging large tumours, or those in which there is a likelihood of spread. All other tumours should be staged at operation.

18.3.2 Treatment

Based on long experience with transitional cell carcinoma of the renal pelvis, radical nephro-ureterectomy appears to be the treatment offering the greatest chance of cure (Johansson and Wahlqvist 1979), at least in the lower-grade tumours (Murphy *et al.* 1981). This means the removal of the kidney and ipsilateral adrenal, Gerota's fascia, the entire ureter, a cuff of bladder surrounding the ureteric orifice and the ipsilateral para-aortic lymph nodes. There are no adequately controlled studies published to back this contention.

In patients with moderately severe renal failure, in whom loss of the affected kidney would precipitate the need for dialysis, or in those with only one kidney, more conservative methods allowing preservation of renal function have been used. These include: partial nephrectomy; local resection at open operation, with and without fulguration (Ziegelbaum *et al.* 1987); fulguration with electrocautery or Neodynium Y.A.G. laser using the ureterorenoscope (Blute *et al.* 1989) or percutaneous techniques (Smith *et al.* 1987); intracavity Mitomycin C or Bacillus Calmette-Guerin (Herr 1985). Although the potential for seeding tumour into the open wound or along the percutaneous tract is a matter of concern, it occurs rarely in practice. With the more widespread use of the ureterorenoscope and Neodynium Y.A.G. laser, it is to be expected that endoscopic resection will assume a greater role in those patients in whom conservative surgery is indicated.

Radiotherapy has a small part in the management of the resectable tumours; given post-operatively in the higher stage cancers, it may reduce the risk of local recurrence (Brookland and Richter 1985).

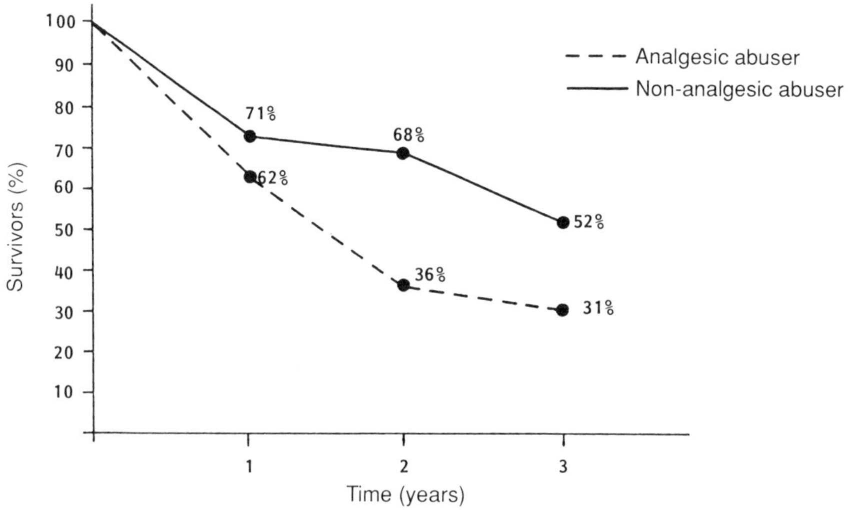

Fig. 18.3 Survival after treatment for renal pelvic cancer in patients who have and have not abused analgesics. Analgesic abuse worsens the prognosis.

Systemic chemotherapy has not been used widely in the treatment of transitional cell cancer of the renal pelvis, and there are no reports of its use in analgesic abusers. Preliminary results using M-VAC (methotrexate, vinblastine, doxorubicin, and cisplatin) have been reported in patients who were not analgesic abusers (Sternberg *et al.* 1985) with significant regression in 71 per cent, and complete clinical remission in 50 per cent. However, impairment of renal function, frequent in the analgesic group, is a contraindication to M-VAC therapy, limiting the role of systemic chemotherapy.

Cystoscopy is an integral part of management because of the increased risk of bladder cancer once a tumour develops in the upper tract. It must be performed at the initial assessment, and then every 6 months until the patient has ceased taking analgesics, stopped smoking, and been tumour free with negative urine cytology for 2 yr.

18.4 Prognosis

The 3-yr survival figures for 37 patients who were, and 18 who were not, analgesic abusers are compared in Fig. 18.3. The trend shown continues out to 5 yr; the prognosis is worse amongst the analgesic abusers.

19
Prevention of analgesic-induced kidney disease

J.H. Stewart

Few diseases other than those of infective aetiology can have had such a fulminating course as analgesic nephropathy; unknown until the early 1950s, the major cause of irreversible renal failure in several Scandinavian countries in the 1960s and Australian states in the 1970s, yet within a decade hardly a significant problem in those same countries. However, there are countries which continue to have a substantial and largely unchanged incidence of this disease—instances are well recorded in western Europe but now are being acknowledged in eastern Europe—and others, chiefly in the third world, where it is just becoming recognized. Moreover, a modern variant, but with a subtly different aetiology, namely kidney disease due to non-steroidal anti-inflammatory drugs (NSAIDs), promises to become more widespread, but is perhaps not as serious for the individual patient, as was analgesic nephropathy 20 years ago.

Although this monograph has concentrated upon disease primarily caused by analgesic drugs, evidence has been presented that both antipyretic-analgesics and NSAIDs significantly contribute to progressive damage and functional impairment in kidneys which are already the seat of disease which may be of quite unrelated aetiology. As there is an impression that this secondary renal injury may occur with smaller exposures than those needed to harm previously healthy kidneys, and with single as well as compound analgesics, its prevention is all the more difficult.

Strategies for disease prevention depend upon some understanding of aetiology, although, as in the case of analgesic-induced kidney diseases, precise knowledge of pathogenesis may not be necessary.

19.1 The aetiology of analgesic-induced kidney disease

This disease illustrates the inherent weaknesses of the epidemiological method, which can but identify what particular circumstances existed during the genesis of the disorder under investigation; and of the experimental research whose conclusions can be secure only in so far as the conditions occurring in life have been reliably reproduced in the laboratory. Agreement between separate investigations undertaken under different conditions strengthens inferences derivable from each method, and in the case of analgesic nephropathy, there is sufficient consensus to arrive at conclusions.

19.1.1 The conclusion based on epidemiological evidence

19.1.1.1 Mixed analgesics

In every country in which analgesic nephropathy has been common, abnormally heavy consumption over a period of years of compound analgesics containing phenacetin has been identified in virtually all cases. However, phenacetin rarely has been used as a single agent, and so it is not possible to judge its potential to induce chronic renal disease in the absence of another antipyretic–analgesic. Moreover, because compound analgesics which have been taken on a large scale usually have contained phenacetin, and persons who have abused non-phenacetin-containing analgesics almost always have earlier taken phenacetin-containing preparations, it has been difficult to determine whether phenacetin is a necessary ingredient of nephrotoxic or carcinogenic preparations. Of combinations not containing phenacetin, most debate centres on paracetamol when taken together with aspirin or phenazone; upon these one must suspend final judgement.

19.1.1.2 Single analgesics and non-steroidal anti-inflammatory drugs

On the whole, single antipyretic-analgesics other than aspirin have not been consumed in the large amounts which have been implicated in nephrotoxicity from compound preparations. The epidemiological data available tends to exonerate single drugs, especially aspirin, in the primary causation of kidney disease, except perhaps in isolated instances. However, the weight of evidence does suggest that they contribute to progression when renal damage is already present.

While there is little formal epidemiological documentation of NSAIDs causing chronic renal failure, there is ample clinical testimony to their harmful effects both as a primary cause of kidney disease and in the progression of renal failure which has other antecedents (Nanra 1989*b*; Sandler *et al.* 1991). These agents differ from the simple antipyretic-analgesics in that on the whole they are taken without other drugs, and in prescribed dosage. That they are nephrotoxic in such circumstances clearly places them in a different category to those substances causing classical analgesic nephropathy.

19.1.1.3 Analgesic associated cancer

As renal pelvic cancer is less common than papillary necrosis, and has causes other than analgesic consumption, the epidemiological evidence for carcinogenicity of specific analgesics is even more restricted. No analgesic can be absolved, although there is little evidence against the NSAIDs. Compound preparations containing phenacetin, and renal papillary necrosis, each have been inculpated (Chapter 17), and the concept that these are promoters rather than initiators of cancer is favoured by the diminishing incidence of urothelioma after cessation of analgesic intake (Chapter 18). It is conceivable that the promoting effect of papillary necrosis is responsible for the predominant occurrence of analgesic-associated cancers in the renal pelvis. Promotion by the drugs themselves might operate throughout the urinary tract, accounting principally for tumours in the bladder and renal parenchyma.

19.1.2 The conclusion based on laboratory evidence

No analgesic can be exonerated from nephrotoxicity on the results of experimental research; and none can be incriminated of initiating urothelial carcinogenesis. The renal papilla is more susceptible to aspirin and the NSAIDs when given alone, than to the other antipyretic-analgesics individually. An evaluation of the potential outcomes of renal medullary metabolism points to the likelihood of drug interactions, notably between aspirin and metabolites of phenacetin (including, and perhaps chiefly, paracetamol), being responsible for the susceptibility of the renal papilla to analgesic toxicity. Laboratory evidence points to phenacetin itself, and renal papillary necrosis whatever its aetiology, being promoters rather than initiators of urothelial cancer.

19.2 Strategies for prevention

It is possible to evaluate the effectiveness of different preventive measures only in societies which have had such a high prevalence of the disease that any regression is readily discernible, or else have kept good records of its occurrence. Such are certain countries in Scandinavia and western Europe, Canada and Australia.

19.2.1 Prohibition of phenacetin (and paracetamol)

Analgesic nephropathy had been reported earlier in the Nordic lands (Denmark, 1957; Sweden, 1961; Finland, 1962) than anywhere except Switzerland (1953). Two factors appear to have influenced the nature of the response by regulatory authorities there—its promptness (in 1961–2) and, unlike in the English-speaking world, the relative absence of extrarenal analgesic toxicity manifestly due to salicylate (Iceland being the exception; Chapter 6). In the circumstances, it is understandable that the least disruptive, and most likely to be effective, measure was taken: namely to make phenacetin and its derivatives (including paracetamol) available only by prescription. In Canada, phenacetin alone was proscribed (in 1973), but manufacturers of proprietary analgesics were in the main dissuaded from replacing it with paracetamol—however, one result in that country was a

5-fold increase in sales of paracetamol as a single agent (Wilson and Gault 1982).

The incidence of terminal and non-terminal kidney disease due to analgesics fell within a few years (Bengtsson 1966; Hood *et al.* 1967; Wilson and Gault 1982), and renal failure due to this cause has become uncommon in Scandinavia (Bengtsson 1979; Brunner *et al.* 1985*a*). A fall in the incidence of analgesic-related renal pelvic carcinoma was evident in Göteborg only from 1970, i.e. 9 yr after limitations were placed on phenacetin and paracetamol sales (Bengtsson 1979).

19.2.2 Restrictions on marketing compound analgesic preparations

Legislation was passed in Australia in 1979 to make all preparations containing more than one ingredient obtainable solely from pharmacies, and phenacetin only by prescription. The delay, 17 yr after recognition of the disease there, and 5 yr from the time a concerted campaign had been launched, was in part due to doubts as to the precise aetiology of analgesic nephropathy, the predominant role of phenacetin having been challenged by experimental evidence that aspirin and, possibly, paracetamol were more nephrotoxic (Chapter 3). Furthermore, in Australia as in Canada, the coexistence of gastric ulcer and anaemia, clinical problems of similar magnitude to kidney disease and clearly due to aspirin, demanded more comprehensive action than simply the elimination of phenacetin. An authoritative case could be made to the regulatory bodies only when a consensus was reached amongst all Australian nephrologists that the problem of chronic analgesic toxicity, whatever its precise aetiology, could be overcome only by curtailing heavy consumption; this was acknowledged to be characteristic of compound, but not of single ingredient, preparations.

During most of the subsequent decade, the efficacy of these measures was not apparent on examination of crude incidence rates for analgesic-induced end stage renal failure (Disney 1991). The explanation lay in the steady widening of criteria for entry into Australian dialysis programs, resulting in acceptance of more late middle aged and elderly patients and those with significant extrarenal disease, particularly cardiovascular. Since analgesic nephropathy is disproportionately represented amongst patients in these categories, the fall in younger cases with this diagnosis, definite by 1984 (Fig. 19.1), was balanced by a rise in the older age groups. The incidence of renal pelvic cancer in women in New South Wales rose until 1983, since when there has been no further increase, but not yet an unequivocal decline (Chapter 17).

19.2.3 Education and lobbying

In Australia and Canada, as in western Europe, there had been a strenuous and largely successful effort to educate both doctors and the public in the dangers of excess analgesic consumption from the time that its medical

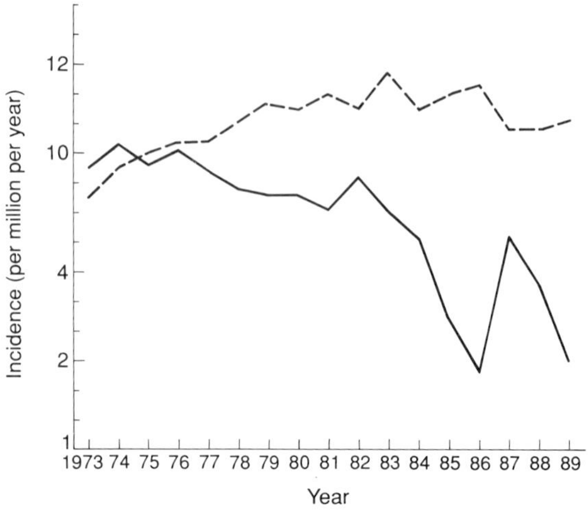

Fig. 19.1 Age standardized (to 'world' population) for all cases in New South Wales of:
——— analgesic nephropathy in persons aged 0–55 years
– – – – cancer of the renal pelvis in women of all ages.

consequences were recognized (Senate Standing Committee on Social Welfare 1977; Wilson and Gault 1982). Additionally, prior to legislation it had been possible to persuade most manufacturers in both countries to remove phenacetin from their analgesics (1967 and 1975 for the two brands most widely sold in Australia); however, not only were the other ingredients (aspirin and either caffeine or codeine) retained but, in Australia unlike in Canada, another agent (salicylamide or paracetamol) was substituted for the phenacetin.

The net effect of these measures was no great reduction in abuse of analgesics in Australia (Senate Standing Committee on Social Welfare 1977). Nevertheless, there was a slow but steady decline in the numbers of patients aged less than 55 yr with analgesic-induced end stage renal failure between 1973 and 1983 in New South Wales (Fig. 19.1). It is of course possible that this was due as much to better conservative treatment of kidney failure as to reduced analgesic consumption.

19.2.4 Forces promoting continuance of analgesic consumption

That education and voluntary restraint alike should have but little effect on analgesic abuse is understandable, even predictable, given the addictive nature of compound analgesic preparations. Moreover, their advertisement as medicaments purporting to relieve, not cause, suffering (e.g. 'Don't share your day with a headache!' and 'Take Vincent's with confidence!') is particularly likely to induce uncritical acceptance of their safety. It is inherently improbable that any business engaged in the manufacture or sale of analgesics for profit would readily make changes to their product, or in their marketing, tending to reduce the level of consumption unless persuaded that there was commercial risk in not doing so.

Placing analgesics, even the compound preparations which are known to be abused, on a drug schedule so as to restrict their sale to pharmacies, was opposed in Australia by *Choice* magazine, speaking for consumers, on the grounds that their price would rise and their availability be curtailed. Civil libertarians argued, in addition, that prohibition of legal sale has proved ineffective in diminishing the problems of alcohol, marijuana, and opiate abuse.

19.3 The reality

Antipyretic–analgesics certainly are habituating, but not so strongly addictive as tobacco, alcohol, or opiates; thus prohibition rarely causes more than temporary and minor symptoms of withdrawal, and the question does not arise of their being sought through illegal channels. Moreover, being sold for the purposes of ameliorating ill-health places upon those involved some responsibility to avoid generating fresh injury. Hence the ready acceptance of legislative measures to restrict their availability in the Nordic and British countries where government is acknowledged to have a role in public health. In continental Europe, with a different tradition of preventive medicine, voluntary measures have been tried for thirty years, but with limited success there as elsewhere.

The most rational approach to prevention of classical analgesic nephropathy would seem to be the prohibition of over-the-counter sale of any antipyretic–analgesic containing more than one ingredient. Rarely are single ingredient preparations abused; and they are decidedly less toxic than preparations which contain both salicylates and phenacetin or its derivatives. If indeed the role of analgesics in cancer is promotion, these measures will lessen, but not eliminate, upper urothelial carcinoma.

19.4 Prevention of secondary renal damage

A challenge for nephrologists in the 1990s will be the prevention of secondary renal damage, particularly from NSAIDs which are relied upon increasingly to remedy arthritic and musculoskeletal pain. The pharmaceutical industry promotes an expectation that symptoms can be alleviated by medication, and the public now presumes that a visit to a doctor will at least provide substantial relief. With no easy alternative to NSAIDs, it will be hard to persuade prescribers to explore different forms of treatment.

Perhaps the most we can expect is that renal function is checked before, and occasionally during, NSAID therapy, and that these drugs will not be used for mildly painful conditions. Our task will prove impossible if, as is occurring in many countries, NSAIDs are to be sold without prescription—nephrologists must join forces with gastroenterologists to ensure that this trend is reversed.

REFERENCES

Abraham, P.A. and Keane, W.F. (1984). Glomerular and interstitial disease induced by non-steroidal anti-inflammatory drugs. *American Journal of Nephrology*, **4**, 1–6.

Abrahams, C. and Levin, N.W. (1967). Experimentally induced analgesic nephropathy. Its pathogenesis. *Medical Proceedings*, **13**, 506–14.

Abrahams, C. and Levinson, C. (1970). Ultrastructure of the renal papilla in experimentally induced analgesic nephritis in rats. *South African Medical Journal*, **44**, 63–5.

Abrahams, C., Rubenstein, A.H., Levin, N.W., and Wunderlich, U. (1964). Experimentally induced analgesic nephritis in rat. *Archives of Pathology*, **78**, 222–30.

Abrahams, C., Van Tonder, H., and Hesse, V. (1976). Abnormal vessels in the urinary tract following analgesic abuse in man. *Archives of Pathology and Laboratory Medicine*, **100**, 630–1.

Abt, A.B. and Gordon, J.A. (1985). Drug-induced interstitial nephritis. Coexistence with glomerular disease. *Archives of Internal Medicine*, **145**, 1063–7.

Adam, W.R., Dawborn, J.K., Price, C.G., Riddell, J., and Story, H. (1970). Anaplastic transitional-cell carcinoma of the renal pelvis in association with analgesic abuse. *Medical Journal of Australia*, **1**, 1108–9.

Adams, F.G. and Murray, R.M. (1975). The radiological diagnosis of analgesic nephropathy. *Clinical Radiology*, **26**, 417–27.

Adams, S.S., Bough, R.G., Cliffe, E.E., Lessel, B., and Mills, R.F.N. (1969). Absorption, distribution and toxicity of ibuprofen. *Toxicology and Applied Pharmacology*, **15**, 310–30.

Adams, D.H., Howie, A.J., Michael, J., McConkey, B., Bacon, P.A., and Adu, D. (1986). Non-steroidal anti-inflammatory drugs and renal failure. *Lancet*, **1**, 57–60.

Akyol, S.M., Thompson, M., and Kerr, D.N.S. (1982). Renal function after prolonged consumption of aspirin. *British Medical Journal*, **284**, 631–2.

Allen, R.C., Petty, R.E., Lirenman, D.S., Malleson, P.N., and Laxer, R.M. (1986). Renal papillary necrosis in children with chronic arthritis. *American Journal of Diseases in Childhood*, **140**, 20–2.

Alt, J.M., Jänig, H., Schurek, H.J., and Stolte, H. (1979). Study of renal protein excretion in chronic pyelonephritis. *Contributions to Nephrology*, **16**, 37–43.

Alt, J.M., Hacke, M., von der Heyde, D., Jänig, H., Junge, P.M., Olbricht, C., and Stolle, H. (1983). Urinary protein excretion in interstitial and tubular kidney disease as characterized by gradient electrophoresis. *Klinische Wochenschrift*, **61**, 641–8.

Alvarez, A.S. and Summerskill, W.H.J. (1958). Gastrointestinal haemorrhage and salicylates. *Lancet*, **2**, 920–5.

Anderson, R.J., Wilson, P.D., Dillingham, M.A., Breckon, R., Schwertschlag, U., and Garcia-Sainz, J.A. (1985). Pertussis toxin reverses prostaglandin E_2 inhibition of arginine-vasopressin (AVP) and forskolin in rabbit collecting tubular epithelium. *Kidney International*, **27**, 252A.

Andersson, B., Larsson, R., Rahimtula, A., and Moldéus, P. (1983). Hydroperoxide-dependent activation of *p*-phenetidine catalyzed by prostaglandin synthase and other peroxidases. *Biochemical Pharmacology*, **32**, 1045–50.

Anderström, C. and Johansson, S.L. (1983). The combined effect of mechanical trauma and phenacetin or sodium saccharin on the rat urinary bladder. *Acta Pathologica, Microbiologica, et Immunologica Scandinavica: Section A, Pathology*, **91**, 381–9.

Anderström, C., Johansson, S.L., and von Schultz, L. (1983). The influence of phenacetin or mechanical perforation on the development of renal pelvic and urinary bladder tumors in FANFT-induced urinary tract carcinogenesis. *Acta Pathologica, Microbiologica, et Immunologica Scandinavica: Section A, Pathology*, **91**, 373–80.

Angervall, L., Lehmann, L., and Lincoln, K. (1962*a*). Induction of interstitial nephritis in rats fed phenacetin and NAPA (*N*-acetyl-*p*-aminophenol). *Acta Pathologica et Microbiologica Scandinavica*, **54**, 274–82.

Angervall, L., Lehmann, L., and Lincoln, K. (1962*b*). On the effect of phenacetin and NAPA (*N*-acetyl-*p*-aminophenol) on the development of bacterial interstitial nephritis in the rat. *Acta Pathologica et Microbiologica Scandinavica*, Suppl. **154**, 61–4.

Angervall, L., Lehmann, L., and Lincoln, K. (1962*c*). On the action of NAPA (*N*-acetyl-*p*-aminophenol) on the induction of interstitial nephritis in rats. *Acta Pathologica et Microbiologica Scandinavica*, **54**, 283–6.

Angervall, L., Lehmann, L., and Bengtsson, U. (1964). The renal concentrating capacity in albino rats after long-term consumption of phenacetin, NAPA (*N*-acetyl-*p*-aminophenol) and acetylsalicylic acid. *Acta Medica Scandinavica*, **175**, 155–60.

Angervall, L., Bengtsson, U., Zetterlund, C.G., and Zsigmond, M. (1969). Renal pelvic carcinoma in a Swedish district with abuse of a phenacetin-containing drug. *British Journal of Urology*, **40**, 401–5.

Anseline, P. and Howarth, V.S. (1977). A case of transitional cell carcinoma of the renal pelvis, clear cell renal carcinoma, and analgesic nephropathy. *Australian and New Zealand Journal of Surgery*, **47**, 521–3.

Antillon, M., Cominelli, F., Reynolds, T.B., and Zipser, R.D. (1989). Comparative acute effects of diflunisal and indomethacin on renal function in patients with cirrhosis and ascites. *American Journal of Gastroenterology*, **84**, 153–5.

Antillon, M., Cominelli, F., Lo, S., Moran, M., Somberg, K., Reynolds, T., and Zipser, R.D. (1990). Effects of oral prostaglandins on indomethacin induced renal failure in patients with cirrhosis and ascites. *Journal of Rheumatology*, **17** (Suppl. 20), 46–9.

Aosima, S. (1940*a*). Der Zusammenhang zwischen Antipyrin und Nierenschädung. *Japanese Journal of Dermatology and Urology*, **47**, 69.

Aosima, S. (1940*b*). Über den Einfluss von Antipyrin auf die Eingeweide des Kaninchens. *Japanese Journal of Dermatology and Urology*, **48**, 82.

Ardaillou, N., Nivez, M.P., Striker, G., and Ardaillou, R. (1983). Prostaglandin synthesis by human glomerular cells in culture. *Prostaglandins*, **26**, 773–84.

Ardaillou, N., Hagege, J., Nivez, M.P., Ardaillou, R., and Schlondorff, D. (1985).

Vasoconstrictor-evoked prostaglandin synthesis in cultured human mesangial cells. *American Journal of Physiology*, **248**, F240–6.

Arger, P.H., Bluth, E.I., Murray, T., and Goldberg, M. (1976). Analgesic abuse nephropathy. *Urology*, **7**, 123–8.

Arisz, L., Donker, A.J., Brentjens, J.R., and van der Hem, G.K. (1976). The effect of indomethacin on proteinuria and kidney function in the nephrotic syndrome. *Acta Medica Scandinavica*, **199**, 121–5.

Armstrong, B., Garrod, A., and Doll, R. (1976). A retrospective study of renal cancer with special reference to coffee and animal protein consumption. *British Journal of Cancer*, **33**, 127–36.

Arnold, L., Collins, C., and Starmer, G.A. (1973*a*). The short-term effects of aspirin on the rat kidney—further observations. *Medical Journal of Australia*, **1**, 678–82.

Arnold, L., Collins, C., and Starmer, G.A. (1973*b*). The short-term effects of acetylsalicylic acid in the rat kidney: further observations. *Nephron*, **10**, 355–75.

Arnold, L., Collins, C., and Starmer, G.A. (1973*c*). The short-term effects of analgesics on the kidney with special reference to acetylsalicylic acid. *Pathology*, **5**, 123–34.

Arnold, L., Collins, C., and Starmer, G.A. (1974). Renal and gastric lesions after phenylbutazone and indomethacin in the rat. *Pathology*, **6**, 303–13.

Arnold, L., Collins, C., and Starmer, G.A. (1976). Further studies of the acute effects of phenylbutazone, oxyphenbutazone and indomethacin on the rat kidney. *Pathology*, **8**, 135–41.

Artinano, M., Etheridge, W.B., Stroehlein, K.B., and Barcenas, C.G. (1986). Progression of minimal-change glomerulopathy to focal glomerulosclerosis in a patient with fenoprofen nephropathy. *American Journal of Nephrology*, **6**, 353–7.

Asal, N.R., Geyer, J.R., Risser, D.R., Lee, E.T., Kadamani, S., and Cherng, N. (1988). Risk factors in renal cell carcinoma. II. Medical history, occupation, multivariate analysis, and conclusions. *Cancer Detection and Prevention*, **13**, 263–79.

Atkinson, L.K., Goodship, T.H.J., and Ward, M.K. (1986). Acute renal failure associated with acute pyelonephritis and consumption of non-steroidal anti-inflammatory drugs. *British Medical Journal*, **292**, 97–8.

Axelsen, R.A. (1973). Spontaneous renal papillary necrosis in the Gunn rat. *Pathology*, **5**, 43–50.

Axelsen, R.A. (1975). The induction of renal papillary necrosis in Gunn rats by analgesics and analgesic mixtures. *British Journal of Experimental Pathology*, **56**, 92–7.

Axelsen, R.A. (1976). Analgesic-induced renal papillary necrosis in the Gunn rat: the comparative nephrotoxicity of aspirin and phenacetin. *Journal of Pathology*, **120**, 145–50.

Axelsen, R.A. (1978). Experimental renal papillary necrosis in the rat: the selective vulnerability of medullary structures to injury. *Virchows Archiv. A. Pathological Anatomy and Histology*, **381**, 79–84.

Axelsen, R.A., and Burry, A.F. (1972). Papillary necrosis in the Gunn rat: rapid induction by analgesics. *Pathology*, **4**, 225–9.

Bach, P.H. (1989). Detection of chemically induced renal injury: the cascade of degenerative morphological and functional changes that follow the primary nephrotoxic insult and evaluation of these changes by *in-vitro* methods. *Toxicology Letters*, **46**, 237–49.

Bach, P.H. (1990). Crystalluria, medullary matrix crystal deposits and bladder calculi associated with an acutely induced renal papillary necrosis. *British Journal of Urology*, **66**, 463–70.

Bach, P.H. and Bridges, J.W. (1984). The role of metabolic activation of analgesics and non-steroidal anti-inflammatory drugs in the development of renal papillary necrosis and upper urothelial carcinoma. *Prostaglandins, Leukotrienes and Medicine*, **15**, 251–74.

Bach, P.H. and Bridges, J.W. (1985). Chemically induced renal papillary necrosis and upper urothelial carcinoma. *CRC Critical Reviews in Toxicology*, **15**, 217–441.

Bach, P.H. and Gregg, N.J. (1988). Experimentally induced renal papillary necrosis and upper urothelial carcinoma. *International Reviews in Experimental Pathology*, **30**, 1–54.

Bach, P.H. and Hardy, T.L. (1985). Relevance of animal models to analgesic associated renal papillary necrosis in humans. *Kidney International*, **28**, 605–13.

Bach, P.H., Grasso, P., Molland, E.A., and Bridges, J.W. (1983). Changes in the medullary glycosaminoglycan histochemistry and microvascular filling during the development of 2-bromoethanamine hydrobromide-induced renal papillary necrosis. *Toxicology and Applied Pharmacology*, **69**, 333–44.

Bach, P.H., Gregg, N.J., and Wachsmuth, E.D. (1987). The application of histochemistry at the light microscopic level to the study of nephrotoxicity. In *Nephrotoxicity in the experimental and clinical situation*, Part 1. (ed. P.H. Bach and E.A. Lock), pp. 19–84. Martinus Nijhoff, Dordrecht.

Bach, P.H., Scholey, D.J., Delacruz, L., Moret, M., and Nichol, S. (1991). Renal and urinary lipid changes associated with an acutely induced renal papillary necrosis. *Food and Chemical Toxicology*, **29**, 211–19.

Bailey, R.R., Neale, T.J., and Little, P.J. (1974). Analgesic nephropathy. *New Zealand Medical Journal*, **79**, 1053–7.

Bakkenist, A.R.J., Platt, H., and Weaver, R. (1981). Oxidation of 4-chloroaniline catalysed by human myeloperoxidase. *Bioorganic Chemistry*, **10**, 324–8.

Bander, S.J. (1985). Reversible renal failure and nephrotic syndrome without interstitial nephritis from zomepirac. *American Journal of Kidney Diseases*, **6**, 233–6.

Banks, R.O. (1990). Effects of endothelin on renal function in dogs and rats. *American Journal of Physiology*, **258**, F775–80.

Bannasch, P. (1986*a*). Preneoplastic lesions as end points in carcinogenicity testing. I. Hepatic preneoplasia. *Carcinogenesis*, **7**, 689–95.

Bannasch, P. (1986*b*). Preneoplastic lesions as end points in carcinogenicity testing. II. Preneoplasia in various non-hepatic tissues. *Carcinogenesis*, **7**, 849–52.

Baran, D.T., Lee, S.W., Jo, O.D., and Avioli, L.V. (1982). Acquired alterations in vitamin D metabolism in the acidotic state. *Calcified Tissue International*, **34**, 165–8.

Barone, J.A., Raia, J.R., and Huang, Y.C. (1988). Evaluation of the effects of multiple-dose activated charcoal on the absorption of orally administered salicylate in a simulated toxic ingestion model. *Annals of Emergency Medicine*, **17**, 34–7.

Bartolone, J.B., Beierschmitt, W.P., Birge, R.B., Hart, S.G.E., Wyand, S., Cohen, S.D., and Khairallah, E.A. (1989). Selective acetaminophen metabolite binding to hepatic and extrahepatic proteins: an *in vivo* and *in vitro* analysis. *Toxicology and Applied Pharmacology*, **99**, 240–9.

Basch, S.H. (1980). Emotional dehiscence after successful renal transplantation. *Kidney International*, **17**, 388–96.

Battegay, R. (1958*a*). Individuelle und soziale Ursachen, Prognose und Prophylaxe der Sucht mit Analgetika. *Schweizerische Medizinische Wochenschrift*, **88**, 89–92.

Battegay, R. (1958*b*). Aktuelle Aspekte der Analgetikasucht. *Nervenarzt*, **29**, 467–8.

Baud, L., Sraer, J., Delarue, F., Bens, M., Balavoine, F., Schlondorff, D. *et al.* (1985). Lipoxygenase products mediate the attachment of rat macrophages to glomeruli *in vitro*. *Kidney International*, **27**, 855–63.

Baum, M., Stirling, G.A., and Dawson, J.L. (1969). Further study into obstructive jaundice and ischaemic renal damage. *British Medical Journal*, **2**, 229–31.

Beaufils, M., Uzan, S., Donsimoni, R., and Colau, J.C. (1985). Prevention of pre-eclampsia by early antiplatelet therapy. *Lancet*, **1**, 840–2.

Becci, P.J., Thompson, H.J., Grubbs, C.J., and Moon, R.C. (1979). A quantitative dosing schedule for the induction of transitional cell carcinomas in female F344 rats with the use of *N*-butyl-*N*-(4-hydroxybutyl)nitrosamine. *Journal of the National Cancer Institute*, **62**, 187–91.

Begley, M., Chadwick, J.M., and Jepson, R.P. (1970). A possible case of analgesic abuse associated with transitional-cell carcinoma of the bladder. *Medical Journal of Australia*, **2**, 1133–4.

Bell, D., Kerr, D.N.S., Swinney, J., and Yeates, W.K. (1969). Analgesic nephropathy. Clinical course after withdrawal of phenacetin. *British Medical Journal*, **3**, 378–82.

Bell, R.L., Kennerly, D.A., Stanford, N., and Majerus, P.W. (1979). Diglyceride lipase: a pathway for archidonate release from human platelets. *Proceedings of the National Academy of Sciences of the United States of America*, **76**, 3238–41.

Bender, W.L., Whelton, A., Beschorner, W.E., Darwish, M.O., Hall-Craggs, M., and Solez, K. (1984). Interstitial nephritis, proteinuria, and renal failure caused by nonsteroidal anti-inflammatory drugs. Immunologic characterization of the inflammatory infiltrate. *American Journal of Medicine*, **76**, 1006–12.

Bengtsson, U. (1962). A comparative study of chronic non-obstructive pyelonephritis and renal papillary necrosis. *Acta Medica Scandinavica*, **172** (Suppl. 388), 1–71.

Bengtsson, U. (1966). Analgesic nephropathy—chronic pyelonephritis. *Proceedings of the 3rd International Congress of Nephrology, Washington*, pp. 291–9. Karger, Basel.

Bengtsson, U. (1974). Phenacetin and renal pelvic carcinoma. *Clinical Nephrology*, **2**, 123–6.

Bengtsson, U. (1979). Prevention of renal disease. *Proceedings of the European Dialysis and Transplant Association*, **16**, 466–74.

Bengtsson, U. (1989). Analgetika-nephropathie—langfristige Erfahrungen aus Schweden. *Zeitschrift für Urologie und Nephrologie*, **82** (Suppl. 1), 121–5.

Bengtsson, U. and Angervall, L. (1970). Analgesic abuse and tumours of the renal pelvis. *Lancet*, **1**, 305

Bengtsson, U., Angervall, L., Ekman, H., and Lehmann, L. (1968). Transitional cell tumors of the renal pelvis in analgesic abusers. *Scandinavian Journal of Urology and Nephrology*, **2**, 145–50.

Bengtsson, U., Angervall, L., Johansson, S., and Wahlqvist, L. (1973). Phenacetin abuse and renal pelvic carcinoma. In *Probleme des phenacetinabusus* (ed. H. Haschek), pp. 221–6. Egermann, Vienna.

Bengtsson, U., Johansson, S., and Angervall, L. (1978). Malignancies of the urinary tract and their relation to analgesic abuse. *Kidney International*, **13**, 107–13.

Benigni, A., Gregorini, G., Frusca, T., Chiabrando, C., Ballerini, S., Valcamonico, A. *et al.* (1989). Effect of low-dose aspirin on fetal and maternal generation of thromboxane by platelets in women at risk for pregnancy-induced hypertension. *New England Journal of Medicine*, **321**, 357–62.

Benowitz, N.L. (1990). Clinical pharmacology of caffeine. *Annual Review of Medicine*, **41**, 277–88.

Berg, K.J. and Talseth, T. (1985). Acute renal effects of sulindac and indomethacin in chronic renal failure. *Clinical Pharmacology and Therapeutics*, **37**, 447–52.

Bernard, A.M., de Russis, R., Amor, A.O., and Lauwerys, R.R. (1988). Potentiation of cadmium nephrotoxicity by acetaminophen. *Archives of Toxicology*, **62**, 291–4.

Berndt, W.O., Hayes, A.W., and Philips, R.D. (1980). Effects of mycotoxins on renal function: mycotoxic nephropathy. *Kidney International*, **18**, 656–64.

Berneis, K. and Studer, A. (1969). Ablagerungen farbiger Lipide in der Haut als Folge von Phenacetinabusus. *Virchows Archiv. B, Zell Pathologie*, **2**, 311–7.

Berneis, K., Kortweg, E., and Mihatsch, M.J. (1983). Characterization of the brown pigment of the mucosa of the urinary tract. *Virchows Archiv. A, Pathological Anatomy and Histology*, **402**, 203–7.

Bernhammer, E. and Krisch, K. (1965). Deacetylation of phenacetin by liver esterase. *Biochemical Pharmacology*, **14**, 863–71.

Beswick, I.P. and Schatzki, P.F. (1960). Experimental renal papillary necrosis. *Archives of Pathology*, **69**, 733–40.

Beun, G.D.M., Leunissen, K.M.L., Van Breda Vriesman, P.J.C., Van Hooff, J.P., and Grave, W. (1987). Isolated minimal change nephropathy associated with diclofenac. *British Medical Journal*, **295**, 182–3.

Beynen, A.C., Buechler, K.F., van der Molen, A.J., and Geelen, M.J.H. (1982). Inhibition of hepatic lipogenesis by salicylate. *Toxicology*, **24**, 33–43.

Billington, B.P. (1960). Gastric ulcer: age, sex, and a curious retrogression. *Australasian Annals of Medicine*, **9**, 111–21.

Billington, B.P. (1963). The Australian gastric ulcer change: interstate variations. *Australasian Annals of Medicine*, **12**, 153–9.

Björck, S., Svalander, C.T., and Aurell, M. (1988). Acute renal failure after analgesic drugs including paracetamol (acetaminophen). *Nephron*, **49**, 45–53.

Blasingham, M.C. and Nasjletti, A. (1980). Differential renal effects of cyclooxygenase inhibition in sodium-replete and sodium-deprived dog. *American Journal of Physiology*, **239**, F360–5.

Blasingham, M.C., Shade, R.E., Share, L., and Nasjletti, A. (1980). The effect of meclofenamate on renal blood flow in the unanesthetized dog: relation to renal prostaglandins and sodium balance. *Journal of Pharmacology and Experimental Therapeutics*, **214**, 1–4.

Bleyer, W.A. and Breckenridge, R.T. (1970). Studies on the detection of adverse drug reactions in the newborn II. The effects of prenatal aspirin on newborn hemostasis. *Journal of the American Medical Association*, **213**, 2049–53.

Blohmé, I. and Johansson, S. (1981). Renal pelvic neoplasms and atypical urothelium in patients with end-stage analgesic nephropathy. *Kidney International*, **20**, 671–5.

Bluemle, L.W. and Goldberg, M. (1968). Renal accumulation of salicylate and phenacetin: possible mechanisms in the nephropathy of analgesic abuse. *Journal of Clinical Investigation*, **47**, 2507–14.

Blute, M.L., Segura, J.W., Patterson, D.E., Benson, R.C., and Zincke, H. (1989). Impact of endourology on diagnosis and management of upper urinary tract urothelial cancer. *Journal of Urology*, **141**, 1298–301.

Bojesen, I. (1974). Quantitative and qualitative analyses of isolated lipid droplets from interstitial cells in renal papillae from various species. *Lipids*, **9**, 835–43.

Bojesen, I.N. (1980). Fatty acid composition and depot function of lipid droplet triacylcylcerols in renomedullary interstitial cells. In *The Renal papilla and hypertension* (ed. A.K. Mandal and S.-O. Bohman), pp. 121–48. Plenum, New York.

Bokelman, D.L., Bagdon, W.J., Mattis, P.A., and Stonier, P.F. (1971). Strain-dependent renal toxicity of a nonsteroidal antiinflammatory agent. *Toxicology and Applied Pharmacology*, **19**, 111–24.

Boletis, J., Williams, A.J., Shortland, J.R., and Brown, C.B. (1989). Irreversible renal failure following mefenamic acid. *Nephron*, **51**, 575–6.

Bolhuis, R.L., Klein, J.C., Kruisbeek, A.M., and Hollander, C.F. (1978). Spontaneous urinary bladder and ureter tumors in the Brown Norway rat. *National Cancer Institute Monograph*, **49**, 301–4.

Bonvalet, J.P., Pradelles, P., and Farman, N. (1987). Segmental synthesis and actions of prostaglandins along the nephron. *American Journal of Physiology*, **253**, F377–87.

Bonventre, J.V., Weber, P.C., and Gronich, J.H. (1988). PAF and PDGF increase cytosolic [Ca^{2+}] and phospholipase activity in mesangial cells. *American Journal of Physiology*, **254**, F87–94.

Boorman, G.A. and Hollander, C.F. (1974). High incidence of spontaneous urinary bladder and ureter tumors in the Brown Norway rat. *Journal of the National Cancer Institute*, **52**, 1005–8.

Boorman, G.A., Burek, J.D., and Hollander, C.F. (1977). Animal model of human disease: carcinoma of the ureter and the urinary bladder. *American Journal of Pathology*, **88**, 251–4.

Borda, E., Chaud, M., Gutnisky, R., Contreras-Ortiz, N., Gimeno, M.F., and Gimeno, A.L. (1983). Relationships between prostaglandins and estrogens on the motility of isolated rings from the rat urinary bladder. *Journal of Urology*, **129**, 1250–3.

Boyd, E.M. (1959*a*). The acute oral toxicity of acetylsalicylic acid. *Toxicology and Applied Pharmacology*, **1**, 229–39.

Boyd, E.M. (1959*b*). The acute oral toxicity of caffeine. *Toxicology and Applied Pharmacology*, **1**, 250–7.

Boyd, E.M. and Bereczky, G.M. (1966). Liver necrosis from paracetamol. *British Journal of Pharmacology*, **26**, 606–14.

Boyd, J.A. and Eling, T.E. (1981). Prostaglandin endoperoxide synthetase-dependent cooxidation of acetaminophen to intermediates which covalently bind *in vitro* to rabbit renal medullary microsomes. *Journal of Pharmacology and Experimental Therapeutics*, **219**, 659–64.

Boyd, E.M. and Hogan, S.E. (1968). The chronic oral toxicity of paracetamol at the range of the LD_{50} (100 days) in albino rats. *Canadian Journal of Physiology and Pharmacology*, **46**, 239–45.

Boyd, E.M., Dolman, M., Knight, L.M., and Sheppard, E.P. (1965). The chronic oral toxicity of caffeine. *Canadian Journal of Physiology and Pharmacology*, **43**, 995–1007.

Boyer, T.D. and Rouff, S.L. (1971). Acetaminophen-induced hepatic necrosis and renal failure. *Journal of the American Medical Association*, **218**, 440–1.

Boyer, T.D., Zia, P., and Reynolds, T.B. (1979). Effect of indomethacin and prostaglandin A_1 on renal function and plasma renin activity in alcoholic liver disease. *Gastroenterology*, **77**, 215–22.

Brater, D.C. (1986). Drug–drug and drug–disease interactions with nonsteroidal anti-inflammatory drugs. *American Journal of Medicine*, **80** (Suppl. 1A), 62–77.

Brater, D.C., Anderson, S., Baird, B., and Campbell, W.B. (1985). Effects of ibuprofen, naproxen, and sulindac on prostaglandins in men. *Kidney International*, **27**, 66–73.

Brattig, N.W., Diao, G.J., and Berg, P.A. (1988). The specificity of the lymphocyte transformation test in a patient with hypersensitivity reactions to pyrazolone compounds. A 10-week follow-up study before and after rechallenge. *European Journal of Clinical Pharmacology*, **35**, 39–45.

Braun, B., Weber, M., Rückel, E., Reuss, J., and Köhler, H. (1983). Sonographische Befunde bei Analgetika-nephropathie. *Deutsche Medizinische Wochenschrift*, **108**, 1230–3.

Brenner, B.M., Ichikawa, I., and Deen, W.M. (1981). Glomerular filtration. In *The kidney*, (2nd edn). (ed. B.M. Brenner and F.C. Rector), pp. 287–327. Saunders, Philadelphia.

Brenner, B.M., Meyer, T.W., and Hostetter, T.H. (1982). Dietary protein restriction and the progressive nature of kidney disease. The role of hemodynamically-mediated glomerular injury in the pathogenesis of progressive glomerulosclerosis in aging, renal ablation, and intrinsic renal disease. *New England Journal of Medicine*, **307**, 652–9.

Breslow, N.E. and Day, N.E. (1980). *Statistical methods in cancer research, Volume I. The analysis of case-control studies.* IARC Scientific Publications No. 32. International Agency for Research on Cancer, Lyon.

Breslow, N.E. and Day, N.E. (1987). *Statistical methods in cancer research. Volume II. The analysis of cohort studies.* IARC Scientific Publications No. 82. International Agency for Research on Cancer, Lyon.

Brezin, J.P., Katz, S.M., Schwartz, A.B., and Chinitz, J.L. (1979). Reversible renal failure and nephrotic syndrome associated with nonsteroidal anti-inflammatory drugs. *New England Journal of Medicine*, **301**, 1271–3.

Briggs, D., Calder, I., Woods, R., and Tange, J. (1982). The influence of metabolic variation on analgesic nephrotoxicity. Experiments with the Gunn rat. *Pathology*, **14**, 349–53.

Brod, J. and Kühn, K. (1973). Chronic pyelonephritis and phenacetin kidney. In *Probleme des Phenacetinabusus* (ed. H. Haschek), pp. 317–24. Egermann, Wien.

Brodie, B.B. and Axelrod, J. (1949). The fate of acetaphenetidin (phenacetin) in man and its metabolites in biological materials. *Journal of Pharmacology and Experimental Therapeutics*, **97**, 58–67.

Brookland, R.K. and Richter, M.P. (1985). The postoperative irradiation of transitional cell carcinoma of the renal pelvis and ureter. *Journal of Urology*, **133**, 952–5.

Brown, D.M. and Hardy, T.L. (1968). Short-term study of the effect of phenacetin, phenazone and amidopyrine on the rat kidney. *British Journal of Pharmacology and Chemotherapy*, **32**, 17–24.

Brown, R.C., Hawtrey, C.E., and Pixley, E.E. (1973). Brush biopsy of the renal pelvis. *American Journal of Roentgenology, Radium Therapeutic and Nuclear Medicine*, **119**, 779–85.

Bruckner, J.V., Khanna, K.L., and Cornish, H.H. (1974). Polychlorinated biphenyl-induced alteration of biologic parameters in the rat. *Toxicology and Applied Pharmacology*, **28**, 189–99.

Brunner, W. and Spühler, O. (1951). Zur Indikation der Dekapsulation und Entnervung der Niere. *Helvetica Chirurgica Acta*, **18**, 339–46.

Brunner, F.P. and Thiel, G. (1986). Klinik der Analgetika Nephropathie. In *Das Analgetika Syndrom* (ed. M.J. Mihatsch), pp. 65–71. Thieme, Stuttgart.

Brunner, F.P., Broyer, M., Brynger, H., Callah, S., Fassbinder, W., Oulès, R. *et al.* (1985*a*). Combined report on regular dialysis and transplantation in Europe, XV, 1984. *Proceedings of the European Dialysis and Transplant Association—European Renal Association*, **22**, 5–53.

Brunner, K., Burger, H.R., Greminger, P., and Streuli, R. (1985*b*). Mefenaminsäure (Ponstan)-induzierte akute interstitielle Nephritis mit reversiblem, schwerem, nicht-oligurischem Nierenversagen. *Schweizerische Medizinische Wochenschrift*, **115**, 1730–4.

Buccianti, C. (1989). Europäische Prospektivstudie zur Analgetika-nephropathie. *Zeitschrift für Urologie und Nephrologie*, **82** (Suppl. 1), 135–42.

Buccianti, C., De Broe, M., and Challah, S. (1987). Combined European study on analgesic nephropathy. In *Prevention in Nephrology* (ed. G. Buccianti), pp. 81–6. Masson Italia, Milano.

Buckalew, V.M. and Schey, H.M. (1986*a*). Analgesic nephropathy: a significant cause of morbidity in the United States. *American Journal of Kidney Diseases*, **7**, 164–8.

Buckalew, V.M. and Schey, H.M. (1986*b*). Renal disease from habitual antipyretic analgesic consumption: an assessment of the epidemiologic evidence. *Medicine* **11**, 291–303.

Burek, J.D. (1978). *Pathology of aging rats*, pp. 101–9. CRC Press, Palm Beach.

Bürgin, M., Schmidt, M., and Reutter, F. (1984). Fokal-segmentale Glomeruloskerose bei Analgetika-nephropathie. *Schweizerische Medizinische Wochenschrift*, **114**, 1118–23.

Burry, A.F. (1966). A profile of renal diseases in Queensland: results of an autopsy survey. *Medical Journal of Australia*, **1**, 826–31.

Burry, A.F. (1967). The evolution of analgesic nephropathy. *Nephron*, **5**, 185–201.

Burry, A. (1978). Pathology of analgesic nephropathy: Australian experience. *Kidney International*, **13**, 34–40.

Burry, A.F. and Hopkins, J. (1977). Phenacetin and analgesic nephropathy. *Medical Journal of Australia*, **1**, 879–82.

Burry, A.F., de Jersey, P., and Weedon, D. (1966). Phenacetin and renal papillary necrosis: results of a prospective autopsy investigation. *Medical Journal of Australia*, **1**, 873–9.

Burry, A.F., Axelson, R.A., and Trolove, P. (1974). Analgesic nephropathy: its present contribution to the renal mortality and morbidity profile. *Medical Journal of Australia*, **1**, 31–6.

Burry, A.F., Cross, R., and Axelsen, R. (1977). Analgesic nephropathy and the renal concentrating mechanism. *Pathology Annual*, **12**, 1–31.

Calder, I.C., Funder, C.C., Green, C.R., Ham, K.N., and Tange, J.D. (1971). Comparative nephrotoxicity of aspirin and phenacetin derivatives. *British Medical Journal*, **4**, 518–21.

Calder, I.C., Yong, A.C., Woods, R.A., Crowe, C.A., Ham, K.N., and Tange, J.D. (1979). The nephrotoxicity of *p*-aminophenol. II. The effect of metabolic inhibitors and inducers. *Chemico-biological Interactions*, **27**, 245–54.

Cameron, J.S. (1983). Effect of the recipient's renal disease on the results of transplantation (other than diabetes mellitus). *Kidney International*, **23** (Suppl. 14), S24–33.

Cameron, J.S. (1988). Allergic interstitial nephritis: clinical features and pathogenesis. *Quarterly Journal of Medicine*, **66**, 97–115.

Campistol, J.M., Galofre, J., Botey, A., Torras, A., and Revert, L. (1989). Reversible membranous nephritis associated with diclofenac. *Nephrology, Dialysis, Transplantation*, **4**, 393–5.

Carlisle, C.H., Penny, R.H.C., Prescott, C.W., and Davidson, H.A. (1968). Toxic effects of phenylbutazone on the cat. *British Veterinary Journal*, **124**, 560–8.

Carmichael, J. and Shankel, S.W. (1985). Effects of nonsteroidal anti-inflammatory drugs on prostaglandins and renal function. *American Journal of Medicine*, **78**, 992–1000.

Carpenter, H.M. and Mudge, G.H. (1981). Acetaminophen nephrotoxicity: studies on renal acetylation and deacetylation. *Journal of Pharmacology and Experimental Therapeutics*, **218**, 161–7.

Carro-Campi, G. (1978). Phenacetin abuse: a review. *Toxicology*, **10**, 311–39.

Carson, J., Notis, W.M., and Orris, E.S. (1990). Colonic ulceration and bleeding during diclofenac therapy. *New England Journal of Medicine*, **323**, 135.

Caruana, R.J. and Semble, E.L. (1984). Renal papillary necrosis due to naproxen. *Journal of Rheumatology*, **11**, 90–1.

Caruso, I., and Porro, G.B. (1980). Gastroscopic evaluation of anti-inflammatory agents. *British Medical Journal*, **280**, 75–8.

Case, R.A.M., Hosker, M.E., McDonald, D.B., and Pearson, J.T. (1954). Tumours of the urinary bladder in workmen engaged in the manufacture and use of certain dyestuff intermediates in the British chemical industry. I. The role of aniline, benzidine, alpha-naphthylamine and beta-naphthylamine. *British Journal of Industrial Medicine*, **11**, 75–104.

Catella, F., Pulgiese, F., Patrignani, P., Filabozzi, P., Ciabattoni, G., and Patrono, C.

(1984). Differential platelet and renal effects of sulfinpyrazone in man. *Clinical Research*, **32**, 239A.

Caterson, R.J. and Duggin, G.G. (1978). Intrarenal distribution of salicylate. *Proceedings of the Australian Society of Medical Research*, **1**, 57.

Caterson, R.J. and Duggin, G.G. (1980). Intrarenal distribution of salicylate. *Clinical and Experimental Pharmacology and Physiology*, **7**, 77–8.

Caterson, R.J., Duggin, G.G., Horvarth, J.S., Mohandas, J., and Tiller, D.J. (1978). Aspirin, protein transacetylation and inhibition of prostaglandin synthetase in the kidney. *British Journal of Pharmacology*, **64**, 353–8.

Champion de Crespigny, P.J., Becker, G.J., Ihle, B.U., Walter, N.M.A., Wright, C.A., and Kincaid-Smith, P. (1988). Renal failure and nephrotic syndrome associated with sulindac. *Clinical Nephrology*, **30**, 52–5.

Chan, L.K., Winearls, C.G., Oliver, D.O., and Dunnill, M.S. (1980). Acute interstitial nephritis and erythroderma associated with diflunisal. *British Medical Journal*, **1**, 84–5.

Chapman, B.L. and Duggan, J.M. (1969). Aspirin and uncomplicated gastric ulcer. *Gut*, **10**, 443–50.

Chatterjee, G.P. (1981). Nephrotic syndrome induced by tolmetin. *Journal of the American Medical Association*, **246**, 1589.

Cheng, H.F., Nolasco, F., Cameron, J.S., Hildreth, G., Neild, G., and Hartley, B. (1989). HLA-DR display by renal tubular epithelium and phenotype of infiltrate in interstitial nephritis. *Nephrology, Dialysis, Transplantation*, **4**, 205–15.

Chernozemsky, I.N., Stoyanov, I.S., Petkova-Bocharova, T.K., Nicolov, I.G. Draganov, I.V. Stoichev, I.I. *et al.* (1977). Geographic correlation between the occurrence of endemic nephropathy and urinary tract tumours in Vratza district, Bulgaria. *International Journal of Cancer*, **19**, 1–11.

Choudhury, S.L., Taylor, S.H., Wieringa, G., Swaminathan, R., and Morgan, D.B. (1983). Sulphinpyrazone and renal function following myocardial infarction. *European Journal of Clinical Pharmacology*, **24**, 747–50.

Christie, D. (1978). 'The analgesic abuse syndrome': an epidemiological perspective. *International Journal of Epidemiology*, **7**, 139–43.

Ciabattoni, G. and Pugliese, F. (1989). Studies of renal eicosanoid synthesis *in vivo* and *in vitro*. In *Renal eicosanoids, advances in experimental medicine and biology*, Vol. 259 (ed. M.J. Dunn, C. Patrono, and G.A. Cinotti), pp. 361–88. Plenum, New York.

Ciabattoni, G., Pugliese, F., Cinotti, G.A., and Patrono, C. (1980). Renal effects of anti-inflammatory drugs. *European Journal of Rheumatology and Inflammation*, **3**, 210–21.

Ciabattoni, G., Cinotti, G.A., Pierucci, A., Simonetti, B.M., Manzi, M., Pugliese, F. *et al.* (1984*a*). Effects of sulindac and ibuprofen in patients with chronic glomerular disease. Evidence for the dependence of renal function on prostacyclin. *New England Journal of Medicine*, **310**, 279–83.

Ciabattoni, G., Porro, G.B., Caruso, I., Fumagalli, M., Pugliese, F., and Patrono, C. (1984*b*). Differential inhibition of prostaglandin (PG) and thromboxane (Tx) synthesis in human tissues by non-steroidal anti-inflammatory drugs (NSADs). *Clinical Research*, **32**, 462A.

Clarkson, A.R. and Lawrence, J.R. (1970). The clinical features of analgesic nephropathy. In *Renal infection and renal scarring* (ed. P. Kincaid-Smith and K.F. Fairley), pp. 375–84. Mercedes, Melbourne.

Claude, J.C., Frentzel-Beyme, R.R., and Kunze, E. (1988). Occupation and risk of cancer of the lower urinary tract among men. A case-control study. *International Journal of Cancer*, **41**, 371–9.

Clausen, E. (1962). Nephrotoxic effects of phenacetin and acetylsalicylic acid in animal experiments. *Acta Medica Scandinavica*, **172**, 419–26.

Clausen, E. (1964). Histological changes in rabbit kidneys induced by phenacetin and acetylsalicylic acid. *Lancet*, **2**, 123–4.

Clausen, E. and Pedersen, J. (1961). Necrosis of the renal papillae in rheumatoid arthritis. *Acta Medica Scandinavica*, **170**, 631–3.

Clèdes, J., Gentric, A., Brière, J., and Leroy, J.P. (1988). Glomérulonéphrite extra-membraneuse (GNEM) au cours d'un traitement par le diclofénac. *Néphrologie*, **9**, 283.

Clissold, S.P. (1986). Paracetamol and phenacetin. *Drugs*, **32** (Suppl. 4), 46–59.

Clive, D.M. and Stoff, J.S. (1984). Renal syndromes associated with nonsteroidal antiinflammatory drugs. *New England Journal of Medicine*, **310**, 563–72.

Cobden, I., Record, C.O., Ward, M.K., and Kerr, D.N.S. (1982). Paracetamol-induced acute renal failure in the absence of fulminant liver damage. *British Medical Journal*, **284**, 21–2.

Cohen, S.M. (1985). Multi-stage carcinogenesis in the urinary bladder. *Food and Chemical Toxicology*, **23**, 521–8.

Cohen, S.M. and Ellwein, L.B. (1989). Cell growth dynamics in bladder carcinogenesis: implications for risk assessment. *Journal of the American College of Toxicology*, **8**, 1103–13.

Cohen, S.M. and Ellwein, L.B. (1990*a*). Proliferative and genotoxic cellular effects in 2-acetylaminofluorene bladder and liver carcinogenesis: biological modeling of the ED01 study. *Toxicology and Applied Pharmacology*, **104**, 79–93.

Cohen, S.M. and Ellwein, L.B. (1990*b*). Cell proliferation in carcinogenesis. *Science*, **249**, 1007–11.

Cohen, S.M., and Friedell, G.H. (1979). Animal model: carcinoma of the urinary bladder, induced in Fischer rats by *N*-[4-(5-nitro-2-furyl)-2-thiazolyl]formamide. *American Journal of Pathology*, **95**, 849–52.

Cohen, S.M., Murasaki, G., Fukushima, S., and Greenfield, R.E. (1982). Effect of regenerative hyperplasia on the urinary bladder: carcinogenicity of sodium saccharin and *N*-[4-(5-nitro-2-furyl)-2-thiazolyl]formamide. *Cancer Research*, **42**, 65–71.

Cohen, S.M., Greenfield, R.E., and Ellwein, L.B. (1983). Multistage bladder carcinogenesis in the urinary bladder. *Environmental Health Perspectives*, **49**, 209–15.

Coldwell, B.B. and Boyd, E.M. (1966). The acute rectal toxicity of acetylsalicylic acid. *Canadian Journal of Physiology and Pharmacology*, **44**, 909–18.

Colin-Jones, D.G. and Maskell, R. (1986). Acute renal failure associated with acute pyelonephritis and consumption of nonsteroidal antiinflammatory drugs. *British Medical Journal*, **292**, 487–8.

Collins, E. (1981). Maternal and fetal effects of acetaminophen and salicylates in pregnancy. *Obstetrics and Gynecology*, **58**, 57–62S.

Collins, E. and Turner, G. (1975). Maternal effects of regular salicylate ingestion in pregnancy. *Lancet*, **2**, 335–8.

Colvin, R.B. and Fang, L.S.T. (1989). Interstitial nephritis. In *Renal pathology with clinical and functional correlations*, Vol. 1 (ed. C.C. Tisher and B.M. Brenner), pp. 728–76. Lippincott, Philadelphia.

Consensus Conference (1984). Analgesic-associated kidney disease. *Journal of the American Medical Association*, **251**, 3123–5.

Cornet, S., Braillon, A., Guilmard, C., Chabrier, P.E., Pirotzky, E., and Braquet, P. (1990). Involvement of endothelin in renal processes. *Hypertension*, **15**, 724–8.

Corpier, C.L., Jones, P.H., Suki, W.N., Lederer, E.D., Quinones, M.A., Schmidt, S.W., and Young, J.B. (1988). Rhabdomyolysis and renal injury with lovastatin use. Report of two cases in cardiac transplant recipients. *Journal of the American Medical Association*, **260**, 239–41.

Corwin, H.L. and Bonventre, J.V. (1984). Renal insufficiency associated with nonsteroidal anti-inflammatory agents. *American Journal of Kidney Diseases*, **4**, 147–52.

Cotran, R.S., Rubin, R.H., and Tolkoff-Rubin, N.E. (1986). Tubulointerstitial diseases. In *The kidney*, (3rd edn) (ed. B.M. Brenner and R.C. Rector), pp. 1143–73. Saunders, Philadelphia.

Cottier, P., Strausak, A., and Hiltbold, P. (1958). Diagnose und Therapie der chronische Pyelonephritis. *Schweizerische Medizinische Wochenschrift*, **88**, 463–8.

Cove-Smith, J.R. and Knapp, M.S. (1973). Sodium handling in analgesic nephropathy. *Lancet*, **2**, 70–2.

Cove-Smith, J.R. and Knapp, M.S. (1978). Analgesic nephropathy: an important cause of chronic renal failure. *Quarterly Journal of Medicine*, **47**, 49–69.

Crowe, C.A., Yong, A.C., Calder, I.C., Ham, K.N., and Tange, J.D. (1979). The nephrotoxicity of *p*-aminophenol. I. The effect on microsomal cytochromes, glutathione and covalent binding in kidney and liver. *Chemico-biological Interactions*, **27**, 235–43.

Cummings, D.M., McGehee, E.H., Dalmady, I.C., and Burke, J.F. (1984). Interstitial nephritis and proteinuria associated with zomepirac. *Clinical Pharmacology*, **3**, 198–200.

Curatolo, P.W. and Robertson, D. (1983). The health consequences of caffeine. *Annals of Internal Medicine*, **98**, 641–53.

Curry, R.W., Robinson, J.D., and Sughrue, M.J. (1982). Acute renal failure after acetaminophen ingestion. *Journal of the American Medical Association*, **247**, 1012–4.

Curt, G.A., Kaldany, A., Whitley, L.G., Crosson, A.W., Rolla, A., Merino, M.J., and D'Elia, J.A. (1980). Reversible rapidly progressive renal failure with nephrotic syndrome due to fenoprofen calcium. *Annals of Internal Medicine*, **92**, 72–3.

Dabbagh, S. and Chesney, R.W. (1985). Acute renal failure related to acetaminophen (paracetamol) overdose without fulminant hepatic disease. *International Journal of Pediatric Nephrology*, **6**, 221–4.

Dalquen, P., Fasel, J., Mihatsch, M.J., Rist, M., and Rutishauser, G. (1980). Phenacetinabusus IV. Sind zytologische Harnuntersuchungen in der Tumorvorsorge bei Phenacetinabusern erfolgversprechend und anwendbar? *Schweizerische Medizinische Wochenschrift*, **110**, 302–6.

Darwish, R., Vaziri, N.D., Gupta, S., Novey, H., Spear, G.S., Licorish, K. *et al.* (1984). Focal renal cortical necrosis associated with zomepirac. *American Journal of Medicine*, **76**, 1113–7.

Daskalopoulos, G., Kronborg, I., Katkov, W., Gonzales, M., Laffi, G., and Zipser, R.D. (1985). Sulindac and indomethacin suppress the diuretic action of furosemide in patients with cirrhosis and ascites: evidence that sulindac affects renal prostaglandins. *American Journal of Kidney Disease*, **6**, 217–21.

Davenport, A. and Finn, R. (1988). Paracetamol (acetaminophen) poisoning resulting in acute renal failure without hepatic coma. *Nephron*, **50**, 55–6.

Davidson, C. (1971). Salicylate metabolism in man. *Annals of the New York Academy of Sciences*, **179**, 249–68.

Davidson, W., Bassist, L., and Shippey, W. (1973*a*). *In vitro* effects of aspirin and phenacetin metabolites on the metabolism of dog renal medulla. *Clinical Research*, **21**, 227.

Davidson, W., Bassist, L., and Shippey, W. (1973*b*). Effect of aspirin and phenacetin metabolites on protein synthesis in dog renal medulla. *Clinical Research*, **21**, 683.

Davies, D.J. (1968). Changes in the renal cortex following experimental medullary necrosis. *Archives of Pathology*, **86**, 377–82.

Davies, D.J., Kennedy, A., and Roberts, C. (1970). The aetiology of renal medullary necrosis: a survey of adults cases in Liverpool. *Journal of Pathology and Bacteriology*, **100**, 257–68.

Dawborn, J.K., Kincaid-Smith, P., and McLaren, J. (1964). The effect of aspirin and phenacetin on ascending infection in the rat kidney. *Australasian Annals of Medicine*, **13**, 217–21.

Dawborn, J.K., Fairley, K.F., Kincaid-Smith, P., and King, W.E. (1966). The association of peptic ulceration, chronic renal disease, and analgesic abuse. *Quarterly Journal of Medicine*, **35**, 69–83.

Dawson, A.G. (1975). Effects of acetylsalicylate on gluconeogenesis in isolated rat kidney tubules. *Biochemical Pharmacology*, **24**, 1407–11.

de Crespigny, P.C., Hewitson, T., Birchall, I., and Kincaid-Smith, P. (1990). Caffeine potentiates the nephrotoxicity of mefenamic acid on the rat renal papilla. *American Journal of Nephrology*, **10**, 311–15.

Deerberg, F., Rehm, S., and Jostmeyer, H.H. (1985). Spontaneous urinary bladder tumours in DA/Han rats: a feasible model of human bladder cancer. *Journal of the National Cancer Institute*, **75**, 1113–21.

De Morias, S.M.F. and Wells, P.G. (1989). Enhanced acetaminophen toxicity in rats with bilirubin glucuronyl transferase deficiency. *Hepatology*, **10**, 163–7.

Denison, H., Kaczynski, J., and Wallerstedt, S. (1987). Paracetamol medication and alcohol abuse: a dangerous combination for the liver and the kidney. *Scandinavian Journal of Gastroenterology*, **22**, 701–4.

Deray, G., Le Hoang, P., Aupetit, B., Achour, A., Rottembourg, J., and Baumelou, A. (1987). Enhancement of cyclosporin A nephrotoxicity by diclofenac. *Clinical Nephrology*, **27**, 213–4.

Desvignes, V., Fialip, J., Palcoux, J.B., and Lavarenne, J. (1988). Rhabdomyolyse et acide niflumique. *Thérapie*, **43**, 429–30.

de Wardener, H.E. and MacGregor, G.A. (1988). Blood pressure and the kidney. In

Diseases of the kidney, (4th edn), (ed. R.W. Schrier and C.W. Gottschalk), pp. 1543–72. Little Brown, Boston.

DeWitt, D.L., el-Harith, E.A., Kraemer, S.A., Andrews, M.J., Yao, E.F., Armstrong, R.L., and Smith, W.L. (1990). The aspirin and heme-binding sites of ovine and marine prostaglandin endoperoxide synthases. *Journal of Biological Chemistry*, **265**, 5192–8.

Diaz-Esquivel, J. and Farmer, S. (1968). The effect of phenacetin on experimental ascending pyelonephritis. *Archives of Pathology*, **85**, 129–32.

Dichgans, J., Diener, H.C., Gerber, W.D., Verspohl, E.J., Kukiolka, H., and Kluck, M. (1984). Analgetika-induzierter Dauerkopfschmerz. *Deutsche Medizinische Wochenschrift*, **10**, 369–73.

Diener, H.-C. (1988*a*). Klinik des Analgetikakopfschmerzes. *Deutsche Medizinische Wochenschrift*, **113**, 472–4.

Diener, H.-C. (1988*b*). Therapie des Analgetika-induzierten Dauerkopfschmerzes. *Deutsche Medizinische Wochenschrift*, **113**, 475–6.

Disney, A.P.S. and Roy, P. (1988). *Eleventh report of the Australia and New Zealand Dialysis and Transplant Registry (ANZDATA).* Australian Kidney Foundation, Adelaide.

Disney, A.P.S. (1991). *Fourteenth report of the Australia and New Zealand Dialysis and Transplant Registry (ANZDATA*). Australian Kidney Foundation, Adelaide.

Dixon, M.F. (1976). Paracetamol hepatotoxicity. *Lancet*, **1**, 35.

Dixon, A.J., Winearls, C.G., and Dunnill, M.S. (1981). Interstitial nephritis. *Journal of Clinical Pathology*, **34**, 616–24.

Donker, A.J. (1983). The effects of indomethacin on renal function and glomerular protein loss. In *Prostaglandins and the kidney: biochemistry, physiology, pharmacology, and clinical applications* (ed. M. Dunn, C. Patrono, and G. Cinotti), pp. 251–62. Plenum, New York.

Donker, A.J.M., Arisz, L., Brentjens, J.R.H., vanderHem, G.K., and Hollemans, H.J.F. (1976). The effect of indomethacin on kidney function and plasma renin activity in man. *Nephron*, **17**, 288–96.

Douglas, R.A. and Johnston, E.D. (1961). Aspirin and chronic gastric ulcer. *Medical Journal of Australia*, **2**, 893–7.

Douglas, A.P., Hamlyn, A.N., and James, O. (1976). Controlled trial of cysteamine in treatment of acute paracetamol (acetaminophen) poisoning. *Lancet*, **1**, 111–5.

Douthwaite, A.H. and Lintott, G.A.M. (1938). Gastroscopic observation of effect of aspirin and certain other substances on the stomach. *Lancet*, **2**, 1222–5.

Doyle, G.D., Campbell, E., Gavin, N., Garrett, P., and Carmody, M. (1983). Phenylbutazone nephrotoxicity—a light and electron microscopic study. *Irish Journal of Medical Sciences*, **152**, 435–9.

Dreisbach, R.H. and Pfeiffer, C. (1943). Caffeine-withdrawal headache. *Journal of Laboratory and Clinical Medicine*, **28**, 1212–9.

Druckrey, H., Preussman, R., Ivanokovic, S., and Schmidt, C.H. (1964). Selektive erzeugung vonblaserkrebs an ratten durch dibutyl- und *N*-butyl-*N*-butanol-(4)-nitrosamin. *Zeitschrift für Krebsforschung*, **66**, 280–90.

Drukker, W., Schwarz, A., and Vanherweghem, J.-L. (1986). Analgesic nephropathy: an underestimated cause of end-stage renal disease. *International Journal of Artificial Organs*, **9**, 219–46.

Dubach, U.C. (1967). *P*-amino-phenol Bestimmung in Urin als Routinmethode zur Erfassung der Phenacetineinnahme. *Deutsche Medizinische Wochenschrift*, **92**, 311–5.

Dubach, U.C., Rosner, B., and Pfister, E. (1983). Epidemiologic study of abuse of analgesics containing phenacetin. Renal morbidity and mortality (1968–1979). *New England Journal of Medicine*, **308**, 357–62.

Dubach, U.C., Rosner, B., and Stürmer, T. (1991). An epidemiologic study of abuse of analgesic drugs. Effects of phenacetin and salicylate on mortality and cardiovascular morbidity (1968–87). *New England Journal of Medicine*, **324**, 155–60.

Ducret, F., Pointet, P., and Pichot, C. (1980). Glomérulonéphrite extramembraneuse au cours d'une polyarthrite rhumatoïde. Rôle possible du diclofénac. *Nouvelle Presse Medicale*, **2**, 387.

Ducret, F., Pointet, P., Martin, D., and Villermet, B. (1982). Insuffisance rénale aiguë réversible induite par le kétoprofène. *Néphrologie*, **3**, 105–6.

Duggan, J.M. (1970*a*). Gastrointestinal haemorrhage, gastric ulcer and aspirin. *Australasian Annals of Medicine*, **19**, 135–8.

Duggan, J.M. (1970*b*). Splenomegaly in analgesic takers. *Medical Journal of Australia*, **2**, 580–3.

Duggan, J.M. (1974). The analgesic syndrome. *Australian and New Zealand Journal of Medicine*, **4**, 365–72.

Duggin, G.G. (1980). Mechanisms in the development of analgesic nephropathy. *Kidney International*, **18**, 553–61.

Duggin, G.G. and Mohandas, J. (1982). Biochemical mechanisms of acetaminophen (paracetamol) induced hepatic and renal toxicity. In *Advances in pharmacology and therapeutics II*, Vol. 5 (ed. H. Yoshida, Y. Hagihara, and S. Ebashi), pp. 77–86. Pergamon, Oxford.

Duggin, G.G. and Mudge, G.H. (1975). Renal tubular transport of paracetamol and its conjugates in the dog. *British Journal of Pharmacology*, **54**, 359–66.

Duggin, G.G. and Mudge, G.H. (1976*a*). Analgesic nephropathy: renal distribution of acetaminophen and its conjugates. *Journal of Pharmacology and Experimental Therapeutics*, **199**, 1–9.

Duggin, G.G. and Mudge, G.H. (1976*b*). Phenacetin: renal tubular transport and intrarenal distribution in the dog. *Journal of Pharmacology and Experimental Therapeutics*, **199**, 10–6.

Duggin, G.G., Caterson, R.J., Mohandas, J., Horvath, J. and Tiller, D. (1980). Biochemical basis of synergistic analgesic toxicity. *Australian and New Zealand Journal of Medicine*, **10**, 129–30.

Dunn, T.B. (1944). Relationship of amyloid infiltration and renal disease in mice. *Journal of the National Cancer Institute*, **5**, 17–28.

Dunn, M.J. (1983). Renal prostaglandins. In *Renal endocrinology*, pp. 1–74. Williams and Wilkins, Baltimore.

Dunn, M.J. (1984). Nonsteroidal antiinflammatory drugs and renal function. *Annual Reviews of Medicine*, **35**, 411–28.

Dunn, M. (1987). The role of arachiodonic acid metabolites in renal homeostasis. Non-steroidal anti-inflammatory drugs, renal function and biochemical, histological and clinical effects and drug interactions. *Drugs*, **33** (Suppl. 1), 56–66.

Dunn, M.J. (1990*a*). Prostaglandins, angiotensin II, and proteinuria. *Nephron*, **55** (Suppl. 1), 30–7.

Dunn. M.J. (1990*b*). The roles of angiotensin II and prostaglandins in the regulation of the glomerular filtration of albumin. *Journal of Hypertension*, 8 (Suppl. 1), S47–52.

Dunn, M.J. and Zambraski, E.J. (1980). Renal effects of drugs that inhibit prostaglandin synthesis. *Kidney International*, **18**, 609–22.

Dworkin, L.D., Ichikawa, I., and Brenner, B.M. (1983). Hormonal modulation of glomerular function. *American Journal of Physiology*, **244**, F95–104.

East, C., Alvizatos, P.A., Grundy, S.M., Jones, P.H., and Farmer, J.A. (1988). Rabdomyolysis in patients receiving lovastatin after cardiac transplantation. *New England Journal of Medicine*, **318**, 47–8.

Eddy, N.B., Halbach, H., Isbell, H., and Seevers, M.H. (1965). Drug dependence: its significance and characteristics. *Bulletin of the World Health Organization*, **32**, 721–33.

Edel, H.H. (1966). Dialysetherapie bei chronischer Pyelonephritis. In *Pyelonephritis, Forschungsergebnisse* (ed. H. Losse and M. Kienetz), pp. 385–90. Thieme, Stuttgart.

Eder, H. (1964). Chronic toxicity studies on phenacetin, *N*-acetyl-*p*-aminophenol (NAPA) and acetylsalicylic acid on cats. *Acta Pharmacologica et Toxicologica*, **21**, 197–204.

Edwards, R.M. (1983). Segmental effects of norepinephrine and angiotension II on isolated renal microvessels. *American Journal of Physiology*, **244**, F526–34.

Edwards, K.D.G., Curtis, E.A., and Stoker, L.M. (1971). One-day renal function testing in normal rats and in cases of experimentally-induced analgesic nephropathy, nephrocalcinosis and nephrotic syndrome. *Nephron*, 8, 235–45.

Edwards, R.M., Jackson, B.A., and Dousa, T.P. (1981). ADH-sensitive cAMP system in papillary collecting duct: effect of osmolality and PGE_2. *American Journal of Physiology*, **240**, F311–18.

Egan, R.W., Gale, P.H., Baptista, E.M., Kennicott, K.L., VandenHeuvel, W.J.A., Walker, R.W. *et al.* (1981). Oxidation reactions by prostaglandin cyclooxygenase-hydroperoxide. *Journal of Biological Chemistry*, **256**, 7352–61.

Eisalo, A., and Talanti, S. (1961). Observations on the effect of phenacetin and *N*-acetyl-*p*-aminophenol on rat kidneys. *Acta Medica Scandinavica*, **169**, 655–60.

Eknoyan, G. (1984). Analgesic nephrotoxicity and renal papillary necrosis. *Seminars in Nephrology*, **4**, 65–76.

Eknoyan, G., Qunibi, W.Y., Grissom, R.T., Tuma, S.M., and Ayus, J.C. (1982). Renal papillary necrosis: an update. *Medicine*, **61**, 55–73.

Eling, T., Boyd, J., Reed, G., Mason, R., and Sivarajah, K. (1983). Xenobiotic metabolism by prostaglandin endoperoxide synthetase. *Drug Metabolism Reviews*, **14**, 1023–53.

Ellwein, L.B. and Cohen, S.M. (1990). The health risks of saccharin revisited. *Critical Reviews in Toxicology*, **20**, 311–26.

Elseviers, M.M. and De Broe, M.E. (1987). Wurde das Problem der Analgetikanephropathie durch die Entfernung des Phenacetins aus analgetischen Mischpräparaten gelöst? *Mitteilungen Klinische Nephrologie*, **16**, 187–93.

Elseviers, M.M. and De Broe, M.E. (1988). Is analgesic nephropathy still a problem in Belgium? *Nephrology, Dialysis, Transplantation*, **3**, 143–9.

Elseviers, M.M. and De Broe, M.E. (1989). Predisposing factor(s): an important issue in the development of analgesic nephropathy. In *Proceedings of the Fourth International Nephrotoxicity Symposium, 'Mechanisms of nephrotoxicity: the basis for early diagnosis, modulation of effects and improved therapeutic management'*. Guildford, 23–8 July.

Elseviers, M.M., Bosteels, V., Cambier, P., De Paepe, M., Godon, J.P., Lins, R. *et al.* (1992). Diagnostic criteria of analgesic nephropathy in patients with end-stage renal failure: results of the Belgian study. *Nephrology, Dialysis, Transplantation*. **7**, 479–86.

Emkey, R.D. and Mills, J.A. (1982). Aspirin and analgesic nephropathy. *Journal of the American Medical Association*, **247**, 55–7.

Englert, H., Simpson, I.J., Gow, P.J., and Bierre, A.R. (1982). Mefanamic acid (Ponstan) induced interstitial nephritis. *New Zealand Medical Journal*, **95**, 516–7.

Eriksson, O. and Johansson, S. (1976). Urothelial neoplasms of the upper urinary tract. *Acta Cytologica*, **20**, 20–5.

Ertürk, E., Price, J.M., Morris, J.E., Cohen, S., Leith, R.S., von Esch, A.M., and Crovetti, A.J. (1967). The production of carcinoma of the urinary bladder in rats by feeding *N*-[4-(5-nitro-2-furyl)-2-thiazolyl]formamide. *Cancer Research*, **27**, 1998–2002.

Ertürk, E., Cohen, S.M., Price, J.M., and Bryan, G.T. (1969). Pathogenesis, histology and transplantability of urinary bladder carcinomas induced in albino rats by oral administration of *N*-[4-(5-nitro-2-furyl)-2-thiazolyl]formamide. *Cancer Research*, **29**, 2219–28.

Esparza, A.R., Kahn, S.I., Garella, S., and Abuelo, J.G. (1981). Spectrum of acute renal failure in nephrotic syndrome with minimal (or minor) glomerular lesions. Role of hemodynamic factors. *Laboratory Investigation*, **45**, 510–21.

Eugène, M., Deray, G., Cacoub, P., Beaufils, H., and Baumelou, A. (1987). Insuffisance rénale aiguë et syndrome néphrotique après traitement par pirprofène. *Revue de Médecine Interne*, **8**, 115.

Fahrenberg, J., Selg, H., and Hampel, R. (1973). *Das Freiburger Persönlichkeits-inventar: FPI.* Hogrefe, Göttingen.

Fairley, K.F. and Birch, D.F. (1982). Hematuria: a simple method for identifying glomerular bleeding. *Kidney International*, **21**, 105–8.

Fairley, K.F. and Kincaid-Smith, P. (1968). Renal papillary necrosis with a normal pyelogram. *British Medical Journal*, **1**, 156–7.

Farber, E. (1976). Hyperplastic areas, hyperplastic nodules, and hyperbasophilic areas as putative precursor lesions. *Cancer Research*, **36**, 2532–3.

Farber, E. (1984). Cellular biochemistry of the stepwise development of cancer with chemicals: G.H.A. Clowes Memorial Lecture. *Cancer Research*, **44**, 5463–74.

Farber, E. and Sporn, M.B. (1976). Symposium: early lesions and the development of epithelial cancer. *Cancer Research*, **36**, 2475–706.

Farmer, E.R. and Heptinstall, R.H. (1970). Chronic non-obstructive pyelonephritis —a reappraisal. In *Renal infection and renal scarring* (ed. P. Kincaid-Smith and K. F. Fairley), pp. 233–7. Mercedes, Melbourne.

Fassett, R.G., Lien, J.W.K., McClure, J., and Mathew, T.H. (1982). Bone disease in analgesic nephropathy. *Clinical Nephrology*, **18**, 273–9.

Fazekas, I.G., Fazekas, A.G., and Bertok, E.F. (1960*a*). Experimental examination of the mechanism of pyramidon effect. Effect of high pyramidon doses on renal function. *Archives Internationales de Pharmacodynamie et de Therapie*, **129**, 35–61.

Fazekas, A.G., Fazekas, I.G., and Rengei, B. (1960*b*). Experimental examination of the mechanism of pyramidon effect. 3. Effect of high pyramidon doses on the glutamic acid-oxaloacetic acid transaminase activity in serum. *Canadian Journal of Biochemistry and Physiology*, **38**, 899–901.

Fazekas, I.G., Fazekas, A.G., and Rengei, B. (1961). Changes in glutamic acid-oxaloacetic acid-transaminase activity in the liver and kidneys on the effect of high doses of pyramidon (aminopyrine). *Canadian Journal of Biochemistry and Physiology*, **39**, 1189–91.

Feinfeld, D.A., Olesnicky, L., Pirani, C.L., and Appel, G.B. (1984). Nephrotic syndrome associated with use of the nonsteroidal anti-inflammatory drugs. Case report and review of the literature. *Nephron*, **37**, 174–9.

Fellers, F.X., Pradilla, A., and Craig, J.M. (1965). The enhancement of salicylate toxicity by Diamox: chemical and morphological analysis. In *Progress in pyelonephritis* (ed. E.H. Kass), pp. 337–46. Davis, Philadelphia.

Fellner, S.K. (1985). Piroxicam-induced acute interstitial nephritis and minimal-change nephrotic syndrome. *American Journal of Nephrology*, **5**, 142–3.

Fellner, S.K. and Tuttle, E.P. (1969). The clinical syndrome of analgesic abuse. *Archives of Internal Medicine*, **124**, 379–82.

Ferguson, I., Johnson, F., Reay, B., and Wigley, R. (1977). Aspirin, phenacetin, and the kidney—a rheumatism clinic study. *Medical Journal of Australia*, **1**, 950–4.

Ferreira, S.H. and Vane, J.R. (1974). New aspects of the mode of action of non-steroid anti-inflammatory drugs. *Annual Review of Pharmacology*, **14**, 57–73.

Finkelstein, A., Fraley, D.S., Stachura, I., Feldman, H.A., Gandy, D.R., and Bourke, E. (1982). Fenoprofen nephropathy. Lipoid nephrosis and interstitial nephritis. A possible T lymphocyte disorder. *American Journal of Medicine*, **72**, 81–7.

Finnigan, D., Burry, A.F., and Smith, I.D.B. (1974). Analgesic consumption in an antenatal clinic survey. *Medical Journal of Australia*, **1**, 761–2.

Fischbach, T. and Lenk, W. (1985*a*). Additional routes in the metabolism of phenacetin. *Xenobiotica*, **15**, 149–64.

Fischbach, T. and Lenk, W. (1985*b*). The metabolism of *N*-hydroxyphacetin *in vitro* and *in vivo*. *Xenobiotica*, **15**, 915–27.

Flinn, S., Gregory, J., McNaughton, L.R., Tristram, S., and Davies, P. (1990). Caffeine ingestion prior to incremental cycling to exhaustion in recreational cyclists. *International Journal of Sports Medicine*, **11**, 188–93.

Flower, R.J. and Vane, J.R. (1972). Inhibition of prostaglandin synthetase in brain explains the anti-pyretic activity of paracetamol (4-acetamidophenol). *Nature*, **240**, 410–11.

Flower, R.J., Moncada, S., and Vane, J.R. (1985). Analgesic-antipyretics and anti-inflammatory agents; drugs employed in the treatment of gout. In *Goodman and Gilman's the pharmacological basis of therapeutics* (7th edn) (ed. A.G. Gilman, L.S. Goodman, T.W. Rall, and F. Murad), pp. 674–715. Macmillan, New York.

Foidart, J.B. and Mahieu, P. (1986). Glomerular mesangial contractility *in vitro* is controlled by an angiotensin–prostaglandin balance. *Molecular and Cellular Endocrinology*, **47**, 163–73.

Fokkens, W. (1979). Phenacetin abuse related to bladder cancer. *Environmental Research*, **20**, 192–8.

Fong, H.J. and Cohen, A.H. (1982). Ibuprofen-induced acute renal failure with acute tubular necrosis. *American Journal of Nephrology*, **2**, 28–31.

Fordham, C.C. and Huffines, W.D. (1967). Splenomegaly, analgesic ingestion and renal disease. *New England Journal of Medicine*, **277**, 749–51.

Fordham, C.C., Huffines, W.D., and Welt, L.G. (1965). Phenacetin-induced renal disease in rats. *Annals of Internal Medicine*, **62**, 738–43.

Forsström, J. (1968). Anemia in chronic pyelonephritis and in renal failure of analgesic abusers. With special reference to signs of microangiopathic hemolytic anemia. *Acta Medica Scandinavica*, Suppl. **487**, 1–63.

Fourie, I.J., Pauw, F.H., and de Bruin, B. (1982). Analgesic nephropathy. Local experience in Bloemfontein. *South African Medical Journal*, **62**, 351–3.

Friberg, P., Meredith, I., Jennings, G., Lambert, G., Fazio, V., and Esler, M. (1990). Evidence for increased renal norepinephrine overflow during sodium restriction in humans. *Hypertension*, **16**, 121–30.

Frick, P.G. (1956). Hemorrhagic diathesis with increased capillary fragility caused by salicylate therapy. *American Journal of Medical Science*, **231**, 402–6.

Friedman, W.F., Hirschklau, M.J., Printz, M.D., Pitlick, P.T., and Kirkpatrick, S.E. (1976). Pharmacologic closure of patent ductus arteriosus in the premature infant. *New England Journal of Medicine*, **295**, 526–9.

Friedreich, N. (1877). Über Nekrose der Nierenpapillen bei Hydronephrose. *Virchows Archiv für Pathologische Anatomie und Physiologie und für Klinische Medizin*, **69**, 308–12.

Frischer, Z., Waltzer, W.C., and Gonder, M.J. (1985). Bilateral transitional cell carcinoma of the renal pelvis in the cancer family syndrome. *Journal of Urology*, **134**, 1197–8.

Frölich, J.C., Nies, A.S., and Schrier, R.W. (ed.) (1981). Prostaglandins and the kidney. *Kidney International*, **19**, 755–880.

Fujitia, J., Ohuchi, N., Ito, H., Reynolds, S.H., Yoshida, O., Nakayama, H., and Kitamura, Y. (1988). Activation of H-ras oncogene in rat bladder tumors induced by *N*-butyl-*N*-(4-hydroxybutyl)nitrosamine. *Journal of the National Cancer Institute*, **80**, 37–43.

Fukushima, S., Hirose, M., Tsuda, H., Shirai, T., Hirao, K., Arai, M., and Ito, N. (1976). Histological classification of urinary bladder cancers in rats induced by *N*-butyl-*N*-(4-hydroxybutyl)nitrosamine. *Gann; Japanese Journal of Cancer Research*, **67**, 81–90.

Furman, K.I., Galsako, G.T.F., Meyers, A.M., and Rabkin, R. (1976). Post-transplantation analgesic dependence in patients who formerly suffered from analgesic nephropathy. *Clinical Nephrology*, **5**, 54–7.

Furman, K.I., Kündig, H., and Lewin, J.R. (1981). Experimental paracetamol nephropathy and pyelonephritis in rats. *Clinical Nephrology*, **16**, 271–5.

Gabriel, R. (1984). Morbidity and mortality of long-term haemodialysis: a review. *Journal of the Royal Society of Medicine*, **77**, 594–601.

Gabriel, R., Caldwell, J., and Hartley, R.B. (1982). Acute tubular necrosis, caused by therapeutic doses of paracetamol? *Clinical Nephrology*, **18**, 269–71.

Gaetani, M., Debeus, R., Vidi, A., and Coppi, G. (1972). Toxicological investigations of 4-prenyl-1,2-diphenyl-3,5-pyrazolidinedione (DA 2370). 3. A comparative short-term study of the toxicity of DA 2370 and other non-steroid anti-inflammatory drugs (phenylbutazone, mefenamic acid, indomethacin and benzydamine) in the rat. *Arzneimittel-Forschung*, **22** (Suppl. 1*a*), 226–34.

Garella, S. and Matarese, R.A. (1984). Renal effects of prostaglandins and clinical adverse effects of nonsteroidal anti-inflammatory agents. *Medicine*, **63**, 165–81.

Gary, N.E., Dodelsen, R., and Eisenger, R.P. (1980). Indomethacin associated acute renal failure. *American Journal of Medicine*, **69**, 135–6.

Gates, T.N. and Temple, A.R. (1989). Analgesic use and chronic renal disease. *New England Journal of Medicine*, **321**, 1125.

Gault, M.H. (1971). Intrarenal gradients of radioactive acetylsalicylic acid (ASA) and inulin. *Clinical Research*, **19**, 808.

Gault, M.H. (1975). The clinical course of patients with analgesic nephropathy. *Canadian Medical Association Journal*, **113**, 204–7.

Gault, M.H. and Wilson, D.R. (1978). Analgesic nephropathy in Canada: clinical syndrome, management, and outcome. *Kidney International*, **13**, 58–63.

Gault, M.H., Rudwal, T.C., Engles, W.D., and Dossetor, J.B. (1968*a*). Syndrome associated with the abuse of analgesics. *Annals of Internal Medicine*, **68**, 906–25.

Gault, M.H., Rudwal, T.C., and Redmond, N.I. (1968*b*). Analgesic habits of 500 veterans: incidence and complications of abuse. *Canadian Medical Association Journal*, **98**, 619–26.

Gault, M.H., Blennerhasset, J., and Muehrcke, R. (1971). Analgesic nephropathy: a clinicopathologic study using electron microscopy. *American Journal of Medicine*, **51**, 740–56.

Gault, M.H., Shahidi, N.T., and Barber, V.E. (1974). Methemoglobin formation in analgesic nephropathy. *Clinical Pharmacology and Therapeutics*, **15**, 521–7.

Gehrig, J.J., Gottheiner, T.I., and Swenson, R.S. (1985). Acquired cystic disease of the end-stage kidney. *American Journal of Medicine*, **79**, 609–20.

Gemborys, M.W. and Mudge, G.H. (1981). Formation and disposition of the minor metabolites of acetaminophen in the hamster. *Drug Metabolism and Disposition*, **9**, 340–51.

Gillies, M. and Skyring, A. (1968). Gastric ulcer, duodenal ulcer and gastric carcinoma: a case-control study of certain social and environmental factors. *Medical Journal of Australia*, **2**, 1132–6.

Gillies, M.A., and Skyring, A. (1969). Gastric and duodenal ulcer. The association between aspirin ingestion, smoking and family history of ulcer. *Medical Journal of Australia*, **2**, 280–5.

Gilman, A. (1964). Analgesic nephrotoxicity; a pharmacological analysis. *American Journal of Medicine*, **36**, 167–73.

Gloor, F. (1960). Über verschiedene Formen der Papillennekrosen der Nieren. *Pathologia et Microbiologia Basel*, **23**, 263–72.

Gloor, F. (1961). Die doppelseitigen chronischen nicht-obstruktiven interstitiellen Nephritiden. *Ergebnisse der Allgemeine Pathologie und Pathologische Anatomie*, **41**, 63–207.

Gloor, F. (1965). Die doppelseitigen chronischen nicht-obstruktiven interstitiellen Nephritiden. *Verhandlungen der Deutschen Gesellschaft für Pathologie*, **49**, 92–106.

Gloor, F. (1974). Unsere heutige Vorstellung über die Morphologie und Pathogenese der Analgetika-nephropathie. *Schweizerischer Medizinische Wochenschrift*, **104**, 785–91.

Gloor, F.J. (1978*a*). Changing concepts in pathogenesis and morphology of analgesic nephropathy as seen in Europe. *Kidney International*, **13**, 27–38.

Gloor, F. (1978*b*). Pathologisch-anatomische Diagnose und Differentialdiagnose der Pyelonephritis. *Radiologe*, **18**, 2–7.

Gloor, F. (1982). Die Kapillarsklerose in den ableitenden Harnwegen bei Schmerzmittel-(Phenacetin)-mißbrauch. *Pathologe*, **3**, 132–6.

Goebel, K.M. and Mueller-Brodmann, W. (1982). Reversible overt nephropathy with Henoch-Schönlein purpura due to piroxicam. *British Medical Journal*, **284**, 311–2.

Goldberg, M. (1986). Analgesic-associated nephropathy: an important cause of chronic renal failure in the United States? *American Journal of Kidney Diseases*, **7**, 162–3.

Goldberg, M., Myers, C.L., Peshel, W., McCarron, D., and Morrison, A.B. (1971). Mechanism of analgesic abuse nephropathy. *Journal of Clinical Investigation*, **50**, 37a.

Goldberger, L.E. and Talner, L.B. (1975). Analgesic abuse syndrome. *Urology*, **5**, 728–32.

Gonwa, T.A., Corbett, W.T., Schey, H.M., and Buckalew, V.M. (1980). Analgesic-associated nephropathy and transitional cell carcinoma of the urinary tract. *Annals of Internal Medicine*, **93**, 249–52.

Gonwa, T.A., Hamilton, R.W., and Buckalew, V.M. (1981). Chronic renal failure and end-stage renal disease in northwest North Carolina. Importance of analgesic-associated nephropathy. *Archives of Internal Medicine*, **141**, 462–5.

Goodwin, J.S. and Ceuppens, J. (1983). Regulation of the immune response by prostaglandins. *Journal of Clinical Immunology*, **3**, 295–315.

Goodwin, J.S. and Webb, D.R. (1980). Regulation of the immune response by prostaglandins. *Clinical Immunology and Immunopathology*, **15**, 106–22.

Gorer, P.A. (1940). Renal lesions found in pure lines of mice. *Journal of Pathology and Bacteriology*, **50**, 25–30.

Grant, D.C., Yoder, I.C., Newhouse, J.H., and Dee, G.J. (1986). Sonography in transitional cell carcinoma of the renal pelvis. *Urological Radiology*, **8**, 1–5.

Green, J., Yoffe, B., Barzilai, D., and Better, O.S. (1985). Reversible acute interstitial nephritis associated with indomethacin. *Israel Journal of Medical Sciences*, **21**, 142–5.

Greenstone, M., Hartley, B., Gabriel, R., and Bevan, G. (1981). Acute nephrotic syndrome with reversible renal failure after phenylbutazone. *British Medical Journal*, **282**, 950–1.

Greer, H.D., Ward, H.P., and Corbin, K.B. (1965). Chronic salicylate intoxication in adults. *Journal of the American Medical Association*, **193**, 555–8.

Gregg, N.J. and Bach, P.H. (1990). 2-bromoethanamine nephrotoxicity in the nude mouse: an atypical targetting for the renal cortex. *International Journal of Experimental Pathology*, **71**, 659–70.

Gregg, N.J., Elseviers, M.M., De Broe, M.E., and Bach, P.H. (1989*a*). Epidemiology and mechanistic basis of analgesic-associated nephropathy. *Toxicology Letters*, **46**, 141–51.

Gregg, N.J., Courtauld, E.A., and Bach, P.H. (1989*b*). High resolution microscopic changes in an acutely induced renal papillary necrosis: morphology and enzyme histochemistry. In *Nephrotoxicity: extrapolation from* in vitro *to* in vivo, *and animals to man* (ed. P.H. Bach and E.A. Lock), pp. 415–21. Plenum, London.

Gregg, N.J., Ijomah, P., Courtauld, E.A., and Bach, P.H. (1989*c*). Upper urothelial carcinoma, using *N*-butyl-*N*-(4-hydroxybutyl)-nitrosamine initiation and an acute papillary necrosis. In *Nephrotoxicity: extrapolation from* in vitro *to* in vivo, *and animals to man* (ed. P.H. Bach and E.A. Lock), pp. 411–4. Plenum, London.

Gregg, N.J., Courtauld, E.A., and Bach, P.H. (1990*a*). Enzyme histochemical changes in an acutely induced renal papillary necrosis. *Toxicologic Pathology*, **18**, 39–46.

Gregg, N.J., Courtauld, E.A., and Bach, P.H. (1990*b*). High resolution light microscopic morphological and microvascular changes in an acutely induced renal papillary necrosis. *Toxicologic Pathology*, **18**, 47–55.

Gregg, N.J., Wilks, M.L., and Bach, P.H. (1991*a*). The mechanistic basis of chemical- and drug-induced nephrotoxicity. In *Histochemistry and immunocytochemistry: applications to pharmacology and toxicology* (ed. P.H. Bach and J.R.J. Baker), pp. 225–54. Chapman Hall, London.

Gregg, N.J., Ijomah, P., Courtauld, E.A., and Bach, P.H. (1991*b*). Two stage model of upper urothelial carcinoma using *N*-butyl-*N*-(4-hydroxybutyl)-nitrosamine initiation and promotion by an acutely-induced renal papillary necrosis. *Cancer Research*, (submitted).

Grenier, F.C., Rollins, T.E., and Smith, W.L. (1981). Kinin-induced prostaglandin synthesis by renal papillary collecting tubule: AVP induces PGE release. *American Journal of Physiology*, **241**, F94–104.

Griffiths, R.R. and Woodson, P.P. (1988). Caffeine physical dependence: a review of the human and laboratory animal studies. *Psychopharmacology*, **94**, 437–51.

Grimlund, K. (1963). Phenacetin and renal damage at a Swedish factory. *Acta Medica Scandinavica*, **174** (Suppl. 405), 1–26.

Grimlund, K. (1973). Phenacetin and renal damage. In *Probleme des Phenacetinabusus* (ed. H. Haschek), pp. 195–201. Egermann, Wien.

Grünfeld, J.P., Kleinknecht, D., and Droz, D. (1988). Acute interstitial nephritis. In *Diseases of the kidney*, Vol. 2 (4th edn) (ed. R.W. Schrier and C.W. Gottschalk), pp. 1461–87. Little Brown, Boston.

Gsell, O. (1974). Nephropathie durch Analgetika. Papillennekrosen und chronische interstitielle Nephritis durch Mißbrauch phenacetinhaltiger Analgetika. *Ergebnisse der Inneren Medizin und Kinderheilkunde*, **35**, 68–175.

Gsell, O., von Rechenberg, H.K., and Miescher, P. (1957). Die primär chronische interstitielle Nephritis; klinische, experimentelle und aetiologische Untersuchungen. *Deutsche Medizinische Wochenschrift*, **82**, 1673–6 and 1718–26.

Gsell, O., Kielholz, P., and Hegg, J.-J. (1961). Phenacetinabusus; Vergleich psychiatrisch und internistisch behandelter Mißbraucher phenacetinhaltiger Analgetika. *Schweizerische Medizinische Wochenschrift*, **91**, 1529–31.

Gsell, O., Dubach, U.C., and Raillard-Peucker, U. (1968). Phenacetinabusus und Nierenleiden. *Deutsche Medizinische Wochenschrift*, **94**, 101–12.

Günther, G.W. (1937). Die Papillennekrosen der Niere bei Diabetes. *Münchener Medizinische Wochenschrift*, **84**, 1695–9.

Hall, P.W. and Dammin, G.J. (1978). Balkan nephropathy. *Nephron*, **22**, 281–300.

Hallesy, D., Shott, L.D., and Hill, R. (1973). Comparative toxicity of naproxen. *Scandinavian Journal of Rheumatology*, Suppl. **2**, 20–8.

Ham, K.N. and Tange, J.D. (1969). Some experimental observations relating to the pathogenesis of renal papillary necrosis. *Australasian Annals of Medicine*, **18**, 199–208.

Hamilton, D.V., Pryor, J.S., and Cardoe, N. (1979). Fenclofenac-induced nephrotic syndrome. *British Medical Journal*, **2**, 391.

Hamlyn, A.N., Douglas, A.P., and James, O. (1978). The spectrum of paracetamol (acetaminophen) overdose: clinical and epidemiological studies. *Postgraduate Medical Journal*, **54**, 400–4.

Handa, S.P. (1980). Renal effects of fenoprofen. *Annals of Internal Medicine*, **93**, 508–9.

Handa, S.P. (1986). Drug-induced acute interstitial nephritis: report of 10 cases. *Canadian Medical Association Journal*, **135**, 1278–81.

Handa, S.P. and Tewari, H.D. (1981). Urinary tract carcinoma in patients with analgesic nephropathy. *Nephron*, **28**, 62–4.

Hannedouche, T., Fournier, J.F., Moore, N., Godin, M., and Fillastre, J.P. (1986). Nephrotic syndrome due to isolated minimal change glomerular disease in a patient taking pirprofen. *Clinical Nephrology*, **25**, 314.

Hardy, T.L. (1970*a*). *N*-phenylanthranilic acid: an agent for inducing and studying renal papillary necrosis in the rat. *British Journal of Experimental Pathology*, **51**, 348–55.

Hardy, T.L. (1970*b*). Partial renal papillectomy and the study of drug induced renal papillary necrosis in the rat. *British Journal of Experimental Pathology*, **51**, 591–6.

Hardy, T.L. (1974). Experimental surgery in the evaluation of drug induced renal toxicity in the rat with particular reference to diphenylamine. *Proceedings of the European Society for the Study of Drug Toxicity*, **15**, 337–44.

Hardy, T.L. and Bach, P.H. (1984). The effect of *N*-phenylanthranilic acid-induced renal papillary necrosis on urinary acidification and renal electrolyte handling. *Toxicology and Applied Pharmacology*, **75**, 265–77.

Hare, W.S.C. and Poynter, J.D. (1974). The radiology of renal papillary necrosis as seen in analgesic nephropathy. *Clinical Radiology*, **25**, 423–43.

Harper, G.S. and Axelsen, R.A. (1982). Salicylate-induced renal papillary necrosis in the Gunn rat. The role of bilirubin. *Laboratory Investigation*, **47**, 258–64.

Harris, K.P.G., Schreiner, G.F., and Klahr, S. (1989). Effect of leukocyte depletion on the function of the postobstructed kidney in rat. *Kidney International*, **36**, 210–5.

Harris, K.P.G., Purkerson, M.L., Yates, J., and Klahr, S. (1990). Lovastatin ameliorates the development of glomerulosclerosis and uremia in experimental nephrotic syndrome. *American Journal of Kidney Diseases*, **15**, 16–23.

Harrow, B.R., Sloane, J.A., and Liebman, N.C. (1963). Roentgenologic demonstration of renal papillary necrosis in sickle-cell trait. *New England Journal of Medicine*, **268**, 969–76.

Hart, S., Calder, I., Ross, B., and Tange, J. (1980). Renal metabolism of paracetamol: studies in the isolated perfused rat kidney. *Clinical Science*, **58**, 379–84.

Hart, S.J., Tontodonati, R., and Calder, I.C. (1981). Reverse phase chromatography of urinary metabolites of paracetamol using ion suppression and ion pairing. *Journal of Chromatography*, **225**, 387–405.

Hart, D., Ward, M., and Lifschitz, M.D. (1987). Suprofen-related nephrotoxicity. A distinct clinical syndrome. *Annals of Internal Medicine*, **106**, 235–8.

Harvald, B. (1963). Renal papillary necrosis. A clinical survey of sixty-six cases. *American Journal of Medicine*, **35**, 481–6.

Haschek, H. (ed.) (1973). *Probleme des Phenacetinabusus*. Egermann, Wien.

Hashimoto, Y., Suzuki, K., and Okada, M. (1974). Induction of bladder tumors by intravesical instillation of butyl-(4-hydroxybutyl)nitrosamine and its principal urinary metabolite butyl-(3-carboxypropyl)nitrosamine in rats. *Gann; Japanese Journal of Cancer Research*, **65**, 69–73.

Hassid, A. (1983). Inhibition of prostaglandin biosynthesis in renal (MDCK) cells by cAMP. *American Journal of Physiology*, **244**, C369–76.

Hawkins, D., Pinkard, R.N., Crawford, I.P., and Farr, R.S. (1969). Structural changes in human serum albumin induced by ingestion of acetylsalicylic acid. *Journal of Clinical Investigation*, **48**, 536–42.

Helber, A., Wambach, G., Böttcher, W., Weller, P., and Schmidt, R. (1980). Hypercholesterolaemia and hypertriglyceridaemia in patients with analgesic nephropathy. *Nephron*, **26**, 111–5.

Hellerstedt, W.L., Johnson, W.J., Ascher, N., Kjellstrand, C.M., Knutson, R., Shapiro, F.L., and Sterioff, S. (1984). Survival rates of 2728 patients with end-stage renal disease. *Mayo Clinic Proceedings*, **59**, 776–83.

Hennis, H.L., Hennigar, G.R., Greene, W.B., Hilton, C.W., and Spector, M. (1982). Intratubular calcium phosphate deposition in acute analgesic nephropathy in rabbits. *American Journal of Pathology*, **106**, 356–63.

Henrich, W.L. (1981). Role of prostaglandins in renin secretion. *Kidney International*, **19**, 822–30.

Henrich, W.L. (1988). Nephrotoxicity of nonsteroidal anti-inflammatory agents. In *Diseases of the kidney* (4th edn) (ed. R.W. Schrier and C.W. Gottschalk), pp. 1319–16. Little Brown, Boston.

Henry, M. and Tange, J.D. (1982). The genesis and ultrastructural appearance of spontaneous renal lesions in the homozygous Gunn rat. *Pathology*, **14**, 355–61.

Henry, M.A. and Tange, J.D. (1983). Ultrastructural appearances of acute renal papillary lesions induced by aspirin. *Journal of Pathology*, **139**, 57–67.

Henry, M.A. and Tange, J.D. (1984). Chronic renal lesions in the uninephrectomized Gunn rat after analgesic mixtures. *Pathology*, **16**, 278–84.

Henry, M.A. and Tange, J.D. (1987). Lesions of the renal papilla induced by paracetamol. *Journal of Pathology*, **151**, 11–9.

Henry, M.A., Sweet, R.S., and Tange, J.D. (1983). A new reproducible experimental model of analgesic nephropathy. *Journal of Pathology*, **139**, 23–32.

Hensler, L. (1957). Die chronische interstitielle Nephritis. *Deutsche Medizinische Wochenschrift*, **82**, 202–4.

Heptinstall, R.H. (1983). Pyelonephritis: pathologic features. In *Pathology of the kidney* (3rd edn) (ed. R.H. Heptinstall), pp. 1323–96. Little Brown, Boston.

Herman, C.J., Vegt, P.D.J., Debruyne, F.M.J., Vooijs, G.P., and Ramaekers, F.C.S. (1985). Squamous and transitional elements in rat bladder carcinomas induced by *N*-butyl-*N*-4-hydroxybutyl-nitrosamine (BBN). A study of cytokeratin expression. *American Journal of Pathology*, **120**, 419–26.

Herr, H.W. (1985). Durable response of a carcinoma in situ of the renal pelvis to topical bacillus Calmette-Guerin. *Journal of Urology*, **134**, 531–2.

Heyman, S.N., Brezis, M., Reubinoff, C.A., Greenfeld, Z., Lechene, C., Epstein, F.H., and Rosen, S. (1988). Acute renal failure with selective medullary injury in the rat. *Journal of Clinical Investigation*, **82**, 401–12.

Heymann, M.A., Rudolph, A.M., and Silverman, N.H. (1976). Closure of the ductus arteriosus in premature infants by inhibition of prostaglandin synthesis. *New England Journal of Medicine*, **295**, 530–3.

Hicks, R.M. (1980). Multistage carcinogenesis in the urinary bladder. *British Medical Bulletin*, **36**, 39–46.

Hicks, R.M. (1983*a*). Effect of promoters on incidence of bladder cancer in experimental animal models. *Environmental Health Perspectives*, **50**, 37–49.

Hicks, R.M. (1983*b*). Pathological and biochemical aspects of tumour promotion. *Carcinogenesis*, **4**, 1209–14.

Hinson, J.A. (1983). Reactive metabolites of phenacetin and acetaminophen: a review. *Environmental Health Perspectives*, **49**, 71–9.

Hiraga, K. and Fujii, T. (1985). Carcinogenicity testing of acetaminophen in F344 rats. *Japanese Journal of Cancer Research (Gann)*, **76**, 79–85.

Hirose, M., Fukushima, S., Hananouchi, M., Shirai, T., Ogiso, T., Takashi, M., and Ito, N. (1976). Different susceptibilities of the urinary bladder epithelium of animal species to three nitroso compounds. *Japanese Journal of Cancer Research (Gann)*, **67**, 175–89.

Hodson, C.J. (1970). Differential diagnosis between atrophic pyelonephritis and analgesic nephropathy. In *Renal infection and renal scarring* (ed. P. Kincaid-Smith and K.F. Fairley), pp. 415–9. Mercedes, Melbourne.

Honn, K.V., Bockman, R.S., and Marnett, L.J. (1981). Prostaglandins and cancer: a review of tumor initiation through tumor metastasis. *Prostaglandins*, **21**, 833–64.

Hood, B., Falkheden, T. and Carlsson, M. (1967). Trends and present pattern of mortality in chronic uremia. *Acta Medica Scandinavica*, **181**, 561–9.

Horisberger, B., Grandjean, E., and Lanz, F. (1958). Untersuchungen über den Medikamentenmißbrauch in einem Großbetrieb der Schweizerischen Uhrenindustrie. *Schweizerische Medizinische Wochenschrift*, **88**, 920–6.

Horvath, J.S., Waugh, R.C., Tiller, D.J., and Duggin, G.G. (1982). The detection of renovascular hypertension: a study of 490 patients by renal angiography. *Quarterly Journal of Medicine*, **51**, 139–46.

Howe, G.R., Burch, J.D., Miller, A.B., Cook, G.M., Esteve, J., Morrison, B. *et al.* (1980). Tobacco use, occupation, coffee, various nutrients, and bladder cancer. *Journal of the National Cancer Institute*, **64**, 701–13.

Høybye, G. and Nielsen, O.E. (1971). Renal pelvic carcinoma in phenacetin abusers. *Scandinavian Journal of Urology and Nephrology*, **5**, 190–2.

Hubert, D., Habibi, B., Krulik, M., and Debray, J. (1984). Anémie hémolytique immunoallergique, thrombopénie et insuffisance rénale aiguë induites par l'aspirine. *Presse Médicale*, **13**, 2567–9.

Hukill, P.B. and Vidone, R.A. (1965). Histochemistry of mucus and other polysaccharides in tumors. I. Carcinoma of the bladder. *Laboratory Investigation*, **14**, 1624–35.

Hultengren, N. (1961). Renal papillary necrosis. A clinical study of 103 cases. *Acta Chirurgica Scandinavica*, Suppl. **277**.

Hultengren, N., Lagergren, C., and Ljungqvist, A. (1965). Carcinoma of the renal pelvis in renal papillary necrosis. *Acta Chrirurgica Scandinavica*, **130**, 314–20.

Humes, J.L., Winter, C.A., Sadowski, S.J., and Kuehl, F.A. Jr. (1981). Multiple sites on prostaglandin cyclooxygenase are determinants in the action of nonsteroidal anti-inflammatory agents. *Proceedings of the National Academy of Sciences of the United States of America*, 78, 2053–6.

Hurault de Ligny, B., Faure, G., Béné, M.C., Kessler, M., and Huriet, C. (1984). Glomérulonéphrite extra-membraneuse au cours du traitement d'une polyarthrite rheumatoide par diclofénac. *Nephrologie*, **5**, 135–6.

Hurault de Ligny, B., Ryckelynck, J.P., Levaltier, B., Gallet, B., and Trunet, P. (1986). Néphropathie interstitielle avec syndrome néphrotique induite par le pirprofène. *Revue de Médecine Interne*, **7**, 525–7.

Husserl, F.E., Lange, R.K., and Kantrow, C.M. (1979). Renal papillary necrosis and pyelonephritis accompanying fenoprofen therapy. *Journal of the American Medical Association*, **242**, 1896–8.

IARC (1980). Phenacetin. In *IARC monographs on the evaluation of the carcinogenic risk of chemicals to humans. Some pharmaceutical drugs*, vol. 24, pp. 135–61. International Agency for Research on Cancer, Lyon.

IARC (1982). Analgesic mixtures containing phenacetin. In *IARC Monographs on the evaluation of carcinogenic risks to humans. Chemicals, Industrial Processes and Industries Associated with Cancer in Humans*, Supplement No. 4. International Agency for Research on Cancer, Lyon.

IARC (1987). Phenacetin (Group 2A) and analgesic mixtures containing phenacetin (Group 1). In *IARC monographs on the evaluation of carcinogenic risks to humans. Overall evaluations of carcinogenicity: an updating of IARC Monographs volumes 1 to 42*, Suppl. 4. International Agency for Research on Cancer, Lyon.

Ibels, L.S., Alfrey, A.C., Huffer, W.E., Craswell, P.W., and Weil, R. (1981). Calcification in endstage kidneys. *American Journal of Medicine*, **71**, 33–7.

Ingham, J.P., Kleerekoper, M., Stewart, J.H., and Posen, S. (1974). Symptomatic skeletal disease in non-terminal renal failure. *Medical Journal of Australia*, **1**, 873–6.

Ingram, S.J. (1979). Naproxen and renal impairment. *British Medical Journal*, **1**, 1216.

Isaka, H., Yoshii, H., Otsuji, A., Koike, M., Nagain, Y., Koura, M. *et al.* (1979). Tumors of Sprague–Dawley rats induced by long-term feeding of phenacetin. *Japanese Journal of Cancer Research (Gann)*, **70**, 29–36.

Ito, N. (1976). Early changes caused by *N*-butyl-*N*-(4-hydroxybutyl) nitrosamine in the bladder epithelium of different animal species. *Cancer Research*, **36**, 2528–31.

Ito, N. and Fukushima, S. (1986). Carcinogenesis, urinary tract, rat. In *Urinary system, monograph on the pathology of laboratory animals* (ed. T.C. Jones, U. Mohr, and R.D. Hunt), pp. 317–21. Springer, Heidelberg.

Ito, N., Hiasa, Y., Tamai, A., Okajima, E., and Kitamura, H. (1969). Histogenesis of urinary bladder tumours induced by *N*-butyl-*N*-(4-hydroxybutyl) nitrosamine. *Japanese Journal of Cancer Research (Gann)*, **60**, 401–10.

Ito, N., Makiura, S., Yokota, Y., Kamamoto, Y., Hiasa, Y., and Sugihara, S. (1971). Effect of unilateral ureter ligation on development of tumors in the urinary system of rats treated with *N*-butyl-*N*-(4–hydroxybutyl) nitrosamine. *Japanese Journal of Cancer Research (Grann)*, **62**, 359–65.

Izumi, Y., Franco-Saenz, R., and Mulrow, P.J. (1985). Effects of prostaglandin synthesis inhibitors on the renin–angiotensin system and renal function. *Hypertension*, **7**, 791–6.

Izzo, J.L. (1989). Sympathoadrenal activity, catecholamines, and the pathogenesis of vasculopathic hypertensive target-organ damage. *American Journal of Hypertension*, **2**, 305–12S.

Jacobs, L.A. and Morris, J.G. (1962). Renal papillary necrosis and the abuse of phenacetin. *Medical Journal of Australia*, **2**, 531–8.

Jacobs, J.B., Arai, M., Cohen, S.M., and Friedell, G.H. (1979). Early lesions in experimental bladder cancer: scanning electron microscopy of cell surface markers. *Cancer Research*, **36**, 2512–7.

Jacobson, H.R. (1988). Ischemic renal disease: an overlooked clinical entity? *Kidney International*, **34**, 729–43.

Jaeger, P., Burckhardt, P., and Wauters, J.P. (1982). Ca–P metabolism is particularly disturbed in analgesic abuse nephropathy (AAN). *Kidney International*, **21**, 903–4.

Jaffe, J.H. (1970). Drug addiction and drug abuse. In *The pharmacological basis of therapeutics* (4th edn) (ed. L.S. Goodman and A. Gilman), pp. 276–313. Macmillan, New York.

Jao, W. (1986). Iatrogenic renal disease as revealed by renal biopsy. *Seminars in Diagnostic Pathology*, **5**, 63–79.

Jasinski, B. and Müller, D. (1950). Zur Pathogenese der toxisch-hämolytischen Anämien nach chronischem Phenacetinabusus. *Schweizerische Medizinische Wochenschrift*, **80**, 681–4.

Jasinski, B. and Wuhrmann, F. (1958). Zur Frage der Schäden infolge Phenacetinabusus. *Schweizerische Medizinische Wochenschrift*, **88**, 1290–2.

Jeffery, W.H. and Lafferty, W.E. (1981). Acute renal failure after acetaminophen overdose: report of two cases. *American Journal of Hospital Pharmacy*, **38**, 1355–8.

Jenkins, D.A.S., Harrison, D.J., MacDonald, M.K., and Winney, R.J. (1988). Mefenamic acid nephropathy: an interstitial and messangial lesion. *Nephrology, Dialysis, Transplantation*, **2**, 217–20.

Jensen, O.M., Knudsen, J.B., McLaughlin, J.K., and Sørensen, B.L. (1988). The Copenhagen case-control study of renal pelvis and ureter cancer: role of smoking and occupational exposures. *International Journal of Cancer*, **41**, 557–61.

Jensen, O.M., Knudsen, J.B., Tomasson, H., and Sørensen, B.L. (1989). The

Copenhagen case-control study of renal pelvis and ureter cancer: role of analgesics. *International Journal of Cancer*, **44**, 965–8.

Joh, K., Aizawa, S., Yamaguchi, Y., Inomata, I., Shibasaki, T., Sakai, O., and Hamaguchi, K. (1990). Drug-induced hypersensitivity nephritis: lymphocyte stimulation testing and renal biopsy in 10 cases. *American Journal of Nephrology*, **10**, 222–30.

Johansson, S.L. (1981). Carcinogenicity of analgesics: long-term treatment of Sprague-Dawley rats with phenacetin, phenazone, caffeine and paracetamol (acetaminophen). *International Journal of Cancer*, **27**, 521–9.

Johansson, S.L. and Anderström, C. (1988). The influence of antipyrene on *N*-[4-(5-nitro-2-furyl)-2-thiazolyl]-formamide-induced urinary tract carcinogenesis. *Carcinogenesis*, **9**, 783–7.

Johansson, S. and Angervall, L. (1976*a*). Urothelial hyperplasia of the renal papillae in female Sprague–Dawley rats induced by long term feeding of phenacetin. *Acta Pathologica et Microbiologica Scandinavica; Section A, Pathology*, **84**, 353–4.

Johansson, S. and Angervall, L. (1976*b*). Urothelial changes of the renal papillae in Sprague–Dawley rats induced by long term feeding of phenacetin. *Acta Pathologica et Microbiologica Scandinavica; Section A, Pathology*, **84**, 375–83.

Johansson, S. and Wahlqvist, L. (1977). Tumours of urinary bladder and ureter associated with abuse of phenacetin-containing analgesics. *Acta Pathologica et Microbiologica Scandinavica; Section A, Pathology*, **85**, 768–74.

Johansson, S. and Wahlqvist, L. (1979). A prognostic study of urothelial renal pelvic tumors. Comparison between the prognosis of patients treated with intrafascial nephrectomy and perifascial nephroureterectomy. *Cancer*, **43**, 2525–31.

Johansson, S., Angervall, L., Bengtsson, U., and Wahlqvist, L. (1974). Uroepithelial tumors of the renal pelvis associated with abuse of phenacetin-containing analgesics. *Cancer*, **33**, 743–53.

Johansson, S., Angervall, L., Bengtsson, U., and Wahlqvist, L. (1976). A clinicopathologic and prognostic study of epithelial tumors of the renal pelvis. *Cancer*, **37**, 1376–83.

Johansson, S.L., Anderström, C., von Schultz, L., and Larsson, P. (1987*a*). Enhancement of *N*-[4-(5-nitro-2-furyl)-2-thiazolyl] formamide-induced carcinogenesis by urinary tract infection in rats. *Cancer Research*, **47**, 559–62.

Johansson, S.L., Anderström, C., and Larsson, P. (1987*b*). The influence of urinary tract infection on the incidence of urinary tract tumors in *N*-[4-(5-nitro-2-furyl)-2-thiazolyl] formamide induced carcinogenesis in male Sprague–Dawley rats. *Cancer Letters*, **37**, 87–98.

Johansson, S.L., Radio, S.J., Saidi, J., and Sakata, T. (1989). The effects of acetaminophen, antipyrine and phenacetin on rat urothelial cell proliferation. *Carcinogenesis*, **10**, 105–11.

Joubert, P.H., Clark, E.C., Otto, A.C., and Pannall, P.R. (1977). Unreliable drug histories, analgesics, and changes in renal function. *South African Medical Journal*, **52**, 107–9.

Juhl, R.P., Van Thiel, D.H., Dittert, L.W., Albert, K.S., and Smith, R.B. (1983). Ibuprofen and sulindac kinetics in alcoholic liver disease. *Clinical Pharmacology and Therapeutics*, **34**, 104–9.

Juusela, H. (1973). Carcinoma of the renal pelvis and its relationship to analgesic abuse. *Annales Chirurgiae et Gynaecologiae Fenniae*, **62**, 386–90.

Kadlubar, F., Miller, J.A., and Miller, E.C. (1977). Hepatic microsomal *N*-glucuronidation and nucleic acid binding of *N*-hydroxy arylamines in relation to urinary bladder carcinogenesis. *Cancer Research*, **37**, 805–14.

Kadlubar, F.F., Frederick, C.B., Weis, C.C., and Zenser, T.V. (1982). Prostaglandin endoperoxide synthetase-mediated metabolism of carcinogenic aromatic amines and their binding to DNA and protein. *Biochemical and Biophysical Research Communications*, **108**, 253–8.

Kaladelfos, G. and Edwards, K.D.G. (1976). Increased prevalence of coronary heart disease in analgesic nephropathy: relation to hypertension, hypertriglyceridemia and combined hyperlipidemia. *Nephron*, **15**, 388–400.

Kasanen, A. and Valleala, P. (1963). Electroencephalographic findings in chronic phenacetin abusers. *Acta Medica Scandinavica*, **173**, 35–40.

Kasiske, B.L. (1987). Relationship between vascular disease and age-associated changes in the kidney. *Kidney International*, **31**, 1153–9.

Kasiske, B.L., Tortorice, K.L., Heim-Duthoy, K.L., Goryance, J.M., and Rao, K.V. (1990). Lovastatin treatment of hypercholesterolemia in renal transplant recipients. *Transplantation*, **49**, 95–100.

Katz, S.M., Capaldo, R., Everts, E.A., and DiGregorio, J. (1981). Tolmetin. Association with reversible renal failure and acute interstitial nephritis. *Journal of the American Medical Association*, **246**, 243–5.

Kaude, J.V., Stone, M., Fuller, T.J., Cade, J.R., Tarrant, D.G., and Juncos, L.J. (1976). Papillary necrosis in kidney transplant patients. *Radiology*, **120**, 69–74.

Kauffman, G. (1989). Aspirin-induced gastric mucosal injury: lessons learned from animal models. *Gastroenterology*, **96**, 606–14.

Kaump, D.H. (1966). Pharmacology of the fenemates. II. Toxicology in animals. In *Fenemates in medicine*, (ed. H. Kendall). *Annals of Physiological Medicine* (Suppl.), pp. 16–23.

Kaysen, G.A., Pond, S.M., Roper, M.H., Menke, D.J., and Marrama, M.A. (1985). Combined hepatic and renal injury in alcoholics during therapeutic use of acetaminophen. *Archives of Internal Medicine*, **145**, 2019–23.

Keaton, M.R. (1988). Acute renal failure in an alcoholic during therapeutic acetaminophen ingestion. *Southern Medical Journal*, **81**, 1163–6.

Keller, F. and Schwarz, A. (1983). Analgesic dilemma in chronic hemodialysis patients. *Pain*, **17**, 99–101.

Keller, H.M., Cottier, H., and Reubi, F. (1961). Fehlen von Nierenveränderungen nach Coli-bazilleninjektionen bei mit phenacetin chronische behandelten Kaninchen. *Schweizerische Medizinische Wochenschrift*, **91**, 1021–5.

Keller, F., Faber, U., and Reeck, S. (1987). Effect and toxicity of bezafibrate in hemodialysis patients. *Clinical Nephrology*, **28**, 159–60.

Kennedy, J.F. (1979). *Proteoglycans—biological and chemical aspects in human life*. Elsevier, Amsterdam.

Kennedy, A. and Saluga, P.G. (1970). Urine cytology in experimental renal toxic injury. *Annals of Rheumatic Diseases*, **29**, 546–52.

Kher, K. and Makker, S. (1987). Acute renal failure due to acetaminophen ingestion without concurrent hepatotoxicity. *American Journal of Medicine*, **82**, 1280–1.

Kielholz, P. (1954). Äetiologie und Therapie der Analgetika- und hypnotikasucht. *Schweizerische Medizinische Wochenschrift*, **84**, 753–6.

Kielholz, P. (1957). Abusus und Sucht mit phenacetinhaltigen Kombinationspräparaten. *Schweizerische Medizinische Wochenschrift*, **87**, 1131–4.

Kimberly, R.P., Bowden, R.E., Keiser, H.R., and Plotz, P.H. (1978*a*). Reduction of renal function by newer nonsteroidal anti-inflammatory drugs. *American Journal of Medicine*, **64**, 804–7.

Kimberly, R.P., Gill, J.R., Bowden, R.E., Keiser, H.R., and Plotz, P.H. (1978*b*). Elevated urinary prostaglandins and the effects of aspirin on renal function in lupus erythematosus. *Annals of Internal Medicine*, **89**, 336–41.

Kincaid-Smith, P. (1967). Pathogenesis of the renal lesion associated with abuse of analgesics. *Lancet*, **1**, 859–62.

Kincaid-Smith, P. (1968). Analgesic nephropathy. *Annals of Internal Medicine*, **68**, 949–53.

Kincaid-Smith, P. (1978). Analgesic nephropathy. *Kidney International*, **13**, 1–4.

Kincaid-Smith, P. (1979). Analgesic nephropathy in Australia. *Contributions to Nephrology*, **16**, 57–64.

Kincaid-Smith, P. (1980). Analgesic abuse and the kidney. *Kidney International*, **17**, 250–60.

Kincaid-Smith, P. (1986*a*). Effects of non-narcotic analgesics on the kidney. *Drugs*, **32** (Suppl. 4), 109–28.

Kincaid-Smith, P. (1986*b*). Renal toxicity of non-narcotic analgesics. At-risk patients and prescribing applications. *Medical Toxicology*, **1** (Suppl. 1), 14–22.

Kincaid-Smith, P. and Fairley, K.F. (ed.) (1970). *Renal infection and renal scarring*. Mercedes, Melbourne.

Kincaid-Smith, P. and Nanra, R.S. (1988). Lithium-induced and analgesic-induced renal diseases. In *Diseases of the kidney* (4th edn) (eds R.W. Schrier and C.W. Gottschalk), pp. 1197–227. Little Brown, Boston.

Kincaid-Smith, P., Saker, B.M., McKenzie, I.F.C., and Muirden, K.D. (1968*a*). Lesions in the blood supply of the papilla in experimental analgesic nephropathy. *Medical Journal of Australia*, **1**, 203–6.

Kincaid-Smith, P., Saker, B.M., and McKenzie, I.F.C. (1968*b*). Lesions in vasa recta in experimental analgesic nephropathy. *Lancet*, **1**, 24.

King, E.B., Vanderlaan, M., Jensen, R.H., Kromhout, L.K., and Hoffman, J.W. (1984). Morphologic changes in rat urothelial cells during carcinogenesis: I. Histologic and cytologic changes. *Cytometry*, **5**, 447–53.

Kirschenbaum, M.A. and Serros, E.R. (1981). Effect of prostaglandin inhibition on glomerular filtration rate in normal and uremic rabbits. *Prostaglandins*, **22**, 245–54.

Kirschenbaum, M.A., Chaudhari, A., Aframian, D., Cherry, J., Kownacki, J.J., and Pae, H. (1985). Prostacyclin (PGI_2) and prostaglandin E_2 (PGE_2) biosynthesis by isolated renal microvessels (MV). *Kidney International*, **27**, 259.

Kitchen, E.A., Boot, J.R., and Dawson, W. (1978). Chemotactic activity of thromboxane A_2, prostaglandins and their metabolites for polymorphonuclear leukocytes. *Prostaglandins*, **16**, 239–44.

Kleinknecht, D., Vanhille, P., Morel-Maroger, L., Kanfer, A., Lemaitre, V., Mery, J.P. *et al.* (1983). Acute interstitial nephritis due to drug hypersensitivity. An up-to-date review with report of 19 cases. *Advances in Nephrology*, **12**, 277–308.

Kleinknecht, D., Landais, P., and Goldfarb, B. (1986). Analgesic and nonsteroidal anti-inflammatory drug-associated acute renal failure: a prospective collaborative study. *Clinical Nephrology*, **25**, 275–81.

Kleinknecht, D., Vanhille, P., and Druet, P. (1988). Néphrites interstitielles aiguës granulomateuses d'origine médicamenteuse. *Presse Médicale*, **17**, 201–5.

Kleinknecht, D., Fleury, D., and Vanhille, P. (1989). Drug-related acute renal failure in the late 1980s: a preventable disease linked to drug misuse. In *Proceedings of Conference on Newer Aspects in the Treatment of Renal Failure*, Geneva, p. 34.

Kleinman, J.G., Breitenfield, R.V., and Roth, D.A. (1980). Acute renal failure associated with acetaminophen ingestion: report of a case and review of the literature. *Clinical Nephrology*, **24**, 201–5.

Köhler, H., Weber, M., Wandel, E., and Schild, H.H. (1987). Analgetika-niere. Bedeutung der bilgebenden Verfahren. *Deutsche Medizinische Wochenschrift*, **112**, 1347–52.

Kokot, F. (1989). Analgetika-nephropathie in Polen. *Zeitschrift für Urologie und Nephrologie*, **82** (Suppl. 1), 150–1.

Kravath, R.E., Abel, G., and Colli, A. (1972). Salicylate poisoning: effect on 2,3-diphosphoglycerate levels in the rat. *Biochemical Pharmacology*, **21**, 2656–8.

Kreisberg, J.I. (1983). Contractile properties of the glomerular mesangium. *Federation Proceedings*, **42**, 3053–7.

Kreisberg, J.I., Karnowsky, M.J., and Levine, L. (1982). Prostaglandin production by homogeneous cultures of rat glomerular epithelial and mesangial cells. *Kidney International*, **22**, 355–9.

Kreisberg, J.I., Venkatachalam, M., and Troyer, D. (1985). Contractile properties of cultured glomerular mesangial cells. *American Journal of Physiology*, **249**, F457–63.

Krikler, D.M. (1967). Paracetamol and the kidney. *British Medical Journal*, **3**, 615–6.

Krishnaswamy, S. and Nanra, R.S. (1976). 'Phenacetin' nephropathy without phenacetin. *Australian and New Zealand Journal of Medicine*, **6**, 88.

Krishnaswamy, S., Wallace, D.C., and Nanra, R.S. (1974). Ischaemic heart disease in analgesic nephropathy. *Australian and New Zealand Journal of Medicine*, **4**, 426.

Krishnaswamy, S., Kuna, K., and Nanra, R.S. (1976). Pattern of changes in renal functions with analgesic abuse. *Australian and New Zealand Journal of Medicine*, **6**, 88.

Kriz, W. and Lever, A.E. (1969). Renal countercurrent mechanisms: structure and function. *American Heart Journal*, **78**, 101–18.

Kudrow, L. (1982). Paradoxical effects of frequent analgesic use. *Advances in Neurology*, **33**, 335–41.

Küng, L.G. (1976). Hypernephroides Karzinom und Karzinome der ableitenden Harnwege nach Phenacetinabusus. *Schweizerische Medizinische Wochenschrift*, **106**, 47–51.

Kunze, E. (1979). Development of urinary bladder cancer in the rat. *Current Topics in Pathology*, **67**, 145–232.

Kunze, E. and Schauer, A. (1971). Enzymhistochemische und autoradiographische Untersuchungen an dibutylnitrosamine-induzierten Harnblasenpapillomen der Ratte. *Zeitschrift für Krebsforschung und Klinische Onkologie*, **75**, 146–60.

Kunze, E. and Schauer, A. (1977). Morphology, classification and histogenesis of *N*-butyl-*N*-(4-hydroxybutyl) nitrosamine-induced carcinomas in the urinary bladder of rats. *Zeitschrift für Krebsforschung und Klinische Onkologie*, **88**, 273–89.

Kunze, E., Rath, G., and Graewe, T. (1987). Effect of phenacetin and caffeine on *N*-butyl-*N*-(4-hydroxybutyl)-nitrosamine-initiated urothelial carcinogenesis in rats. *Urologia Internationalis*, **42**, 108–14.

Kunzendorf, U., Keller, F., Schwietzer, G., Sorensen, R., and Distler, A. (1990). Control of renovascular hypertension by renal embolization. *American Journal of Nephrology*, **10**, 339–43.

Küster, G. and Ritz, E. (1989). Analgesic abuse and hypertension. *Lancet*, **2**, 1105.

Ladewig, D. (1979). Abusus und Abhängigkeit von nicht-narkotischen Analgetika und Sedativa. *Nervenarzt*, **50**, 212–8.

Ladewig, D., Miest, P., Dubach, U.C., Ettlin, C., and Hobi, V. (1978). Use and abuse of non-narcotic analgesics. *Drug and Alcohol Dependence*, **3**, 435–42.

Ladewig, D., Dubach, U.C., Ettlin, C., and Hobi, V. (1979). Zur Psychologie des Analgetikakonsums bei berufstätigen Frauen. Ergebnisser einer epidemiologischen Prospektivstudie. *Nervenarzt*, **50**, 219–24.

Laffi, G., LaVilla, G., Pinzani, M., Ciabattoni, G., Patrignani, P., and Mannelli, M. *et al.* (1986). Altered renal and platelet arachidonic acid metabolism in cirrhosis. *Gastroenterology*, **90**, 274–82.

Lai, F.M., Lai, K.N., and Chong, Y.W. (1987). Papillary necrosis associated with rifampicin therapy. *Australian and New Zealand Journal of Medicine*, **17**, 68–70.

Lalich, J.J., Paik, W.C.W., and Pradhan, B. (1974). Epithelial hyperplasia in the renal papilla of rats. Induction in animals fed excess sodium chloride. *Archives of Pathology*, **97**, 29–32.

Lancet (1981). Aspirin or paracetamol? *Lancet*, **2**, 287–9.

Landmann-Suter, R. and Dubach, U.C. (1975). Phenacetin und Nierenschädigung. Verlaufskontrolle bei langjährigen Schmerzmittelmißbrauch. *Deutsche Medizinische Wochenschrift*, **100**, 1451–6.

Lang, P., Santelli, G., Benarbia, S., Moritz, S., Charpentier, B., and Fries, D. (1986). Etude immunopathologique d'une néphropathie interstitielle aiguë induite par la clométacine. *Presse Médicale*, **15**, 915–8.

Lapetina, E.G. (1982). Regulation of arachidonic acid production: role of phospholipases C and A_2. *Trends in Pharmacological Sciences*, **3**, 115–8.

Larsen, K. and Møller, C.E. (1959). A renal lesion caused by abuse of phenacetin. *Acta Medica Scandinavica*, **164**, 53–71.

Latini, R., Corletti, C., de Gaetano, G., Dejana, E., Galletti, F., Urso, R., and Marzot, M. (1986). Comparative bioavailability of aspirin from buffered, enteric coated and plain preparations. *International Journal of Clinical Pharmacology, Therapeutics and Toxicology*, **24**, 313–18.

Lavaud, S., Mamez, B., Lavaud, F., Birembaut, B., Toupance, O., Brunois, J.P., and Chanard, J. (1984). Insuffisance rénale aiguë par hypersensibilité à la clométacine. *Néphrologie*, **5**, 131–4.

Lawson, D.H. (1973). Analgesic consumption and impaired renal function. *Journal of Chronic Diseases*, **26**, 39–45.

Lawson, A.A.H. and Maclean, N. (1966). Renal disease and drug therapy in rheumatoid arthritis. *Annals of the Rheumatic Diseases*, **25**, 441–9.

Lechat, P., Levillain, R., Dechezlepretre, S., and Cluzan, R. (1974). Mise en évidence de la néphrotoxicité aiguë de la glafénine chez le rat. *Thérapie*, **29**, 567–73.

Lee, H.A., Davidson, A.R., and Burston, J. (1974). Analgesic nephropathy in Wessex: a clinico-pathological survey. *Clinical Nephrology*, **2**, 197–207.

Leist, M.H., Gluskin, L.E., and Payne, J.A. (1985). Enhanced toxicity of acetaminophen in alcoholics: report of three cases. *Journal of Clinical Gastroenterology*, **7**, 55–9.

Leistenschneider, W. and Ehmann, R. (1973). Nierenbeckenkarzinom nach Phenacetinabusus. *Schweizerische Medizinische Wochenschrift*, **103**, 433–9.

Leonards, J.R. (1963). The influence of solubility on the rate of gastrointestinal absorption of aspirin. *Clinical Pharmacology and Therapeutics*, **4**, 476–9.

Leung, S.F., Delzell, E., Dreyer, N.A., and Rothman, N.A. (1984). Analgesics and kidney disease. *International Journal of Epidemiology*, **15**, 454–5.

Levy, G., Procknal, J.A., and Garrettson, L.K. (1975). Distribution of salicylate between neonatal and maternal serum at diffusion equilibrium. *Clinical Pharmacology and Therapeutics*, **18**, 210–14.

Lévy, M., Prieur, A.M., Gubler, M.C., Hayem, F., Manigne, P., Cheron, G., and Naiudet, P. (1987). Renal involvement in juvenile chronic arthritis: clinical and pathologic features. *American Journal of Kidney Diseases*, **9**, 138–46.

Lewis, R.B. and Schulman, J.D. (1973). Influence of acetylsalicylic acid, an inhibitor of prostaglandin synthesis, on the duration of human gestation and labour, *Lancet*, **2**, 1159–61.

Lewis, C.T., Molland, E.A., Marshall, V.R., Tresidder, G.C., and Blandy, J.P. (1975). Analgesic abuse, ureteric obstruction, and retroperitoneal fibrosis. *British Medical Journal*, **2**, 76–8.

Licht, A., Alpert, B.E., Bourgoignie, J., and Schlondorff, D. (1981). The effect of prostaglandin synthetase inhibitors on renal function: studies in normal rats during sodium or water diuresis and in rats with chronic renal insufficiency *Prostaglandins*, **22**, 1–10.

Lijinsky, W. (1988). Importance of animal experiments in carcinogenesis research. *Environmental and Molecular Mutagenesis*, **11**, 307–14.

Lin, J.H. and Levy, G. (1983). Renal clearance of inorganic sulfate in rats: effect of acetaminophen-induced depletion of endogenous sulfate. *Journal of Pharmaceutical Sciences*, **72**, 213–17.

Lindeneg, O., Fischer, S., Pedersen, J., and Nissen, N.I. (1959). Necrosis of the renal papillae and prolonged abuse of phenacetin. *Acta Medica Scandinavia*, **165**, 321–8.

Lindsley, C.B. and Warady, B.A. (1990). Nonsteroidal anti-inflammatory drugs. Renal toxicity. Review of pediatric issues. *Clinical Pediatrics*, **29**, 10–3.

Lindvall, N. (1960). Renal papillary necrosis. A roentgenographic study of 155 cases. *Acta Radiologica (Stockholm)*, **192** (Suppl.), 1–153.

Lindvall, N. (1978). Radiological changes of renal papillary necrosis. *Kidney International*, **13**, 93–106.

Lins, R.L., Verpooten, G.A., De Clerck, D.S., and De Broe, M.E. (1986). Urinary indices in acute interstitial nephritis. *Clinical Nephrology*, **26**, 131–3.

Lomax-Smith, J. and Seymour, A.E. (1980*a*). Unsuspected analgesic nephropathy in transitional cell carcinoma of the upper tract: a morphological study. *Histopathology*, **4**, 255–69.

Lomax-Smith, J.D. and Seymour, A.E. (1980*b*). Neoplasia in analgesic nephropathy. A urothelial field change. *American Journal of Surgical Pathology*, **4**, 565–72.

Lomvardias, S., Pinn, V.W., Wadhwa, M.L., Koshy, K.M., and Heller, M. (1981). Nephrotic syndrome associated with sulindac. *New England Journal of Medicine*, **304**, 424.

Lorenzen, I. and Schwartz, M. (1960). Phenacetin-induced hæmolysis in patients with chronic nephritis and phenacetin abuse. *Acta Medica Scandinavica*, **168**, 461–6.

Lornoy, W., Becaus, I., De Vleeschouwer, M., Morelle, V., Fonteyne, E., Thienpont, L., and Mestdagh, J. (1986). Renal cell carcinoma, a new complication of analgesic nephropathy. *Lancet*, **1**, 1271–2.

Losse, H., Westerboer, S., and Gast, K.U. (1966). Bedeutung der Peritoneal- bzw. Hämodialysein der Therapie der chronische Pyelonephritis. In *Pyelonephritis, Forschungsergebnisse* (ed. H. Losse and M. Kienitz), pp. 358–66. Thieme, Stuttgart.

Lote, C.J. and Haylor, J. (1989). Eicosanoids in renal function. *Prostaglandins, Leukotrienes and Essential Fatty Acids*, **36**, 203–17.

Lum, G.M., Aisenbrey, G.A., Dunn, M.J., Berl, T., Schrier, R.W., and McDonald, K.M. (1977). *In vivo* effect of indomethacin to potentiate the renal medullary cyclic AMP response to vasopressin. *Journal of Clinical Investigation*, **59**, 8–13.

Lusvarghi, E., Bonucchi, D., Vandelli, L., Minari, M., Malmusi, G., and Savi, N. (1987). Analgesic abuse: epidemiologic evidence in the district of Modena. In *Prevention in Nephrology* (ed. G. Buccianti), pp. 64–7. Masson, Milano.

McAnally, J.F., Winchester, J.F., and Schreiner, G.E. (1983). Analgesic nephropathy. An uncommon cause of end-stage renal disease. *Archives of Internal Medicine*, **143**, 1897–9.

McArthur, J.N., Dawkins, P.D., and Smith, M.J.H. (1971). The displacement of *L*-tryptophan and dipeptides from bovine albumin *in vitro* and from human plasma *in vivo* by antirheumatic drugs. *Journal of Pharmacy and Pharmacology*, **29**, 393–8.

McCarthy, J.T., Schwartz, G.L., Blair, T.J., Pierides, A.M., and Van Den Berg, C.J. (1982). Reversible nonoliguric acute renal failure associated with zomepirac therapy. *Mayo Clinic Proceedings*, **57**, 351–4.

McCormick, D.L., Ronan, S.S., Becci, P.J., and Moon, R.C. (1981*a*). Influence of total dose and dose schedule on induction of urinary bladder cancer in the mouse by *N*-butyl-*N*-(4-hydroxybutyl)-nitrosamine. *Carcinogenesis*, **2**, 251–4.

McCormick, D.L., Becci, P.J., and Moon, R.C. (1981*b*). Inhibition of mammary and urinary bladder carcinogenesis by a retinoid and a maleic anhydride-divinyl ether copolymer (MVE-2). *Carcinogenesis*, **3**, 1473–7.

McCoy, R.N., Fried, T.A., Osgood, R.W., and Stein, J.H. (1985). Release of prostaglandin E_2 (PGE_2) by a single isolated perfused glomerulus. *Kidney International*, **27**, 297.

McCredie, M. (1989). Analgesic use and chronic renal disease. *New England Journal of Medicine*, **321**, 1125–6.

McCredie, M. and Stewart, J.H. (1988). Does paracetamol cause urothelial cancer or renal papillary necrosis? *Nephron*, **49**, 296–300.

McCredie, M., Ford, J.M., Taylor, J.S., and Stewart, J.H. (1982*a*). Analgesics and cancer of the renal pelvis in New South Wales. *Cancer*, **49**, 2617–25.

McCredie, M., Stewart, J.H., and Mahony, J.F. (1982*b*). Is phenacetin responsible for analgesic nephropathy in New South Wales? *Clinical Nephrology*, **17**, 134–40.

McCredie, M., Stewart, J.H., Ford, J.M., and MacLennan, R.A. (1983*a*). Phenacetin-containing analgesics and cancer of the bladder or renal pelvis in women. *British Journal of Urology*, **55**, 220–4.

McCredie, M., Stewart, J.H., and Ford, J.M. (1983*b*). Analgesics and tobacco as risk factors for cancer of the ureter and renal pelvis in men. *Journal of Urology*, **130**, 28–30.

McCredie, M., Stewart, J.H., Carter, J.J., Turner, J., and Mahony, J.F. (1986). Phenacetin and papillary necrosis: independent risk factors for renal pelvic cancer. *Kidney International*, **30**, 81–4.

McCredie, M., Ford, J.M., and Stewart, J.H. (1988). Risk factors for cancer of the renal parenchyma. *International Journal of Cancer*, **42**, 13–16.

McCredie, M., Stewart, J.H., Mathew, T.H., Disney, A.P.S., and Ford, J.M. (1989). The effect of withdrawal of phenacetin-containing analgesics on the incidence of kidney and urothelial cancer and renal failure. *Clinical Nephrology*, **31**, 35–9.

McCredie, M., Coates, M.S., Ford, J.M., Disney, A.P.S., Auld, J.J., and Stewart, J.H. (1990). Geographical distribution of cancers of the kidney and urinary tract and analgesic nephropathy in Australia and New Zealand. *Australian and New Zealand Journal of Medicine*, **20**, 684–8 and 694.

McCutcheon, A.D. (1962). Renal damage and phenacetin. *Medical Journal of Australia*, **2**, 543–6.

McGiff, J.C. (1981). Prostaglandins, prostacyclin and thromboxanes. *Annual Review of Pharmacology and Toxicology*, **21**, 479–509.

McIver, M.A. and Hobbs, J.B. (1975). The failure of high doses of aspirin to produce renal lesions in pigs. *Medical Journal of Australia*, **1**, 197–9.

Macklin, A.W. and Szot, R.J. (1980). Eighteen month oral study of aspirin, phenacetin and caffeine, in C57BL/6 mice. *Drug and Chemical Toxicology*, **3**, 135–63.

Macklon, A.F., Craft, A.W., Thompson, M., and Kerr, D.N.S. (1974). Aspirin and analgesic nephropathy. *British Medical Journal*, **1**, 597–600.

McLaughlin, J.K., Blot, W.J., Mandel, J.S., Schuman, L.M., Mehl, E.S., and Fraumeni, J.F. (1983). Etiology of cancer of the renal pelvis. *Journal of the National Cancer Institute*, **71**, 287–91.

McLaughlin, J.K., Mandel, J.S., Blot, W.J., Schuman, L.M., Mehl, E.S., and Fraumeni, J.F. (1984). A population-based case-control study of renal cell carcinoma. *Journal of the National Cancer Institute*, **72**, 275–84.

McLaughlin, J.K., Mandel, J.S., Mehl, E.S., and Blot, W.J. (1991). Comparison of next-of-kin with self-respondents regarding questions on cigarette, coffee, and alcohol consumption. *Epidemiology*, **1**, 408–12.

MacLean, D., Peters, T.J., Brown, R.A.G., McCathie, M., Baines, G.F., and Robertson, P.G.C. (1968). Treatment of acute paracetamol poisoning. *Lancet*, **2**, 849–52.

Maclure, M. and MacMahon, B. (1985). Phenacetin and cancers of the urinary tract. *New England Journal of Medicine*, **313**, 1479.

McMurtry, J.R., Snodgrass, W.R., and Mitchell, J.R. (1978). Renal necrosis, glutathione depletion, and covalent binding after acetaminophen. *Toxicology and Applied Pharmacology*, **46**, 87–100.

McQueen, C.A., Way, B.M., and Williams, G.M. (1987). Biotransformation of aromatic amines to DNA-damaging products by urinary bladder organ cultures. *Carcinogenesis*, **8**, 401–4.

Magil, A.B. (1983). Drug-induced acute interstitial nephritis with granulomas. *Human Pathology*, **14**, 36–41.

Maher, J.F. (1984). Analgesic nephropathy. Observations, interpretations, and perspective on the low incidence in America. *American Journal of Medicine*, **76**, 345–8.

Maher, J.F. (1986). Renal failure in America is infrequently due to analgesic abuse. *American Journal of Kidney Diseases*, **7**, 169–73.

Mahony, J.F., Stewart, J.H., McCarthy, S.W., Storey, B.G., and Sheil, A.G.R. (1974). The effect of age and primary renal disease upon survival on renal replacement therapy. *Australian and New Zealand Journal of Medicine*, **4**, 437.

Mahony, J.F., Storey, B.G., Ibañez, R.C., and Stewart, J.H. (1977). Analgesic abuse, renal parenchymal disease and carcinoma of the kidney or ureter. *Australian and New Zealand Journal of Medicine*, **7**, 463–9.

Mandel, J.S. (1989). Analgesic use and chronic renal disease. *New England Journal of Medicine*, **321**, 1125.

Marasco, W.A., Gikas, P.W., Azziz-Baumgartner, R., Hyzy, R., Elredge, C.J., and Stross, J. (1987). Ibuprofen-associated renal dysfunction. Pathophysiologic mechanisms of acute renal failure, hyperkalemia, tubular necrosis, and proteinuria. *Archives of Internal Medicine*, **147**, 210–16.

Markovic, B. (1971). Recherches expérimentales sur le rôle de la phénacétin dans la pathogénèse des néphropathies interstitielles chroniques. *Archiv Union Medicale du Balkan*, **9**, 591–8.

Marnett, L.J. (1981). Polycyclic aromatic hydrocarbon oxidation during prostaglandin biosynthesis. *Life Sciences*, **29**, 531–46.

Marnett, L.J. and Eling, T.E. (1984). Co-oxidation during prostaglandin biosynthesis: a pathway for the metabolic activation of xenobiotics. *Reviews of Biochemical Toxicology*, **5**, 135–72.

Marnett, L.J., Reed, G.A., and Johnson, J.T. (1977). Prostaglandin synthetase dependent benzo[a]pyrene oxidation: products of the oxidation and inhibition of their formation by antioxidants. *Biochemical and Biophysical Research Communications*, **79**, 569.

Marnett, L.J., Reed, G.A., and Dennison, D.J. (1978). Prostaglandin synthetase dependent activation of 7,8-dihydro-7,8-dihydroxy-benzo[a]pyrene to mutagenic derivatives. *Biochemical and Biophysical Research Communications*, **82**, 210–6.

Marrocco, F.S., Leekam, R.N., Matzinger, M., and Gray, R.R. (1986). Displaced calcium as a sign of transitional cell carcinoma in analgesic nephropathy. *Journal of the Canadian Association of Radiology*, **37**, 122–4.

Marsepoil, T., Levesque, P. Agard, D., Dubeaux, P., and Blin, F. (1987). Hépatonéphrite due au piroxicam. *Gastroentérologie Clinique et Biologique*, **11**, 712–3.

Marshall, P.J., Kulmacz, R.J., and Lands, W.E.M. (1987). Constraints on prostaglandin biosynthesis in tissues. *Journal of Biological Chemistry*, **262**, 3510–17.

Marti, H.R. (1958). Die Anämie bei chronischem Phenacetinabusus. *Schweizerische Medizinische Wochenschrift*, **88**, 1054–6.

Maruta, T., Swanson, D.W., and Finlayson, R.E. (1979). Drug use and dependency in patients with chronic plain. *Mayo Clinic Proceedings*, **54**, 241–4.

Matsuda, K., Ohnishi, K., Misaka, E., and Yamazaki, M. (1983). Decrease of urinary prostaglandin E_2 and prostaglandin $F_{2\alpha}$ excretion by nonsteroidal anti-inflammatory drugs in rats. Relationship to anti-inflammatory activity. *Biochemical Pharmacology*, **32**, 1347–52.

Mattingley, G., Gregg, N.J., and Bach, P.H. (1991). The response of the pelvic and ureteric epithelial cells to an acutely-induced renal papillary necrosis. *Toxicologic Pathology*, (submitted).

Mease, P.J., Ellsworth, A.J., Killen, P.D., and Wilkens, R.F. (1982). Zomepirac, interstitial nephritis, and renal failure. *Annals of Internal Medicine*, **97**, 454.

Mehta, A., White, K.H., and Nanra, R.S. (1977). Significance of proteinuria in analgesic nephropathy. *Australian and New Zealand Journal of Medicine*, **7**, 200–1.

Meier-Hirschi, V. (1980). Zusammenhänge zwischen dem Analgetika-abusus und der Persönlichkeitsstruktur berufstätiger Frauen. *Medizinische Dissertation*, Basel.

Melicow, M.M. (1945). Tumors of the urinary drainage tract; urothelial tumors. *Journal of Urology*, **54**, 186–93.

Mené, P., and Cinotti, G.A. (1989). Paracrine and autocrine functions of glomerular mesangial cells. *Journal of Endocrinological Investigation*, **12**, 497–509.

Mené, P. and Dunn, M.J. (1990). Prostaglandins and rat glomerular mesangial cell proliferation. *Kidney International*, **37**, 1256–62.

Mené, P., Simonson, M.S., and Dunn, M.J. (1989*a*). Physiology of the mesangial cell. *Physiological Reviews*, **69**, 1347–424.

Mené, P., Simonson, M.S., and Dunn, M.J. (1989*b*). Phospholipids in signal transduction of mesangial cells. *American Journal of Physiology*, **256**, F375–86.

Michultka, D.M., Blanchard, E.B., Appelbaum, K.A., Jaccard, J., and Dentinger, M.P. (1989). The refractory headache patient—II. High medication consumption (analgesic rebound) headache. *Behavioural Research and Therapy*, **27**, 411–20.

Miescher, P. and Studer, A. (1961). Further animal experiments on the problem of the pathogenesis of interstitial nephritis. *Schweizerische Medizinische Wochenschrift*, **91**, 939–43.

Miescher, P., Schnyder, U., and Krech, U. (1959). Zur Pathogenese der 'interstitiellen Nephritis' bei Abusus phenacetinhaltiger analgetika. Tierexperimentelle Untersuchungen. *Schweizerische Medizinische Wochenschrift*, **88**, 432–7.

Mignon, F., Méry, J.P., Mougenot, B., Ronco, P., Roland, J., and Morel-Maroger, L. (1984). Granulomatous interstitial nephritis. *Advances in Nephrology*, **13**, 219–45.

Mihatsch, M.J. (ed.) (1986). *Das Analgetika-syndrom. Folgen des langjährigen Schmerzmittelmißbrauches. Grundlagen-klinik-prävention.* Thieme, Stuttgart.

Mihatsch, M.J. (1989). Analgetika-nephropathie und Harnwegstumoren. *Zeitschrift für Urologie und Nephrologie*, **82** (Suppl. 1), 13–35.

Mihatsch, M.J. and Knüsli, C. (1982). Phenacetin abuse and malignant tumours. An autopsy study covering 25 years (1953–1977). *Klinische Wochenschrift*, **60**, 1339–49.

Mihatsch, M.J., Torhorst, J., Amsler, B., and Zollinger, H.U. (1978). Capillarosclerosis of the lower urinary tract in analgesic (phenacetin) abuse. An electron microscope study. *Virchows Archiv. A. (Pathological Anatomy and Histology)*, **381**, 41–7.

Mihatsch, M.J., Torhorst, J., Steinmann, E., Hofer, H., Stickelberger, M., Bianchi, L. *et al.* (1979). The morphological diagnosis of analgesic (phenacetin) abuse. *Pathology Research and Practice*, **164**, 68–79.

Mihatsch, M.J., Hofer, H.O., Gutzwiler, F., Brunner, F.P., and Zollinger, H.U. (1980*a*). Phenacetinabusus I. Häufigkeit, pro-kopf-Verbrauch und Folgekosten. *Schweizerische Medizinische Wochenschrift*, **110**, 108–15.

Mihatsch, M.J., Manz, T., Knüsli, C., Hofer, H.O., Rist, M., Guetg, R. *et al.* (1980*b*). Phenacetinabusus III. Maligne Harnwegtumoren bei Phenacetinabusus in Basel 1963–1977. *Schweizerische Medizinische Wochenschrift*, **110**, 255–64.

Mihatsch, M.J., Hofer, H.O., Korteweg, F., and Zollinger, H.U. (1982*a*). Phenacetinabusus V. Häufigkeit der Phenacetinabuser im Basler Autopsiegut 1978–1980. *Schweizerische Medizinische Wochenschrift*, **112**, 1245–8.

Mihatsch, M.J., Kernen, R., and Zollinger, H.U. (1982*b*). Phenacetinabusus VI. Eine Autopsiestatistik unter besonderer Berücksichtigung extrarenaler Befunde. *Schweizerische Medizinische Wochenschrift*, **112**, 1383–8.

Mihatsch, M.J., Hofer, H.O., Gudat, F., Knüsli, C., Torhorst, J., and Zollinger, H.U. (1983*a*). Capillary sclerosis of the urinary tract and analgesic nephropathy. *Clinical Nephrology*, **20**, 285–301.

Mihatsch, M.J., Saehelin, H.B., Musfeld, D., Perret, E., and Oberholzer, M. (1983*b*). Phenacetin-abusus: kardiovaskuläre Risikofaktoren. *Nieren-und Hochdruckkrankheiten*, **12**, 83–92.

Mihatsch, M.J., Theil, G., Basler, V., Ryffel, B., Landmann, J., von Overbeck, J., and Zollinger, H.U. (1985). Morphological patterns in cyclosporin-treated renal transplant recipients. *Transplantation Proceedings*, **17**, 101–16.

Millar, J., Péloquin, R., and de Leeuw, N.K.M. (1972). Phenacetin-induced hemolytic anemia. *Canadian Medical Association Journal*, **106**, 770–5.

Miller, A.L., Worsley, L.R., and Chu, P.K. (1970). Brown urine as a clue to phenacetin intoxication. *Lancet*, **2**, 1102–4.

Miller, M.J.S., Bednar, N.M., and McGiff, J.C. (1984). Renal metabolism of sulindac: functional implications. *Journal of Pharmacology and Experimental Therapeutics*, **231**, 449–56.

Mitchell, J.R., Jollow, D.J., Potter, W.Z., Davis, D.C., Gillette, J.R., and Brodie,

B.B. (1973*a*). Acetaminophen-induced hepatic necrosis. I. Role of drug metabolism. *Journal of Pharmacology and Experimental Therapeutics*, **187**, 185–94.

Mitchell, J.R., Jollow, D.J., Potter, W.Z., Gillette, J.R., and Brodie, B.B. (1973*b*). Acetaminophen-induced hepatic necrosis. IV. Protective role of glutathione. *Journal of Pharmacology and Experimental Therapeutics*, **187**, 211–17.

Mitchell, J.R., McMurtry, R.J., Statham, C.N., and Nelson, S.D. (1977). Molecular basis for several drug-induced nephropathies. *American Journal of Medicine*, **62**, 518–26.

Mitchell, H., Muirden, K.D., and Kincaid-Smith, P. (1982). Indomethacin-induced renal papillary necrosis in juvenile chronic arthritis. *Lancet*, **2**, 558–9.

Mitnick, P.D. and Klein, W.J. (1984). Piroxicam-induced renal disease. *Archives of Internal Medicine*, **144**, 63–4.

Mobley, T.L., Coyle, J.K., Al-Hussaini, M., and McDonald, D.F. (1966). The role of chronic mechanical irritation in experimental urothelial tumourigenesis. *Investigative Urology*, **3**, 325–33.

Moel, D.I., Safirstein, R.L., McEvoy, R.C., and Hsueh, W. (1987). Effect of aspirin on experimental diabetic nephropathy. *Journal of Laboratory and Clinical Medicine*, **110**, 300–7.

Moeschlin, S. (1957). Phenacetinsucht und -schäden. Innenkörperanämien und interstitielle Nephritis. *Schweizerische Medizinische Wochenschrift*, **87**, 123–8.

Moeschlin, S. (1958). Phenacetinabusus und Phenacetinschäden in der Schweiz (anaemia haemolytica und nephritis interstitialis). In *Phenacetinabusus und Nierenschädigung* (ed. H. Sarre, A. Moench, and R. Kluthe), pp. 53–77. Thieme, Stuttgart.

Mohandas, J., Duggin, G.G., Horvath, J.S., and Tiller, D.J. (1981*a*). Metabolic oxidation of acetaminophen (paracetamol) mediated by cytochrome P-450 mixed function oxidase and prostaglandin endoperoxide synthetase in rabbit kidney. *Toxicology and Applied Pharmacology*, **61**, 252–9.

Mohandas, J., Duggin, G.G., Horvath, J.S., and Tiller, D.J. (1981*b*). Regional differences in peroxidatic activation of paracetamol (acetaminophen) mediated by cytochrome P450 and prostaglandin endoperoxide synthetase in rabbit kidney. *Research Communications in Chemical Pathology and Pharmacology*, **34**, 69–80.

Mohandas, J., Marshall, J.J., Duggin, G.G., Horvath, J.S., and Tiller, D.J. (1984). Differential distribution of glutathione-related enzymes in rabbit kidney. Possible implications in analgesic nephropathy. *Biochemical Pharmacology*, **33**, 1801–7.

Moldéus, P. and Rahimtula, A. (1980). Metabolism of paracetamol to a glutathione conjugate catalyzed by prostaglandin synthetase. *Biochemical and Biophysical Research Communications*, **96**, 469–75.

Moldéus, P., Andersson, B., Rahimtula, A., and Berggren, M. (1982). Prostaglandin synthetase catalyzed activation of paracetamol. *Biochemical Pharmacology*, **31**, 1363–8.

Molland, E.A. (1976). Aspirin damage in the rat kidney in the intact animal and after unilateral nephrectomy. *Journal of Pathology*, **120**, 43–8.

Molland, E.A. (1978). Experimental renal papillary necrosis. *Kidney International*, **13**, 5–14.

Molland, E.A. (1982). Renal papillary necrosis produced by long-term fat-free diet.

In *Nephrotoxicity, pathogenesis and assessment* (ed. P.H. Bach, F.W. Bonner, J.W. Bridges, and E.A. Lock), pp. 200–5. Wiley Heyden, Chichester.

Mommsen, S. and Aagaard, J. (1983). Tobacco as a risk factor in bladder cancer. *Carcinogensis*, **4**, 335–8.

Monnin, E., Bories, P., Canaud, B., Béraud, J.J., Boldet, P., Mirouze, J., and Michel, H. (1984). Insufficance rénale aiguë et hépatite à la clométacine. *Gastroenterologie Clinique et Biologique*, **8**, 264–8.

Moss, A.H., Riley, R., Murgo, A., and Skaff, L.A. (1986). Over-the-counter ibuprofen and acute renal failure. *Annals of Internal Medicine*, **105**, 303.

Mourad, G., Mimran, A., Baldet, P., and Barjon, P. (1982). Insuffisance rénale aiguë réversible et syndrome néphrotique induits par le fénoprofène. *Néphrologie*, **3**, 65–8.

Mudge, G.H. (1985). Pathogenesis of nephrotoxicity: pharmacological principles. In *Renal heterogeneity and target cell toxicity* (ed. P.H. Bach and E.A. Lock), pp. 1–12. Wiley, Chichester.

Mudge, G.H., Gemborys, M.W., and Duggin, G.G. (1978). Covalent binding of metabolites of acetaminophen to kidney protein and depletion of renal glutathione. *Journal of Pharmacology and Experimental Therapeutics*, **206**, 218–26.

Muir, C., Waterhouse, J., Mack, T., Powell, J., and Whelan, S. (ed) (1987). *Cancer incidence in five continents*, Vol. V. IARC Scientific Publication No. 88. IARC, Lyon.

Muirhead, E.E. (1980). The renomedullary antihypertensive system and its putative hormone(s). In *Hypertension* (2nd edn) (ed. J. Genest, O. Kuchel, P. Hamet, and M. Cantin), pp. 394–407. McGraw Hill, New York.

Muirhead, E.E., Vanatta, J., and Grollman, A. (1950). Papillary necrosis of the kidney; clinical and experimental correlation. *Journal of the American Medical Association*, **142**, 627–31.

Müller, T. and Kielholz, P. (1957). Erhebungen über Analgetikamißbrauch in der Schweiz. *Schweizerische Aerztezeitung*, 6 Juli 1957.

Munck, A., Lindlar, F., and Masshoff, W. (1970). Die Pigmentierung der Nierenpapillen und der Schleimhaut der ableitenden Harnwege bei der chronischen sklerosierenden interstitiellen Nephritis ('Phenacetinniere'). *Virchows Archiv. A. Pathological Anatomy and Histopathology*, **349**, 323–31.

Munn, E., Lynn, K.L., and Bailey, R.R. (1982). Renal papillary necrosis following regular consumption of non-steroidal anti-inflammatory drugs. *New Zealand Medical Journal*, **95**, 213–4.

Murasaki, G., Greenfield, R.E., and Cohen, S.M. (1982). Alterations in the rat kidney associated with sodium saccharin feeding. *Toxicology Letters*, **12**, 251–8.

Murphy, D.M., Zincke, H., and Furlow, W.L. (1981). Management of high grade transitional cell cancers of the upper urinary tract. *Journal of Urology*, **125**, 25–9.

Murray, R.M. (1972). Analgesic nephropathy: removal of phenacetin from proprietary analgesics. *British Medical Journal*, **4**, 131–2.

Murray, R.M. (1973*a*). The origins of analgesic nephropathy. *British Journal of Psychiatry*, **123**, 99–106.

Murray, R.M. (1973*b*). Dependence on analgesics in analgesic nephropathy. *British Journal of Addiction*, **68**, 265–72.

Murray, R.M. (1978). Genesis of analgesic nephropathy in the United Kingdom. *Kidney International*, **13**, 50–7.

Murray, M.D. and Brater, D.C. (1990). Adverse effects of nonsteroidal anti-inflammatory drugs on renal function. *Annals of Internal Medicine*, **112**, 559–60.

Murray, T. and Goldberg, M. (1975). Chronic interstitial nephritis: etiologic factors. *Annals of Internal Medicine*, **82**, 453–9.

Murray, T.G. and Goldberg, M. (1978). Analgesic-associated nephropathy in the U.S.A.: epidemiologic, clinical and pathogenetic features. *Kidney International*, **13**, 64–71.

Murray, G., Wylie, R.G., Hill, G.S., Ramsden, P.W., and Heptinstall, R.H. (1972). Experimental papillary necrosis of the kidney. I. Morphologic and functional data. *American Journal of Pathology*, **67**, 285–302.

Murray, R.M., Lawson, D.H., and Linton, A.L. (1971*a*). Analgesic nephropathy: clinical syndrome and prognosis. *British Medical Journal*, **1**, 479–82.

Murray, R.M., Greene, J.G., and Adams, J.H. (1971*b*). Analgesic abuse and dementia, *Lancet*, **2**, 242–5.

Murray, T.G., Stolley, P.D., Anthony, J.C., Schinnar, R., Hepler-Smith, E., and Jeffreys, J.L. (1983). Epidemiologic study of regular analgesic use and end-stage renal disease. *Archives of Internal Medicine*, **143**, 1687–93.

Murray, M.D., Brater, D.C., Tierney, W.M., Hui, S.L., and McDonald, C.J. (1990). Ibuprofen-associated renal impairment in a large general internal medicine practice. *American Journal of Medical Sciences*, **299**, 222–9.

Mustonen, J., Pasternack, A., Helin, H., Pystynen, S., and Tuominen, T. (1984). Renal biopsy in acute renal failure. *American Journal of Nephrology*, **4**, 27–31.

Nakanishi, K., Fukushima, S., Shibata, M., Shirai, T., Ogiso, T., and Ito, N. (1978). Effect of phenacetin and caffeine on the urinary bladder of rats treated with *N*-butyl-*N*-(4-hydroxybutyl)nitrosamine. *Japanese Journal of Cancer Research (Gann)*, **69**, 395–400.

Nakanishi, K., Kurata, Y., Oshima, M., Fukushima, S., and Ito, N. (1982). Carcinogenicity of phenacetin: long-term feeding study in $B6C3F_1$ mice. *International Journal of Cancer*, **29**, 439–44.

Nanra, R.S. (1976*a*). Pathology, aetiology and pathogenesis of analgesic nephropathy. *Australian and New Zealand Journal of Medicine*, **6** (Suppl. 1), 33–7.

Nanra, R.S. (1976*b*). Analgesic nephropathy. *Medical Journal of Australia*, **1**, 745–8.

Nanra, R.S. (1980). Clinical and pathological aspects of analgesic nephropathy. *British Journal of Clinical Pharmacology*, **10** (Suppl. 2), 359–68S.

Nanra, R.S. (1983). Renal effects of antipyretic analgesics. *American Journal of Medicine*, **75** (Suppl. 5A), 70–81.

Nanra, R.S. (1989*a*). Evolution of the analgesic syndrome (AS) following legislation restricting analgesic sales. *Kidney International*, **35**, 752.

Nanra, R.S. (1989*b*). Renal papillary necrosis (RPN) and chronic interstitial nephritis (CIN) with nonsteroidal anti-inflammatory drugs (NSAIDs)—comparison with the analgesic syndrome. *Kidney International*, **35**, 752.

Nanra, R.S. and Kincaid-Smith, P. (1970). Papillary necrosis in rats caused by aspirin and aspirin-containing mixtures. *British Medical Journal*, **3**, 559–61.

Nanra, R.S. and Kincaid-Smith, P. (1972). Chronic effect of analgesics on the kidney. *Progress in Biochemical Pharmacology*, **7**, 285–323.

Nanra, R.S. and Kincaid-Smith, P. (1973*a*). Experimental renal papillary necrosis (RPN) with non-steroid anti-inflammatory analgesics. In *Probleme des phenacetin-abusus* (ed. H. Haschek), pp. 67–88. Egermann, Wien.

Nanra, R.S. and Kincaid-Smith, P. (1973*b*). Experimental and clinical analgesic nephropathy with aspirin. In *Probleme des Phenacetinabusus* (ed. H. Haschek), pp. 89–114. Egermann, Wien.

Nanra, R.S. and Kincaid-Smith, P. (1975). Renal papillary necrosis in rheumatoid arthritis. *Medical Journal of Australia*, **1**, 194–7.

Nanra, R.S. and Kincaid-Smith, P. (1986). Experimental renal effects of analgesics, rat. In *Monographs on the pathology of laboratory animals—urinary system* (ed. T.C. Jones, U. Mohr, and R.D. Hunt), pp. 254–61. Springer, New York.

Nanra, R.S. and Nanra, S.K. (1988). The proteinuria in analgesic nephropathy (AN) is glomerular. *Kidney International*, **33**, 141–2.

Nanra, R.S., Chirawong, P., and Kincaid-Smith, P. (1971). Renal papillary necrosis in rats produced by aspirin, APC and other analgesics. In *Renal infection and renal scarring* (ed. P. Kincaid-Smith and K.F. Fairley), pp. 347–58. Mercedes, Melbourne.

Nanra, R.S., Chirawong, P., and Kincaid-Smith, P. (1973). Medullary ischaemia in experimental analgesic nephropathy—the pathogenesis of renal papillary necrosis. *Australian and New Zealand Journal of Medicine*, **3**, 580–6.

Nanra, R.S., Stuart-Taylor, J., De Leon, A.H., and White, K.H. (1978*a*). Analgesic nephropathy: etiology, clinical syndrome, and clinicopathologic correlations in Australia. *Kidney International*, **13**, 79–92.

Nanra, R.S., Howard, M., and Daniel, V. (1978*b*). Secondary gout in analgesic nephropathy. *Australian and New Zealand Journal of Medicine*, **8**, 237.

Nanra, R.S., Daniel, V., and Howard, M. (1980). Analgesic nephropathy induced by common proprietary mixtures. *Medical Journal of Australia*, **1**, 486–7.

Nanra, R.S., Daniel, V., Howard, M., and Gupta, J.W. (1981*a*). Physiological changes in experimental analgesic nephropathy. In *Proceedings of the VIIIth International Congress of Nephrology*, Athens, p. 187.

Nanra, R.S., Daniel, V., Howard, M., Murugasu, R., and White, K.H. (1981*b*). Uroepithelial hyperplasia and carcinoma in experimental analgesic nephropathy. In *Proceedings of the VIIIth International Congress of Nephrology*, Athens, p. 188.

Näntö, V., Kasanen, A., and Lehtonen, A. (1964). Urinary excretion of amino acids and acid mucopolysaccharides in rats during phenacetin feeding; preliminary report. *Annales Medicinae Experimentalis et Biologiae Fenniae*, **42**, 88–92.

Neilson, E.G. (1989). Pathogenesis and therapy of interstitial nephritis. *Kidney International*, **35**, 1257–70.

Nelson, S.D. (1982). Metabolic activation and drug toxicity. *Journal of Medicinal Chemistry*, **25**, 753–65.

Nelson, S.D., Forte, A.J., Vaishnar, Y., Mitchell, J.R., and Hinson, J.A. (1981*a*). The formation of arylating and alkylating metabolites of phenacetin in hamsters and hamster liver microsomes. *Molecular Pharmacology*, **19**, 140–5.

Nelson, S.D., Dahlin, D.C., Rauckman, E.J., and Rosen, G.M. (1981*b*). Peroxidase-mediated formation of reactive metabolites of acetaminophen. *Molecular Pharmacology*, **20**, 195–9.

Nery, R. (1971). The possible role of *N*-hydroxylation in the biological effects of phenacetin. *Xenobiotica*, **1**, 339–43.

New Zealand Rheumatism Association Study (1974). Aspirin and the kidney. *British Medical Journal*, **1**, 593–6.

Newman, J. and Hicks, R.M. (1981). Surface ultrastructure of the epithelia lining the normal human lower urinary tract. *British Journal of Experimental Pathology*, **52**, 232–51.

Newton, J.F., Kuo, C.H., Gemborys, M.W., Mudge, G.H., and Hook, J.B. (1982). Nephrotoxicity of *p*-aminophenol, a metabolite of acetaminophen, in the Fischer 344 rat. *Toxicology and Applied Pharmacology*, **65**, 336–44.

Newton, J.F., Yoshimoto, M., Bernstein, J., Rush, G.F., and Hook, H.B. (1983*a*). Acetaminophen nephrotoxicity in the rat. I. Strain differences in nephrotoxicity and metabolism. *Toxicology and Applied Pharmacology*, **69**, 291–306.

Newton, J.F., Bailie, M.B., and Hook, J.B. (1983*b*). Acetaminophen nephrotoxicity in the rat. Renal metabolic activation *in vitro*. *Toxicology and Applied Pharmacology*, **70**, 433–44.

Nicholls, A.J., Shortland, J.R., and Brown, C.B. (1985). Mefenamic acid nephropathy—a spectrum of renal lesions. *Proceedings of the European Dialysis and Transplantation Association*, **22**, 991–6.

Nissen, N.I. and Pedersen, J. (1957). Pyelonefritis og fenacetin. *Ugeskrift Laegere*, **119**, 1639–40.

Nitzsche, T. and Bock, K.D. (1970). Verlaufsbeobachtungen bei Kranken mit Nephropathie nach Analgetika-abusus. *Deutsche Medizinische Wochenschrift*, **95**, 927–34.

Nordenfeldt, O. (1972). Death from renal failure in abusers of phenacetin containing drugs. *Acta Medica Scandinavica*, **191**, 11–6.

Nordenfeldt, O. and Ringertz, N. (1961). Phenacetin takers dead with renal failure. 27 Men and 3 women. *Acta Medica Scandinavica*, **170**, 385–402.

Norman, D.J., Illingworth, D.R., Munson, J., and Hosenpud, J. (1988). Myolysis and acute renal failure in a heart-transplant recipient receiving lovastatin. *New England Journal of Medicine*, **318**, 46–7.

O'Donohoe, M.K., Donohoe, J., and Corrigan, T.P. (1990). Acute renal failure of renovascular origin: cure by aortorenal reconstruction after 25 days of anuria. *Nephron*, **56**, 92–3.

Offerman, G. (1979). Bedeutung der Bestimmung von Parathormonpeptiden zur Charakterisierung der renalen Osteopathie. In *Renale Osteopathie* (ed. R.D. Hesch and R. Hehrmann), pp. 59–69. Thieme, Stuttgart.

Ólafsson, Ó., Gudmundsson, K.R., and Brekkan, Á. (1966). Migraine, gastritis and renal papillary necrosis. A syndrome in chronic nonobstructive pyelonephritis. *Acta Medica Scandinavica*, **179**, 121–8.

Oliver, J.A., Sciacca, R.R., Pinto, J., and Cannon, P.J. (1981). Participation of the prostaglandins in the control of renal blood flow during acute reduction of cardiac output in the dog. *Journal of Clinical Investigation*, **67**, 229–37.

Omachi, R.S., Robbie, D.E., Handler, J.S., and Orloff, J. (1974). Effects of ADH and other agents on cyclic AMP accumulation in toad bladder epithelium. *American Journal of Physiology*, **226**, 1152–7.

Onwubalili, J.K. (1983). Oliguric renal failure associated with benoxaprofen. *Nephron*, **35**, 279–80.

Orell, S.R., Nanra, R.S., and Ferguson, N.W. (1979). Renal pelvic carcinoma in the Hunter Valley. *Medical Journal of Australia*, **2**, 524 and 555–7.

Orphali, S.L.J., Shols, G.W., Hagewood, J., Tesluk, H., and Palmer, J.M. (1986). Familial transitional cell carcinoma of renal pelvis and upper ureter. *Urology*, **27**, 394–6.

Paganini-Hill, A., Chao, A., Ross, R.K., and Henderson, B.E. (1989). Aspirin use and chronic diseases: a cohort study of the elderly. *British Medical Journal*, **299**, 1247–50.

Pagniez, D., Gosset, D., Hardouin, P., Noël, C., Delvallez, L., and Dequiedt, P. (1988). Evolution vers la hyalinose segmentaire et focale d'un syndrome néphrotique à lésions glomérulaires minimes chez une patiente traitée par le sulindac. *Néphrologie*, **9**, 90–1.

Palvio, D.H.B., Falk, E., and Andersen, J.C. (1985). Non-epithelial basement membrane thickening in the urinary tract associated with phenacetin abuse. *Virchows Archiv. A. Pathological Anatomy and Histopathology*, **408**, 173–82.

Palvio, D.H.B., Andersen, J.C., and Falk, E. (1987). Transitional cell tumors of the renal pelvis and ureter associated with capillarosclerosis indicating analgesic abuse. *Cancer*, **59**, 972–6.

Papadopoulos, I., Figge, M., Weissbach, L., and Merkel, K.H. (1987). Diagnosis of urothelial tumour by ureterorenoscopy. *European Urology*, **13**, 296–9.

Patmas, M.A., Wilborn, S.L., and Shankel, S.W. (1984). Acute multisystem toxicity associated with the use of nonsteroidal anti-inflammatory drugs. *Archives of Internal Medicine*, **144**, 519–21.

Patrignani, P., Filabozzi, P., and Patrono, C. (1982). Selective cumulative inhibition of platelet thromboxane production by low-dose aspirin in healthy subjects. *Journal of Clinical Investigation*, **69**, 1366–72.

Patrono, C. (1989). Renal prostaglandins: biochemistry and functional significance in man. *Contributions to Nephrology*, **69**, 55–66.

Patrono, C. and Dunn, M.J. (1987). The clinical significance of inhibition of renal prostaglandin synthesis. *Kidney International*, **32**, 1–12.

Patrono, C. and Pierucci, A. (1986). Renal effects of nonsteroidal anti-inflammatory drugs in chronic glomerular disease. *American Journal of Medicine*, **81** (Suppl. 2B), 71–83.

Patrono, C., Ciabattoni, G., Pinca, E., Pugliese, F., Castrucci, G., De Salvo, A. *et al.* (1980). Low-dose aspirin and inhibition of thromboxane B_2 production in healthy subjects. *Thrombosis Research*, **17**, 317–27.

Patrono, C., Ciabattoni, G., Patrignani, P., Pugliese, F., Filabozzi, P., Catella, F. *et al.* (1985*a*). Clinical pharmocology of platelet cyclooxygenase inhibition. *Circulation*, **72**, 1177–84.

Patrono, C., Ciabattoni, G., Remuzzi, G., Gotti, E., Bombardieri, S., Di Munno, O. *et al.* (1985*b*). Functional significance of renal prostacyclin and thromboxane A_2 production in patients with systemic lupus erythematosus. *Journal of Clinical Investigation*, **76**, 1011–8.

Patrono, C., Ciabattoni, G., Filabozzi, P., Catella, F., Forni, L., Segni, M. *et al.*

(1985*c*). Drugs, prostaglandins, and renal function. *Advances in Prostaglandin, Thromboxane, and Leukotriene Research*, **13**, 131–9.

Patrono, C., Ciabattoni, G., Simonetti, B.M., and Pierucci, A. (1986). Alterations of renal arachidonate metabolism in chronic glomerular disease. *Advances in Prostaglandin, Thromboxane, and Leukotriene Research*, **16**, 199–204.

Pecqueux, J.C., Schwarz, A., Dieckmann, K.P., and Offermann, G. (1990). Cancer incidence in patients on chronic dialysis and in renal transplant recipients. *Urology International*, **45**, 290–2.

Pedersen, A.K., and FitzGerald, G.A. (1984). Dose-related kinetics of aspirin. Presystemic acetylation of platelet cyclooxygenase. *New England Journal of Medicine*, **311**, 1206–11.

Pedersen, A.K. and FitzGerald, G.A. (1985). Cyclooxygenase inhibition, platelet function, and metabolite formation during chronic sulfinpyrazone dosing. *Clinical Pharmacology and Therapeutics*, **37**, 36–42.

Peters, G., Baechtold-Fowler, N., Bonjour, J.P., Chométy-Diézi, F., Filloux, B., Guidoux, R. *et al.* (1972). General and renal toxicity of phenacetin, paracetamol and some anti-mitotic agents in the rat. *Archiv für Toxikologie*, **28**, 225–69.

Petrulis, A.S., Aikawa, M., and Dunn, M.J. (1981). Prostaglandin and thromboxane synthesis by rat glomerular epithelial cells. *Kidney International*, **20**, 469–74.

Phillips, B.M., Hartnagel, R.E., Leeling, J.L., and Gurtoo, H.L. (1976). Does aspirin play a role in analgesic nephropathy? *Australian and New Zealand Journal of Medicine*, **6** (Suppl. 1), 48–53.

Pierides, A.M., Alvarez-Ude, F., Kerr, D.N.S., and Skillen, A.W. (1975). Clofibrate-induced muscle damage in patients with chronic renal failure. *Lancet*, **2**, 1279–82.

Pillans, P. and Hall, C. (1985). Paracetamol-induced acute renal failure in the absence of severe liver damage. *South African Medical Journal*, **67**, 791–2.

Piper, J.M., Tonascia, J., and Matanoski, G.M. (1985). Heavy phenacetin use and bladder cancer in women aged 20 to 49 years. *New England Journal of Medicine*, **313**, 292–5.

Piper, J.M., Matanoski, G.M., and Tonascia, J. (1986). Bladder cancer in young women. *American Journal of Epidemiology*, **123**, 1033–42.

Pirani, C.L., Valeri, A., D'Agati, V., and Appel, G.B. (1987). Renal toxicity of nonsteroidal anti-inflammatory drugs. *Contributions to Nephrology*, **55**, 159–75.

Pirson, Y. and van Ypersele de Strihou, C. (1986). Renal side effects of nonsteroidal anti-inflammatory drugs: clinical relevance. *American Journal of Kidney Diseases*, **8**, 338–44.

Pletscher, A., Studer, A., and Miescher, P. (1958). Experimentelle Untersuchungen über Erythrocyten- und Organveränderungen durch *N*-acetyl-*p*-aminophenol und Phenacetin. *Schweizerische Medizinische Wochenschrift*, **88**, 1214–6.

Pommer, W., Offerman, G., Schultze, G., Krause, P.H., and Molzahn, M. (1983). Akute interstitielle Nephritis durch Medikamente. *Deutsche Medizinische Wochenschrift*, **108**, 783–8.

Pommer, W., Glaeske, G., and Molzahn, M. (1986). The analgesic problem in the Federal Republic of Germany: analgesic consumption, frequency of analgesic nephropathy and regional differences. *Clinical Nephrology*, **26**, 273–8.

Pommer, W., Bronder, E., Greiser, E., Helmert, U., Jesdinsky, H.J., Klimpel, A. *et al.* (1989). Regular analgesic intake and the risk of end-stage renal failure. *American Journal of Nephrology*, 9, 403–12.

Porpáczy, P. (1979). Ursachen und Folgen langjähriger Einnahme phenacetinhaltiger Analgetika aus der Sicht des Urologen. *Wiener Klinische Wochenschrift*, **91** (Suppl. 104), 1–17.

Porpáczy, P. and Schmidt, W. (1973). Mehrjährige Verlaufskontrolle bei urologischen Patienten mit Phenacetinabusus. In *Probleme des Phenacetinabusus* (ed. H. Haschek), pp. 185–9. Egermann, Wien.

Porpáczy, P. and Schramek, P. (1981). Analgesic nephropathy and phenacetin-induced transitional cell carcinoma—analysis of 300 patients with long-term consumption of phenacetin-containing drugs. *European Urology*, **7**, 349–54.

Potter, W.Z., Davis, D.C., Mitchell, J.R., Jollow, D.J., Gillette, J.R., and Brodie, B.B. (1973). Acetaminophen-induced hepatic necrosis. III. Cytochrome P-450-mediated covalent binding *in vivo*. *Journal of Pharmacology and Experimental Therapeutics*, **187**, 203–10.

Poynter, J.D. and Hare, W.S.C. (1974). Necrosis *in situ*: a form of renal papillary necrosis seen in analgesic nephropathy. *Radiology*, **111**, 69–76.

Prát, V. (1989). Einige Angaben zur analgetischen Nephropathie in der Tschechoslowakei. *Zeitschrift für Urologie und Nephrologie*, **82** (Suppl. 1), 148–9.

Precht, K., Teige, J., and Brinbaum, M. (1989). Analgetika-verbrauch in Berlin-DDR und in ausgewählten Bezirken der DDR. *Zeitschrift für Urologie und Nephrologie*, **82** (Suppl. 1), 152–7.

Prescott, L.F. (1965). Effects of acetylsalicylic acid, phenacetin, paracetamol, and caffeine on renal tubular epithelium. *Lancet*, **2**, 91–6.

Prescott, L.F. (1966). Analgesic abuse and renal disease in North-East Scotland. *Lancet*, **2**, 1143–5.

Prescott, L.F. (1980). Kinetics and metabolism of paracetamol and phenacetin. *British Journal of Clinical Pharmacology*, **10** (Suppl. 2), 291–8S.

Prescott, L.F. (1982*a*). Analgesic nephropathy: a reassessment of the role of phenacetin and other analgesics. *Drugs*, **23**, 75–149.

Prescott, L.F. (1982*b*). Assessment of nephrotoxicity. *British Journal of Clinical Pharmacology*, **13**, 303–11.

Prescott, L.F., Steel, R.F., and Ferrier, W.R. (1970). The effects of particle size on the absorption of phenacetin in man. A correlation between plasma concentration of phenacetin and effects on the central nervous system. *Clinical Pharmacology and Therapeutics*, **11**, 496–504.

Prescott, L.F., Sutherland, G.R., Park, J., and Smith, I.J. (1976). Cysteamine, methionine and penicillamine in the treatment of paracetamol poisoning. *Lancet*, **1**, 109–13.

Proudfoot, A.T. and Wright, N. (1990). Acute paracetamol poisoning. *British Medical Journal*, **3**, 557–8.

Pugliese, F. and Ciabattoni, G. (1982). Investigation of arachidonic acid metabolism by radioimmunosassay. In *Prostaglandins and the kidney* (ed. M.J. Dunn, C. Patrono, and G.A. Giuotti), pp. 83–98. Plenum, New York.

Pugliese, F. and Ciabattoni, G. (1984). The role of prostaglandins in the control of renal function: renal effects of non steroidal anti-inflammatory drugs. *Clinical and Experimental Rheumatology*, **2**, 345–52.

Pugliese, F. and Ciabattoni, G. (1987). Differential inhibition of the synthesis of prostaglandins and thromboxane in human tissues by non-steroidal anti-inflammatory drugs commonly used in therapy. *British Journal of Clinical Practice*, **41** (Suppl. 49), 41–9.

Pugliese, F., Sato, M., Williams, S., Aikawa, M., Hassid, A., and Dunn, M. (1983). Rabbit and rat renal papillary collecting tubule cells in culture: the interactions of arginine vasopressin, prostaglandins and cyclic AMP. *Advances in Prostaglandin, Thromboxane, and Leukotriene Research*, **11**, 517–23.

Purnell, J. and Burry, A.F. (1967). Analgesic consumption in a country town. *Medical Journal of Australia*, **2**, 389–91.

Puvaneswary, M. and Segasothy, M. (1988). Analgesic nephropathy: ultrasonic features. *Australian Radiology*, **32**, 247–50.

Quintanilla, A. and Delgado, C. (1966). Effect of phenacetin on the GFR, PAH clearance and the reabsorption of Na, K and PO_4 in the dog kidney. *Proceedings of the Third International Pharmacology Congress*, p. 134. Sao Paolo.

Quintanilla, A. and Kessler, R.H. (1973). Direct effects of salicylate on renal function in the dog. *Journal of Clinical Investigation*, **52**, 3143–53.

Raab, W.P. (1969). Acetylsalicylic acid and the kidneys. *Helvetica Medica Acta*, **34**, 498–502.

Raab, W.P. (1970). Renal enzyme excretion following ingestion of salicylates, increased by caffeine. *Helvetica Medica Acta*, **35**, 290–5.

Raaflaub, J. and Dubach, U.C. (1969). Dose-dependent change in the pattern of phenacetin metabolism in man and its possible significance in analgesic nephropathy. *Klinische Wochenschrift*, **47**, 1286–7.

Raaflaub, J., and Dubach, U.C. (1975). A study on the pharmacokinetics of phenacetin in man. *European Journal of Clinical Pharmacology*, **8**, 24.

Raftery, M.J., Forman, P., Farrington, K. Sweny, P., and Moorhead, J.F. (1985). Fenclofenac induced interstitial nephritis confirmed by inadvertent rechallenge. *British Medical Journal*, **290**, 1178–9.

Rahman, M.A., Stork, J.E., and Dunn, M.J. (1987). The roles of eicosanoids in experimental glomerulonephritis. *Kidney International*, **22** (Suppl. 32), 40–8.

Ramsay, A.G. and White, D.F. (1965). Phenacetin nephropathy. *Canadian Medical Association Journal*, **92**, 55–9.

Ramsay, A.G., D'Agati, V., Dietz, P.A., Svahn, D.A., and Pirani, C.L. (1983). Renal functional recovery 47 days after renal artery occlusion. *American Journal of Nephrology*, **3**, 325–8.

Randerath, E. (1958). Kritik an dem Begriff 'Phenacetinnephritis'. In *Phenacetinabusus und Nierenschädigung* (ed. H. Sarre, A. Moench, and R. Kluthe), pp. 20–5, Thieme, Stuttgart.

Rathert, P., Melchior, H., and Lutzeyer, W. (1975). Phenacetin: a carcinogen for the urinary tract? *Journal of Urology*, **113**, 653–7.

Ratner, S.J. (1982). Zomepirac and renal failure. *Annals of Internal Medicine*, **96**, 793.

Raymond, K.H. and Lifschitz, M.D. (1986). Effect of prostaglandins on renal salt and water excretion. *American Journal of Medicine*, **80** (Suppl. 1A), 22–33.

Reeves, W.B., Foley, R.J., and Weinman, E.J. (1984). Renal dysfunction from non-steroidal anti-inflammatory drugs. *Archives of Internal Medicine*, **144**, 1943–4.

Reeves, W.B., Foley, R.J., and Weinman E.J. (1985). Nephrotoxicity from nonsteroidal anti-inflammatory drugs. *Southern Medical Journal*, **78**, 318–22.

Regester, R.F. (1980). Nephrotic syndrome and renal failure associated with use of nonsteroidal anti-inflammatory drugs. *Journal of the Tennessee Medical Association*, **73**, 709–11.

Reimann, I.W., Golbs, E., Fischer, C., and Frölich, J.C. (1985). Influence of intravenous acetylsalicylic acid and sodium salicylate on human renal function and lithium clearance. *European Journal of Clinical Pharmacology*, **29**, 435–41.

Reubi, M.F. (1954). Le diagnostique de la pyélonéphrite chronique. *Journal d'Urologie Medicale et Chirurgicale*, **60**, 816–30.

Reubi, F. (1958). Zur Frage der sogenannten 'Saridonnephritis'. In *Phenacetinabusus und Nierenschädigung* (ed. H. Sarre, A. Moench, and R. Kluthe), pp. 95–9. Thieme, Stuttgart.

Reynolds, T.B. and Edmondson, H.A. (1963). Chronic renal disease and heavy use of analgesics. *Journal of the American Medical Association*, **184**, 435–44.

Rice, J.M. and Frith, C.H. (1981). The nature of organ specificity in chemical carcinogenesis. *Basic Life Sciences*, **24**, 1–21.

Riegger, G.A.J., Elsner, D., and Kromer, E.P. (1989). Circulatory and renal control by prostaglandins and renin in low cardiac output in dogs. *American Journal of Physiology*, **256**, H1079–86.

Roberts, D.G., Gerber, J.G., Barnes, J.S., Zerbe, G.O., and Nies, A.S. (1985). Sulindac is not renal sparing in man. *Clinical Pharmacology and Therapeutics*, **38**, 258–65.

Robertson, C.E., Ford, M.J., Van Someren, V., Dlugolecka, M., and Prescott, L.F. (1980). Mefenamic acid nephropathy. *Lancet*, **2**, 232–3.

Robinson, M.J., Nichols, A., and Taitz, L. (1967). Nephrotoxic effect of acute sodium salicylate intoxication in the rat. *Archives of Pathology*, **84**, 224–6.

Robinson, J., Malleson, P., Lirenman, D., and Carter, J. (1990). Nephrotic syndrome associated with nonsteroidal anti-inflammatory drug use in two children, *Pediatrics*, **85**, 844–7.

Roman, R.J. and Lechene, C. (1981). Prostaglandin E_2 and F_{2a} reduces urea reabsorption from the rat collecting duct. *American Journal of Physiology*, **241**, F53–60.

Roman, R.J. and Lianos, E. (1990). Influence of prostaglandins on papillary blood flow and pressure-natriuretic response. *Hypertension*, **15**, 29–35.

Rosenmann, E., Dishon, T., and Boss, J.H. (1972). Urinary excretion of kidney antigens in rats consuming analgesics. *Pathologia Europaea*, **7**, 161–6.

Rosner, I. (1976). Experimental analgesic nephropathy. *CRC Critical Reviews in Toxicology*, **4**, 331–52.

Ross, N.S. and Hoppel, C.L. (1987). Partial muscle carnitine palmitoyl transferase-A deficiency. Rhabdomyolysis associated with transiently decreased muscle carnitine content after ibuprofen therapy. *Journal of the American Medical Association*, **257**, 62–5.

Ross, D., Larsson, R., Andersson, B., Nilsson, U., Lindquist, T., Lindeke, B., and Moldéus, P. (1985). The oxidation of *p*-phenetidine by horseradish peroxidase and prostaglandin synthetase and the fate of glutathione during such oxidations. *Biochemical Pharmacology*, **34**, 343–51.

Ross, R.K., Paganini-Hill, A., Landolph, J., Gerkins, V., and Henderson, B.E. (1989). Analgesics, cigarette smoking, and other risk factors for cancer of the renal pelvis and ureter. *Cancer Research*, **49**, 1045–8.

Rossi, E., Ferraccioli, G.F., Cavalieri, F., Menta, R., Dall'Aglio, P.P., and Migone, L. (1985). Diclofenac-associated acute renal failure. Report of 2 cases. *Nephron*, **40**, 491–3.

Rossi, E., Menta, R., and Cambi, V. (1988). Partially reversible chronic renal failure due to long-term use of non-steroidal antiinflammatory drugs. *Nephrology, Dialysis, Transplantation*, **3**, 469–70.

Roth, G.J. and Majerus, P.W. (1975). The mechanism of the effect of aspirin on human platelets: I. Acetylation of a particulate fraction protein. *Journal of Clinical Investigation*, **56**, 624–32.

Roth, G.J. and Siok, C.J. (1978). Acetylation of the NH_2-terminal serine of prostaglandin synthetase by aspirin. *Journal of Biology and Chemistry*, **253**, 3782–4.

Roth, J.L.A., Valdes-Dapena, A., Piese, P., and Buchman, E. (1963). Topical action of salicylates in gastrointestinal erosion and hemorrhage. *Gastroenterology*, **44**, 146–58.

Roth, G.J., Stanford, N.S., and Majerus, P.W. (1975). Acetylation of prostaglandin synthase by aspirin. *Proceedings of the National Academy of Science of the United States of America*, **72**, 3073–6.

Rowland, M.P., Riegelman, S. Harris, P.A., and Sholfkoff, S.D. (1972). Absorption kinetics of aspirin in man following oral administration of an aqueous solution. *Journal of Pharmaceutical Science*, **61**, 379–85.

Rudolf, A.M. (1981). The effects of nonsteroidal antiinflammatory compounds on fetal circulation and pulmonary function. *Obstetrics and Gynecology*, **58**, 63–7S.

Rumack, B.H. (1983). Acetaminophen overdose. *American Journal of Medicine*, **75** (Suppl. 5A), 104–12.

Rumack, B.H., Peterson, R.C., Koch, G.G., and Amara, I.A. (1981*a*). Acetaminophen overdose. 662 cases with evaluation of oral acetylcysteine treatment. *Archives of Internal Medicine*, **141**, 380–5.

Rumack, C.M., Guggenheim, M.A., Rumack, B.H., Peterson, R.G., Johnson, M.L., and Braithwaite, W.R. (1981*b*). Neonatal intracranial hemorrhage and maternal use of aspirin. *Obstetrics and Gynecology*, **58**, 52–6S.

Rumpf, K.W., Albers, R., and Scheler, F. (1976). Clofibrate-induced myopathy syndrome. *Lancet*, **1**, 249.

Rupp, D.J., Seaton, R.D., and Wiegman, T.B. (1983). Acute polyuric renal failure after aspirin intoxication. *Archives of Internal Medicine*, **143**, 1237–8.

Rush, G.F., Smith, J.H., Newton, J.F., and Hook, J.B. (1984). Chemically induced nephrotoxicity: role of metabolic activation. *CRC Critical Reviews in Toxicology*, **13**, 99–160.

Russ, G.R., Horgan, B.A., Mathew, T.H., Brown, H., Mills, L., and Kirkland, J.A. (1982). Beta 2-microglobulin excretion and urinary cytology in analgesic nephropathy. *Clinical Nephrology*, **18**, 148–53.

Sabatini, S., Koppera, S., Manaligod, J., Arruda, J.A.L., and Kurtzman, N.A. (1983). Role of urinary concentrating ability in the generation of toxic papillary necrosis. *Kidney International*, **23**, 705–10.

Saker, B.M. and Kincaid-Smith, P. (1969). Papillary necrosis in experimental analgesic nephropathy. *British Medical Journal*, **1**, 161–2.

Salazar, F.J., Bolterman, R., Fiksen-Olsen, M.J., Quesada, T., and Romero, J.C. (1988). Role of prostaglandins in mediating the renal effects of atrial natriuretic factor. *Hypertension*, **12**, 274–8.

Salvati, P., Ferti, C., Ferrario, R.G., Lamberti, E., Duzzi, L., Bianchi, G. *et al.* (1990). Role of enhanced glomerular synthesis of thromboxane A_2 in progressive kidney disease. *Kidney International*, **38**, 447–58.

Salvetti, A., Pedrinelli, R., Magagna, A., and Ugenti, P. (1982). Differential effects of selective and non-selective prostaglandin-synthesis inhibition on the pharmocological responses to captopril in patients with essential hypertension. *Clinical Science*, **63**, 261–3S.

Sandler, D.P. and Weinberg, C.R. (1989). Analgesic use and chronic renal disease. *New England Journal of Medicine*, **321**, 1126–7.

Sandler, D.P., Smith, J.C., Weinberg, C.R., Buckalew, V.M., Dennis, V.W., Blythe, W.B., and Burgess, W.P. (1989). Analgesic use and chronic renal disease. *New England Journal of Medicine*, **320**, 1238–43.

Sandler, D.P., Burr, F.R., and Weinberg, C.R. (1991). Nonsteroidal anti-inflammatory drugs and the risk for chronic renal disease *Annals of Internal Medicine*, **115**, 165–72.

Sanerkin, N.G. (1966). Chronic phenacetin nephropathy. (With particular reference to the relationship between renal papillary necrosis and 'chronic interstitial nephritis'). *British Journal of Urology*, **38**, 361–70.

Sarma, P.S.A. (1989). Fatal acute renal failure after piroxicam. *Clinical Nephrology*, **31**, 54.

Sarnacki, C.T., McCormack, L.J., Kiser, W.S., Hazard, J.B., McLaughlin, T.C., and Belovich, D.M. (1971). Urinary cytology and the clinical diagnosis of urinary tract malignancy: a clinicopathological study of 1,400 patients. *Journal of Urology*, **106**, 761–4.

Sattler, T.A., Dimitrov, T., and Hall, P.W. (1977). Relation between endemic (Balkan) nephropathy and urinary-tract tumours. *Lancet*, **1**, 278–80.

Schabert, P., Nagel, R., and Leistenschneider, W. (1973). Zur Frage der Koincidenz von Tumoren der oberen Harnwege mit chronischer Einnahme analgetische Substanzen. In *Probleme des Phenacetinabusus* (ed. H. Haschek), pp. 257–61. Egermann, Wien.

Scharschmidt, L.A. and Dunn, M.J. (1983). Prostaglandin synthesis by rat glomerular mesangial cells in culture. Effects of angiotension II and arginine vasopressin. *Journal of Clinical Investigation*, **71**, 1756–64.

Scharschmidt, L.A., Lianos, E., and Dunn, M.J. (1983). Arachidonate metabolites and the control of glomerular function. *Federation Proceedings*, **42**, 3058–63.

Scharschmidt, L., Simonson, M., and Dunn, M.J. (1986). Glomerular prostaglandins, angiotensin II, and nonsteroidal anti-inflammatory drugs. *American Journal of Medicine*, **81** (Suppl. 2B), 30–42.

Schaub, F., Bühlmann, A., and Maier, C. (1953). Nebenerscheinungen und Folgen des chronischen Phenacetinabusus. *Schweizerische Medizinische Wochenschrift*, **83**, 626–9.

Scheidegger, S. (1958). Pathologisch-anatomischer Beitrag zur Frage der chronischen interstitiellen Nephritis im Anschluss an Abusus von phenacetinhaltigen Analgetika. *Bulletin der Schweizerischen Akademie der Medizinischen Wissenschaften*, **14**, 139–53.

Schlondorff, D. (1986). Renal prostaglandin synthesis. Sites of production and specific actions of prostaglandins. *American Journal of Medicine*, **81** (Suppl. 2B), 1–11.

Schlondorff, D. and Ardaillou, R. (1986). Prostaglandins and other arachidonic acid metabolites in the kidney. *Kidney International*, **29**, 108–19.

Schlondorff, D., Carvounis, C.P., Jacoby, M., Satriano, J.A., and Levine, S.D. (1981). Multiple sites for interaction of prostaglandin and vasopressin in toad urinary bladder. *American Journal of Physiology*, **241**, F625–31.

Schlondorff, D., Satriano, J.A., and Schwartz, G.J. (1985). Synthesis of prostaglandin E_2 in different segments of isolated collecting tubules from adult and neonatal rabbits. *American Journal of Physiology*, **248**, F134–44.

Schmidt, L. (1958). Hinweis auf Kombinationspräparate. In *Phenacetinabusus und Nierenschädigung* (ed. H. Staub), p. 27. Thieme, Stuttgart.

Schmidt, M., Bürgin, M., and Gloor, F. (1983). *Fokal-segmentale Glomerulose bei Analgetika-nephropathie (morphologisch-klinische Korrelationen)*. Dissertation, Universität Basel.

Schmitz, P.G., Kasiske, B.L., O'Donnell, M.P., and Keane, W.F. (1989). Lipids and progressive renal injury. *Seminars in Nephrology*, **9**, 354–69.

Schneider, P.D. (1986). Nonsteroidal anti-inflammatory drugs and acute cortical necrosis. *Annals of Internal Medicine*, **105**, 303–4.

Schnermann, J., and Briggs, J.P. (1981). Participation of renal cortical prostaglandins in the regulation of glomerular filtration rate. *Kidney International*, **19**, 802–15.

Schnitzer, B. and Smith, E.B. (1966). Effects of the metabolites of phenacetin on the rat. *Archives of Pathology*, **81**, 264–7.

Schnitzer, B., Smith, E.B., and Golden, A. (1965). The effects of phenacetin and its contaminant on the kidney of the rat. *American Journal of Pathology*, **46**, 917–27.

Schoen, R.T. and Vender, R.J. (1989). Mechanisms of nonsteroidal anti-inflammatory drug-induced gastric damage. *American Journal of Medicine*, **86**, 449–58.

Schor, N., Ichikawa, I., and Brenner, B.M. (1981). Mechanisms of action of various hormones and vasoactive substances on glomerular ultrafiltration in the rat. *Kidney International*, **20**, 442–51.

Schourup, K. (1957). Necrosis of the renal papillae. Post mortem series. *Acta Pathologica et Microbiologica Scandinavica*, **41**, 462–78.

Schourup, K., Ørskov, I., Ørskov, R., and Bartels, E.D. (1963). Phenacetin as the cause of kidney damage in rabbits. *Danish Medical Bulletin*, **10**, 85–9.

Schreiner, G.E., McAnally, J.R., and Winchester, J.F. (1981). Clinical analgesic nephropathy. *Archives of Internal Medicine*, **141**, 349–57.

Schwartzman, M. and D'Agati, V. (1987). Spontaneous relapse of naproxen-related nephrotic syndrome. *American Journal of Medicine*, **82**, 329–32.

Schwarz, A. (1987). Analgesic-associated nephropathy. *Klinische Wochenschrift*, **65**, 1–16.

Schwarz, A. and Offermann, G. (1989). Vorteile und Risiken der Nierentransplantation von verwandten Spendern. *Klinische Wochenschrift*, **67**, 929–35.

Schwarz, A., Faber, U., Borner, K., Keller, F., Offermann, G., and Molzahn, M. (1984). Reliability of drug history in analgesic users. *Lancet*, **2**, 1163–4.

Schwarz, A., Pommer, W., Keller, F., Kühn-Freitag, G., Offermann, G., and Molzahn, M. (1985*a*). Morbidity of patients with analgesic-associated nephropathy and end-stage renal failure. *Proceedings of the European Dialysis and Transplant Association*, **21**, 311–6.

Schwarz, A., Pommer, W., Kühn-Freitag, G., Keller, F., Molzahn, M., and Offermann, G. (1985*b*). Merkmale der terminalen Analgetika-nephropathie. *Schweizerische Medizinische Wochenschrift*, **115**, 790–5.

Schwarz, A., Kraft, D., Keller, F., Gawlik, D., and Offermann, G. (1987). Aluminium load in patients with analgesic nephropathy. *Mineral and Electrolyte Metabolism*, **13**, 141–6.

Schwarz, A., Faber, U., Glaeske, G., Keller, F., Offermann, G., Pommer, W., and Molzahn, M. (1986). Analgesic nephropathy in West Germany. *Lancet*, **1**, 210.

Schwarz, A., Keller, F., Kunzendorf, U., Kühn-Freitag, G., Heinemeyer, G., Pommer, W., and Offermann, G. (1988*a*). Characteristics and clinical course of hemodialysis patients with analgesic-associated nephropathy. *Clinical Nephrology*, **29**, 299–306.

Schwarz, A., Krause, P.H., Keller, F., Offermann, G., and Mihatsch, M.J. (1988*b*). Granulomatous interstitial nephritis after nonsteroidal anti-inflammatory drugs. *American Journal of Nephrology*, **8**, 410–6.

Schwarz, A., Kunzendorf, U., Keller, F., and Offerman, G. (1989). Progression of renal failure in analgesic-associated nephropathy. *Nephron*, **53**, 244–9.

Schweingruber, R. (1955). Probleme der chronischen Vergiftung mit kombinierten Phenacetinpräparaten. *Schweizerische Medizinische Wochenschrift*, **85**, 1162–7.

Sedor, J.R., Davidson, E.W., and Dunn, M.J. (1986). Effects of non-steroidal anti-inflammatory drugs in healthy subjects. *American Journal of Medicine*, **81** (Suppl. 2B), 58–70.

Seedat, Y.K., Naicker, S., Rawat, R., and Parsoo, I. (1984). Racial differences in the causes of end-stage renal failure in Natal. *South African Medical Journal*, **65**, 956–8.

Seeff, L.B. (1981). Drug-induced chronic liver disease, with emphasis on chronic active hepatitis. *Seminars in Liver Disease*, **1**, 104–15.

Seeff, L.B., Cuccherini, B.A., Zimmerman, H.J., Adler, E., and Benjamin, S.B. (1986). Acetaminophen hepatotoxicity in alcoholics. A therapeutic misadventure. *Annals of Internal Medicine*, **104**, 399–404.

Segasothy, M., Kong Chiew Tong, B., Kamal, A., Murad, Z., and Suleiman, A.B. (1984). Analgesic nephropathy associated with paracetamol. *Australian and New Zealand Journal of Medicine*, **14**, 23–6.

Segasothy, M., Suleiman, A.B., Puvaneswary, M., and Rohana, A. (1988). Paracetamol: a cause for analgesic nephropathy and end-stage renal disease. *Nephron*, **50**, 50–4.

Senate Standing Committee on Social Welfare. (1977). Analgesics. In *Drug problems in Australia—an intoxicated society?*, pp. 107–26. Australian Government, Canberra.

Sennesael, J., Van Den Houte, K., and Verbeelen, D. (1986). Reversible membranous glomerulonephritis associated with ketoprofen. *Clinical Nephrology*, **26**, 213–5.

Shah, G.M., Muhalwas, K.K., and Winer, R.L. (1981). Renal papillary necrosis due to ibuprofen. *Arthritis and Rheumatism* **24**, 1208–10.

Shamsuddin, M.R., Mason, R.G., Ritchey, J.M., Honig, G.R., and Klotz, I.M. (1974). Site of acetylation of sickle cell hemoglobin by aspirin. *Proceedings of the National Academy of Sciences of the United States of America*, **12**, 4693–7.

Shapiro, S., Siskind, V., Monson, R.R., Heinonen, O.P., Kaufman, D.W., and Slone, D. (1976). Perinatal mortality and birth-weight in relation to aspirin taken during pregnancy. *Lancet*, **1**, 1375–6.

Sheehan, H.L. and Davis, J.C. (1959*a*). Experimental hydronephrosis. *Archives of Pathology*, **68**, 185–225.

Sheehan, H.L. and Davis, J.C. (1959*b*). Renal ischæmia and good reflow. *Journal of Pathology and Bacteriology*, **78**, 351–77.

Shelley, J.H. (1967). Phenacetin, through the looking glass. *Clinical Pharmacology and Therapeutics*, **8**, 427–71.

Shelley, J.H. (1978). Pharmacological mechanisms of analgesic nephropathy. *Kidney International*, **13**, 15–26.

Sherwood, T., Swales, J.D., and Tange, J.D. (1971). Experimental renal papillary necrosis: progressive changes on intravenous urography. *Investigative Radiology*, **6**, 239–44.

Shimamura, T. and Bonk, K. (1976). Repair of the injured renal papillary tissue in rats. *Investigative Urology*, **14**, 111–14.

Shimamura, T. and Trojanowski, S. (1976). Effects of repeated deprivation of drinking water on the structure of renal medulla in rats. *American Journal of Pathology*, **84**, 87–92.

Shimamura, T., Aogaichi, M., and Liu, C.Y. (1974). Drug-induced renal medullary necrosis. II. Mode of calcification in the kidney. *Experimental and Molecular Pathology*, **20**, 109–14.

Shpilberg, O., Douer, D., Ehrenfeld, M., Engelberg, S., and Ramot, B. (1990). Naproxen-associated fatal acute renal failure in multiple myeloma. *Nephron*, **55**, 448–9.

Simonson, M.S. and Dunn, M.J. (1990). Endothelin-1 stimulates contraction of rat glomerular mesangial cells and potentiates ß adrenergic-mediated cyclic adenosine monophosphate accumulation. *Journal of Clinical Investigation*, **85**, 790–7.

Smith, P.K. (1958). *Acetophenetidin: a critical bibliographic review*. Interscience, New York.

Smith, G.E. and Griffiths, L.A. (1976). Comparative metabolic studies of phenacetin and structurally related compounds in the rat. *Xenobiotica*, **6**, 217–36.

Smith, P.K., Gleason, H.L., Stoll, C.G., and Ogorzalek, S. (1946). Studies on the pharmacology of salicylates. *Journal of Pharmacology and Experimental Therapeutics*, **87**, 237–55.

Smith, J.M., Roberts, W.O., Hall, S.M., White, T.A., and Gilbertson, A.A. (1978).

Late treatment of paracetamol poisoning with mercaptamine. *British Medical Journal*, **1**, 331–3.
Smith, A.D., Orihuela, E., and Crowley, A.R. (1987). Percutaneous management of renal pelvic tumors; a treatment option in selected cases. *Journal of Urology*, **137**, 852–6.
Sneader, W. (1985). *Drug discovery: the evolution of modern medicines*. Wiley, Chichester.
Sorensen, A.W.S. (1966). Is the relation between analgesics and renal disease coincidental and not causal? *Nephron*, **3**, 366–76.
Spühler, O. (1953). Probleme der interstitiellen Nephritis. *Schweizerische Medizinische Wochenschrift*, **83**, 145–8.
Spühler, O. and Zollinger, H.U. (1950). Die chronische interstitielle Nephritis. *Helvetica Medica Acta*, **17**, 564–7.
Spühler, O. and Zollinger, H.U. (1953). Die chronische interstitielle Nephritis. *Zeitschrift für Klinische Medizin*, **151**, 1–50.
Sraer, J., Foidart, D., Chansel, P., Mahieu, B., Kouznetzova, R., and Ardaillou, R. (1979). Prostaglandin synthesis by mesangial and epithelial glomerular cultured cells. *FEBS Letters*, **15**, 420–4.
Sraer, J., Ardaillou, N., Sraer, J.D., and Ardaillou, R. (1982). *In vitro* prostaglandin synthesis by human glomeruli and papillae. *Prostaglandins*, **23**, 855–64.
Stachura, I., Jayakumar, S., and Bourke, E. (1983). T and B lymphocyte subsets in fenoprofen nephropathy. *American Journal of Medicine*, **75**, 9–16.
Stacy, D.L., Scott, J.W., and Granger, J.P. (1990). Control of renal function during intrarenal infusion of endothelin. *American Journal of Physiology*, **258**, F1232–6.
Staub, H. (1958). In *Phenacetinabusus und Nierenschädigung* (ed. H. Sarre, A. Moench, and R. Kluthe), pp. 47–9. Thieme, Stuttgart.
Stavanc, I. and Favre, H. (1986). Nephrotic syndrome and acute renal failure associated with aspirin. *British Medical Journal*, **292**, 1050.
Steele, T.W. and Edwards, K.D.G. (1970). Abnormalities of urinary concentrating, acidifying and sodium conserving abilities induced by excess analgesic intake in rats. *Australasian Annals of Medicine*, **19**, 412–3.
Steele, T.W. and Edwards, K.D.G. (1971). Analgesic nephropathy. Changes in various parameters of renal function following cessation of analgesic abuse. *Medical Journal of Australia*, **1**, 181–7.
Steele, T.W., Gyory, A.Z., and Edwards, K.D.G. (1969). Renal function in analgesic nephropathy. *British Medical Journal*, **2**, 213–6.
Steele, T.W., Hung, E.C.Y., and Edwards, K.D.G. (1971). Hypercalcuria and reduced daily excretion of citrate, potassium and hydrogen ions induced by excess intake of analgesics in rats. *Medical Journal of Australia*, **1**, 170–1.
Steffens, J. and Nagel, R. (1988). Tumours of the renal pelvis and ureter. Observations in 170 patients. *British Journal of Urology*, **61**, 277–83.
Sternberg, C.N., Yagoda, A., Scher, H.I., Watson, R.C., Ahmed, T., Weiselberg, L.R. *et al.* (1985). Preliminary results of M-VAC (methotrexate, vinblastine, doxorubicin and cisplatin) for transitional cell carcinoma of the urothelium. *Journal of Urology*, **133**, 403–7.
Stewart, J.H. (1978). Analgesic abuse and renal failure in Australasia. *Kidney International*, **13**, 72–8.

Stewart, J.H. and Gallery, E.D.M. (1976). Analgesic abuse and kidney disease. *Australian and New Zealand Journal of Medicine*, **6**, 498–508.

Stiller, D. and Rauscher, H. (1971). Irreversible preneoplastic defect in alkaline phosphatase in cancerization of transitional epithelium. *Experimental Pathology*, **5**, 255–8.

Stillman, M.T., Davidman, M., and Abraham, P.A. (1982). Fenoprofen associated nephrotic syndrome with renal insufficiency. *Arthritis and Rheumatism*, **25**, S136.

Stokes, J.B. (1981). Integrated actions of renal medullary prostaglandins in the control of water excretion. *American Journal of Physiology*, **240**, F471–80.

Stokes, J.B. (1985). Modulation of vasopressin-induced water permeability of the cortical collecting tubule by endogenous and exogenous prostaglandins. *Mineral Electrolytes and Metabolism*, **11**, 240–8.

Stork, J.E., Rahman, M.A., and Dunn, M.J. (1986). Eicosanoids in experimental and human renal disease. *American Journal of Medicine*, **80** (Suppl. 1A), 34–45.

Studer, A. (1965). Attempts to induce renal lesions in the experimental animal by analgesics. In *Progress in pyelonephritis* (ed. E.H. Kass), pp. 307–311. Davis, Philadelphia.

Studer, A. and Schärer, K. (1965). Langfristige Phenacetinbelastung am Hund mit Berücksichtigung der Leber- und nierenpigmentierung. *Schweizerische Medizinische Wochenschrift*, **95**, 933–41.

Studer, A. and Zbinden, G. (1955). Experimenteller Beitrag zur Frage von Nierenschäden bei Abusus von phenacetinhaltigen Schmerzmitteln. *Experientia*, **11**, 450–1.

Studer, A., Zbinden, G., Schärer, K., and Fust, B. (1958*a*). Tierexperimentelle Untersuchungen zur Frage der interstitiellen Nephritis bei Mißbrauch phenacetinhaltiger Schmerzmittel. *Bulletin der Schweizerischen Akademie der Medizinischen Wissenschaften*, **14**, 154–65.

Studer, A., Zbinden, G., and Fust, B. (1958*b*). Weitere tierexperimentelle Untersuchungen zur Frage Schmerzmittelmißbrauch und interstitiellen Nephritis. *Schweizerische Medizinische Wochenschrift*, **88**, 469–70.

Stummvoll, H.K. and Breitenfellner, P. (1989). Terminale Niereninsuffizienz durch Analgetika-nephropathie Verhältnisse in Österreich. *Zeitschrift für Urologie und Nephrologie*, **82** (Suppl. 1), 158–64.

Stygles, V. and Iuliucci, J. (1981). Structural and functional alterations in the kidney following intake of nonsteroidal anti-inflammatory analgesics. In *Toxicology of the kidney* (ed. J.B. Hook), pp. 151–78. Raven, New York.

Svendsen, U.G., Gerstoft, J., Hansen, T.M., Christensen, P., and Lorenzen, I. (1984). The renal excretion of prostaglandins and changes in plasma renin during treatment with either sulindac or naproxen in patients with rheumatoid arthritis and thiazide treated heart failure. *Journal of Rheumatology*, **11**, 779–82.

Swainson, C.P. and Griffiths, P. (1985). Acute and chronic effects of sulindac on renal function in chronic renal disease. *Clinical Pharmacology and Therapeutics*, **37**, 298–300.

Szafranowa, H. (1970). Wplyw kwasu acetylosalicylowego (ASA) na zaburzona czynność nerek w doświadczalnym uszkodzeniu kanilków nerkowych. *Patologia Polska*, **21**, 609–18.

Takayama, S. and Kuwabara, N. (1982). Long-term study on the effect of caffeine in Wistar rats. *Japanese Journal of Cancer Research (Gann)*, **73**, 365–71.

Tan, S.Y., Shapiro, R., Franco, R., Stockard, H., and Mulrow, P.J. (1979). Indomethacin-induced prostaglandin inhibition with hyperkalemia. A reversible cause of hyporeninemic hypoaldosteronism. *Annals of Internal Medicine*, **90**, 783–5.

Taraba, I. (1989). Analgetika-nephropathie in Ungarn. *Zeitschrift für Urologie und Nephrologie*, **82** (Suppl. 1), 165–7.

Tarloff, J.B., Goldstein, R.S., and Hook, J.B. (1988). Strain differences in acetaminophen nephrotoxicity in rats: role of pharmacokinetics. *Toxicology*, **56**, 167–77.

Taylor, J.S. (1972). Carcinoma of the urinary tract and analgesic abuse. *Medical Journal of Australia*, **1**, 407–9.

Tepavčevic, P., Fellel, D., Glogovčan, N., Cvetkov, N., Budakov, P., Curic, S. *et al.* (1986). Analgetička nefropatija u regionima Vojvodine. *Medicinski Prelged.*, **39**, 421–4.

ter Borg, E.J., de Jong, P.E., Meijer, S., and Kallenberg, C.G. (1989). Renal effects of indomethacin in patients with systemic lupus erythematosus. *Nephron*, **53**, 238–43.

Terragno, N.A., Terragno, D.A., and McGiff, J.C. (1977). Contribution of prostaglandins to the renal circulation in conscious, anesthetized and laparatomized dogs. *Circulation Research*, **40**, 590–5.

Terragno, N.A., Terragno, D., Early, J.A., Roberts, M.A., and McGiff, J.C. (1978). Endogenous prostaglandin synthesis inhibitor in the renal cortex. Effects on production of prostacyclin by renal blood vessels. *Clinical Science and Molecular Medicine*, **55** (Suppl. 4), 199–202s.

Thiel, G., Tamm, M., Bock, A., and Brunner, F.P. (1989). Klinisches Bild und Verlauf der Analgetika-nephropathie. *Zeitschrift für Urologie und Nephrologie*, **82** (Suppl. 1), 49–62.

Thiele, E.H. (1974). An *in vivo* pyelonephritis assay for screening therapeutic agents. *Journal of Antibiotics*, **27**, 31–41.

Thieler, H. and Sicker, P. (1989). Analgetika-verbrauch im Bezirk Erfurt. *Zeitschrift für Klinische Medizin*, **44**, 1403–6.

Thieler, H., Hottenrott, B., Marx, M., Voigt, D., Winkelmann, L., Oltmanns, U. *et al.* (1990). Die Analgetika-nephropathie unter den chronischen Dialysepatienten im nördlichen Thüringen. *Nieren- und Hochdruchkrankheiten*, **4**, 148–57.

Thölen, H. (1958). Interstitielle Nephritis. In *Phenacetinabusus und Nierenschädigung* (ed. H. Sarre, A. Moench, and R. Kluthe), pp. 101–7. Thieme, Stuttgart.

Thölen, H., Voegtli, J., Renschler, H., and Schaeffer, A. (1956). Ein Beitrag zur Genese der interstitiellen Nephritis. *Schweizerische Medizinische Wochenschrift*, **86**, 946–9.

Thomsen, B.S., From, A., Jacobsen, I.A., Starklint, H., and Pedersen, P.C. (1983). Acute renal failure possibly associated with fenoprofen therapy. *Arthritis and Rheumatism*, **26**, 234–5.

Thomson, B.J., Jenkins, D.A.S., Allan, P.L., Elton, R.A., and Winney, R.J. (1986). Acquired cystic disease of the kidney in patients with end-stage chronic renal failure: a study of prevalence and aetiology. *Nephrology, Dialysis, Transplantation*, **1**, 38–43.

Thurau, K. (1964). Renal hemodynamics. *American Journal of Medicine*, **36**, 698–719.

Tiltman, A.J. and Friedell, G.H. (1971). The histogenesis of experimental bladder cancer. *Investigative Urology*, **9**, 218–26.

Tolins, J.P. and Seel, P. (1987). Ibuprofen-induced interstitial nephritis and the nephrotic syndrome. *Minnesota Medicine*, **70**, 509–11.

Tolman, E.L., Fuller, B.L., Marinan, B.A., Capetola, R.J., Levinson, S.L., and Rosenthale, M.E. (1983). Tissue selectivity and variability of effects of acetaminophen on arachidonic acid metabolism. *Prostaglandins, Leukotrienes and Medicine*, **12**, 347–56.

Torhorst, J. (1976). Nierenschädigung durch Analgetika: pathologische Anatomie und Morphogenese. *Nephrologie in Klinik und Praxis*, **3**, 134–9.

Torhorst, J., Rohr, H.P., Zollinger, H.U., Studer, A., and Tranzer, J.P. (1967). Ultrastrukturelle Veränderungen der proximalen Tubuluszelle von Rattennieren nach Phenacetinüberbelastung. *Virchows Archiv. A. Pathological Anatomy and Histology*, **342**, 70–84.

Torikai, S. and Kurokawa, K. (1983). Effect of PGE_2 on vasopressin-dependent cell cAMP in isolated single nephron segments. *American Journal of Physiology*, **245**, F58–66.

Trèves, R., Gastine, H., Richard, A., Hugon, J., Varnoux, M., Gay, R., and Desproges-Gotteron, P. (1983). Responsabilité de l'ibuprofen dans une méningite aseptique et une insuffisance rénale aiguë au cours d'un lupus érythémateux disséminé. *Revue du Rhumatisme et des Maladies Osteo-Articulares*, **50**, 75–6.

Trnavský, K. and Rovenský, J. (1972). Stúdium nefrotoxicity antireumatik. I. Vplyv niektorých nesteroidných antireumatik na enzýmy v moči. *Fysiatrickya Reumatologicky Vestnik*, **50**, 166–71.

Turner, G. and Collins, E. (1975). Fetal effects of regular salicylate ingestion in pregnancy. *Lancet*, **2**, 338–9.

Uehlinger, E. (1958). Die pathologische Anatomie der interstitiellen Nephritis. In *Phenacetinabusus und Nierenschädigung* (eds. H. Sarre, A. Moench, and R. Kluthe), pp. 1–12. Thieme, Stuttgart.

Uemura, M., Tsujii, T., Fukui, H., Kita, K., Takaya, A., Tsukamoto, N. *et al.* (1986). Urinary prostaglandins and renal function in chronic liver diseases. *Scandinavian Journal of Gastroenterology*, **21**, 75–81.

Urban, H. (1964). Schäden am zentral Nervensystem durch Mißbrauch phenacetinhaltiger Mischpräparate. *Deutsche Medizinische Wochenschrift*, **89**, 223–9.

Uzan, S., Beaufils, M., Breart, G., Bazin, B., Capitant, C., and Paris, J. (1991). Prevention of fetal growth retardation with low dose aspirin: findings of the EPREDA trial. *Lancet*, **1**, 1427–31.

Vallès, M. and Tovar, J.L. (1987). Salsalate and minimal-change nephrotic syndrome. *Annals of Internal Medicine*, **107**, 116.

van Dusseldorp, M. and Katan, M.B. (1990). Headache caused by caffeine withdrawal among moderate coffee drinkers switched from ordinary to decaffeinated coffee: a 12 week double blind trial. *British Medical Journal*, **300**, 1558–9.

van Dusseldorp, M., Katan, M.B., and Demacker, P.N.M. (1990). Effect of decaffeinated versus regular coffee on serum lipoproteins. A 12-week double-blind trial. *American Journal of Epidemiology*, **132**, 33–40.

Van den Bosch, H. (1980). Intracellular phospholipases A. *Biochimica Biophysica Acta*, **604**, 191–246.

Vane, J.R. (1978) The mode of action of aspirin-like drugs. *Agents and Actions*, **8**, 430–1.

Vanherweghem, J.-L., and Even-Adin, D. (1982). Epidemiology of analgesic nephropathy in Belgium. *Clinical Nephrology*, **17**, 129–33.

Vaughan, E.D. (1985). Renovascular hypertension. *Kidney International*, **27**, 811–27.

Velo, G.P. and Milanino, R. (1990). Nongastrointestinal adverse reactions to NSAID. *Journal of Rheumatology*, **17** (Suppl. 20), 42–5.

Venning, V., Dixon, A.J., and Oliver, D.O. (1980). Mefenamic acid nephropathy. *Lancet*, **2**, 745–6.

Vereerstraeten, P., Thoua, Y., Goldman, M., Schandene, L., Vanherweghem, J.L., and Toussaint, C. (1982). Syndrome néphrotique et azotémie réversibles, associés à l'administration d'alclofénac. *Praxis*, **71**, 1222–5.

Veronese, M.E., McLean, S., D'Souza, C.A., and Davies, N.W. (1985). Formation of reactive metabolites of phenacetin in humans and rats. *Xenobiotica*, **15**, 929–40.

Vesell, E.S. (1979). The antipyrine test in clinical pharmacology: conceptions and misconceptions. *Clinical Pharmacology and Therapeutics*, **26**, 275–86.

Viau, C., Bernard, A., Lauwerys, R., and Maldague, P. (1984). Cadmium, analgesics, and the chronic progressive nephrosis in the female Sprague–Dawley rat. *Archives of Toxicology*, **55**, 247–9.

Vinci, G. (1914). Sur l'action des substances caféiques. Les modifications histologiques du rein determinées par la caféine. *Archives Italiennes de Biologie*, **61**, 401–42.

Vivaldi, E. (1968). Effect of chronic administration of analgesics on resistance to experimental infection of the urinary tract in rats. *Nephron*, **5**, 202–9.

Vogt, P., Frei, U., Repp, H., Bunzendahl, H., Oldhafer, K., and Pichlmayr, R. (1990). Malignant tumours in renal transplant recipients receiving cyclosporin: survey of 598 first-kidney transplantations. *Nephrology, Dialysis, Transplantation*, **5**, 282–8.

von Bruchlausen F. and Baumann, J. (1982). Inhibitory actions of deacetylation products of phenacetin and paracetamol on prostaglandin synthetases in neuronal and glial cell lines and rat renal medulla. *Life Sciences*, **30**, 1783–91.

Vracko, R. (1974). Basal lamina scaffold-anatomy and significance for maintenance of orderly tissue structure. *American Journal of Pathology*, **77**, 314–46.

Vriesendorp, R., de Zeeuw, D., de Jong, P.E., Donker, A.J.M., Pratt, J.J., and van der Hem, G.K. (1986*a*). Reduction of urinary protein and prostaglandin E_2 excretion in the nephrotic syndrome by non-steroidal anti-inflammatory drugs. *Clinical Nephrology*, **25**, 105–10.

Vriesendorp, R., Donker, A.J.M., de Zeeuw, D., de Jong, P.E., and van der Hem, G.K. (1986*b*). Antiproteinuric effect of naproxen and indomethacin: a double-blind crossover study. *American Journal of Nephrology*, **5**, 236–42.

Vriesendorp, R., Donker, A.J.M., de Zeeuw, D., de Jong, P.E., van der Hem, G.K., and Brentjens, J.R.H. (1986*c*). Effects of non-steroidal anti-inflammatory drugs on proteinuria. *American Journal of Medicine*, **81** (Suppl. 2B), 84–94.

Wahlqvist, L. (1980). Chemical carcinogenesis—a review and personal observations with special reference to the role of tobacco and phenacetin in the production of urothelial tumors. In *Bladder tumors and other topics in urological oncology* (ed. M. Pavone-Macaluso, P.H. Smith, and F. Edsmyr). Plenum, New York.

Wainscoat, J.S. and Finn, R. (1974). Possible role of laxatives in analgesic nephropathy. *British Medical Journal*, **4**, 697–8.

Wallenburg, H.C.S. and Rotmans, N. (1987). Prevention of recurrent idiopathic fetal growth retardation by low-dose aspirin and dipyridamole. *American Journal of Obstetrics and Gynecology*, **157**, 1230–5.

Walshe, J.J. and Venuto, R.C. (1979). Acute oliguric renal failure induced by indomethacin: possible mechanism. *Annals of Internal Medicine*, **91**, 47–9.

Wanner, C., Hörl, W.H., Luley, C.H., and Weiland, H. (1991). Effects of HMG-Co A reductase inhibitors in hypercholesterolemia in patients on hemodialysis. *Kidney International*, **39**, 754–60.

Warren, G.V., Korbet, S.M., Schwartz, M.M., and Lewis, E.J. (1989). Minimal change glomerulopathy associated with nonsteroidal anti-inflammatory drugs. *American Journal of Kidney Diseases*, **13**, 127–30.

Wasser, W.G., Goldstein, M.H., Barba, F., and Churg, J. (1982). Persistent renal failure following administration of naproxen. *Mount Sinaï Journal of Medicine*, **49**, 127–9.

Waterhouse, J., Muir, C., Shanmugaratnam, K., and Powell, J. (1982). *Cancer incidence in five continents*, Vol. IV, IARC Scientific Publication No. 42. IARC, Lyon.

Waters, W.E., Elwood, P.C., and Asscher, A.W. (1973). Community survey of analgesic consumption and kidney function in women. *Lancet*, **1**, 341–4.

Weber, M., Braun, B., and Köhler, H. (1985). Ultrasonic findings in analgesic nephropathy. *Nephron*, **39**, 216–22.

Welch, R.M. and Conney, A.H. (1965). A simple method for the quantitative determination of *N*-acetyl-*p*-aminophenol (APAP) in urine. *Clinical Chemistry*, **12**, 1064–7.

Wendland, M.L., Wagoner, R.D., and Holley, K.E. (1980). Renal failure associated with fenoprofen. *Mayo Clinic Proceedings*, **55**, 103–7.

Wessling, A. (1987). Over-the-counter sales of drugs in Sweden 1976–1983. *European Journal of Clinical Pharmacology*, **33**, 1–6.

Whelton, A., Bender, W.L., Vaghaiwalla, F., Hall-Craggs, M., and Solez, K. (1983). Sulindac and renal impairment. *Journal of the American Medical Association*, **249**, 2892–3.

Whelton, A., Stout, R.L., Spilman, P.S., and Klassen, D.K. (1990). Renal effects of ibuprofen, piroxicam and sulindac in patients with asymptomatic renal failure. A prospective, randomized, crossover comparison. *Annals of Internal Medicine*, **112**, 568–76.

WHO (1979). *Mycotoxins*. Environmental Health Criteria No. 11. World Health Organization, Geneva.

Wilkinson, S.P., Moodie, H., Arroyo, V.A., and Williams R. (1977). Frequency of renal impairment in paracetamol overdose compared with other causes of acute liver damage. *Journal of Clinical Pathology*, **30**, 141–3.

Williams, R.D. (1991). Renal, perirenal, and ureteral neoplasms. In *Adult and pediatric urology*, (2nd edn), (ed. J.Y. Gillenwater, J.T. Grayback, S.S. Howards, and J.W. Duckett), pp. 571–614. Mosby, St Louis.

Williams, G.M. and Weisburger, J.H. (1986). Chemical carcinogens. In *Casarett and Doull's toxicology: the basic science of poisons*, 3rd edn (ed. C.D. Klassen, M.O. Amdur, and J. Doull), pp. 99–173. Macmillan, New York.

Willman, C.L. and Fenoglio-Preiser, C.M. (1987). Oncogenes, suppressor genes, and carcinogenesis. *Human Pathology*, **18**, 895–902.

Wilson, D.R. and Gault, M.H. (1982). Declining incidence of analgesic nephropathy in Canada. *Canadian Medical Association Journal*, **127**, 500–2.

Windeck, R. and Bock, K.D. (1983). Irreversibles Nierenversagen einer transplantierten Niere ausgelöst durch Ketoprofen? *Deutsche Medizinische Wochenschrift*, **108**, 720–1.

Wing, A.J., Brunner, F.P., Geerlings, W., Broyer, M., Brynger, H., Fassbinder, W. *et al.* (1989). Contribution of toxic nephropathies to end-stage renal failure in Europe: a report from the EDTA-ERA registry. *Toxicology Letters*, **46**, 281–92.

Wise R.W., Zenser, T.V., and Davis, B.B. (1983). Prostaglandin H synthase metabolism of the urinary bladder carcinogens benzidine and ANFT. *Carcinogenesis*, **4**, 285–9.

Wiseman, E.H. and Reinert, H. (1975). Anti-inflammatory drugs and renal papillary necrosis. *Agents and Actions*, **5**, 322–5.

Wolters, J. and van Breda Vriesman, P.J. (1985). Minimal change nephropathy and interstitial nephritis associated with diclofenac. *Netherlands Journal of Medicine*, **28**, 311–4.

Woodbury, D.M. (1970). Analgesic-antipyretics, anti-inflammatory agents and inhibitors of uric acid synthesis. In *The pharmacological basis of therapeutics* (ed. L.S. Goodman and A. Gilman), pp. 314–47. Macmillan, New York.

Woods, K.L. and Michael, J. (1981). Mefenamic acid nephropathy. *British Medical Journal*, **282**, 1471.

Wu, M.J., Kumar, K.S., Kulkarni, G., and Kaiser, H. (1987). Multiple myeloma in naproxen-induced acute renal failure. *New England Journal of Medicine*, **317**, 170–1.

Yu, M.C., Mack, T.M., Hanisch, R., Cicioni, C., and Henderson, B.E. (1986). Cigarette smoking, obesity, diuretic use, and coffee consumption as risk factors for renal cell carcinoma. *Journal of the National Cancer Institute*, **77**, 351–6.

Zambraski, E.J. and Dunn, M.J. (1984). Importance of renal prostaglandins in control of renal function after chronic ligation of the common bile duct in dogs. *Journal of Laboratory and Clinical Medicine*, **103**, 549–59.

Zambraski, E.J., Atkinson, D.C., and Diamond, J. (1988*a*). Effects of salicylate vs. aspirin on renal prostaglandins and function in normal and sodium-depleted dogs. *Journal of Pharmacology and Experimental Therapeutics*, **247**, 96–103.

Zambraski, E.J., Guidotti, S.M., Atkinson, D.C., and Diamond, J. (1988*b*). Salicylic acid causes a diuresis and natriuresis in normal and common bile-duct-ligated cirrhotic miniature swine. *Journal of Pharmacology and Experimental Therapeutics*, **247**, 983–8.

Zech, P., Geitner, S., Birraux, B., Colon, S., Deteix, P., and Leitienne, P. (1982). Insuffisance rénale aiguë et syndrome néphrotique secondaires à la prise de fénoprofène. *Nouvelle Presse Médicale*, **11**, 2227.

Zenser, T.V., Mattammal, M.B., Herman, C.A., Joshi, S., and Davis, B.B. (1978). Effect of acetaminophen on prostaglandin E_2 and prostaglandin $F_{2\alpha}$ synthesis in the renal inner medulla of rat. *Biochimica et Biophysica Acta*, **542**, 486–95.

Zenser, T.V., Mattammal, M.B., and Davis, B.B. (1979*a*). Cooxidation of benzidine by renal medullary prostaglandin cyclooygenase. *Journal of Pharmacology and Experimental Therapeutics*, **211**, 460–4.

Zenser, T.V., Mattammal, M.B., Brown, W.W., and Davis, B.B. (1979*b*). Cooxygenation by prostaglandin cyclooxygenase from rabbit inner medulla. *Kidney International*, **16**, 688–94.

Zenser, T.V., Mattammal, M.B., Rapp, N.S., and Davis, B.B. (1983*a*). Effect of aspirin on metabolism of acetaminophen and benzidine by renal inner medulla prostaglandin hydroperoxidase. *Journal of Laboratory and Clinical Medicine*, **101**, 58–65.

Zenser, T.V., Cohen, S.M., Mattammal, M.B., Wise, R.W. Rapp, N.S., and Davis, B.B. (1983*b*). Prostaglandin hydroperoxidase-catalyzed activation of certain *N*-substituted aryl renal and bladder carcinogens. *Environmental Health Perspectives*, **49**, 33–41.

Ziegelbaum, M., Novick, A.C., Streem, S.B., Montie, J.E., Pontes, J.E., and Straffon, R.A. (1987). Conservative surgery for transitional cell carcinoma of the renal pelvis. *Journal of Urology*, **138**, 1146–9.

Zimran, A., Kramer, M., Plaskin, M., and Hershko, C. (1985). Incidence of hyperkalaemia induced by indomethacin in a hospital population. *British Medical Journal*, **291**, 107–8.

Zipser, R.D., Hoefs, J.C., Speckart, P.F., Zia, P.K., and Horton R. (1979). Prostaglandins: modulators of renal function and pressor resistance in chronic liver disease. *Journal of Clinical Endocrinology and Metabolism*, **48**, 895–900.

Zoja, C., Benigni, A., Renzi D., Piccinelli, A., Perico, N., and Remuzzi G. (1990). Endothelin and eicosanoid synthesis in cultured mesangial cells. *Kidney International*, **37**, 927–33.

Zollinger, H.U. (1955). Chronische interstitielle Nephritis bei Abusus von phenazetinhaltigen Analgetika (Saridon usw). *Schweizerische Medizinische Wochenschrift*, **84**, 747.

Zollinger, H.U. (1966). *Niere und ablietende Harnwege*. Springer, Berlin.

Zollinger, H.U. and Spühler, O. (1950). Die nicht-eitrige, chronische interstitielle Nephritis. *Schweizerische Zeitschrift Allergie und Pathologie*, **13**, 807–11.

INDEX

Oxford Monographs on Clinical Nephrology

SUBSCRIPTION INFORMATION

This major new series will provide clinical nephrologists with up-to-date reviews of areas of importance in their everyday work. The series will build into an indispensable resource with two to three volumes published each year.

If you would like to subscribe to the series please complete the card at the end of this book and return it to us.

Our subscription service guarantees that:

- Each volume will be conveniently delivered to you as soon as it becomes available.
- Each book will be sent on approval (14 days UK, 28 days Europe, 15 days USA).
- You keep only the books you want.
- There is no minimum number of books to buy.
- You will receive early information on new and forthcoming titles.
- You are free to cancel your subscription at any time.

When future volumes are sent to you, you simply pay the invoice enclosed (by £ sterling cheque or credit card) **or** return the book and invoice within the approval period.

USA Residents

Residents in the USA should complete the personal details on the card, sign, and mail to Barbara Wasserman, Oxford University Press, 200 Madison Avenue, New York, NY 10016.

Canadian Residents

For Canadian subscription service information, please complete the personal details on the card, sign, and mail to Catherine Belcastro, Direct Mail Coordinator, Oxford University Press Canada, 70 Wynford Drive, Don Mills, Ontario, M3C 1J9.

Australian Residents

Residents in Australia should complete the personal details on the card and mail to Shelley Muir, Oxford University Press, GPO Box 2784Y, Melbourne 3001.

We regret that this service is, at present, not available outside the UK, Europe, North America, and Australia.

Oxford Monographs on Clinical Nephrology

SUBSCRIPTION INFORMATION

This major new series will provide clinical nephrologists with up-to-date reviews of areas of importance in their everyday work. The series will build into an indispensable resource with two to three volumes published each year.

If you would like to subscribe to the series please complete the card at the end of this book and return it to us.

Our subscription service guarantees that:

- Each volume will be conveniently delivered to you as soon as it becomes available.
- Each book will be sent on approval (14 days UK, 28 days Europe, 15 days USA).
- You keep only the books you want.
- There is no minimum number of books to buy.
- You will receive early information on new and forthcoming titles.
- You are free to cancel your subscription at any time.

When future volumes are sent to you, you simply pay the invoice enclosed (by £ sterling cheque or credit card) **or** return the book and invoice within the approval period.

USA Residents

Residents in the USA should complete the personal details on the card, sign, and mail to Barbara Wasserman, Oxford University Press, 200 Madison Avenue, New York, NY 10016.

Canadian Residents

For Canadian subscription service information, please complete the personal details on the card, sign, and mail to Catherine Belcastro, Direct Mail Coordinator, Oxford University Press Canada, 70 Wynford Drive, Don Mills, Ontario, M3C 1J9.

Australian Residents

Residents in Australia should complete the personal details on the card and mail to Shelley Muir, Oxford University Press, GPO Box 2784Y, Melbourne 3001.

We regret that this service is, at present, not available outside the UK, Europe, North America, and Australia.